Hypnosis in the
Relief of Pain

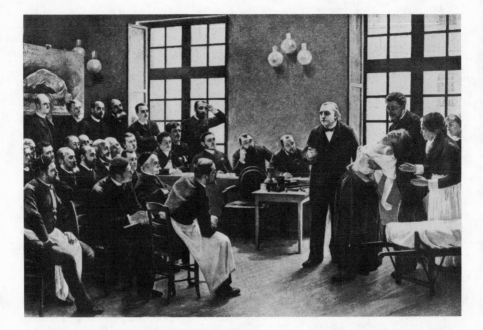

Jean-Martin Charcot (1835–1893), the leading neurologist of his day, made hypnosis respectable as a topic for scientific investigation. This painting by Brouillet shows him demonstrating a patient before his colleagues at the Salpêtrière in Paris. Behind him is Joseph Babinski, one of his favorites. Others identifiable in the audience include Charles Féré, Gilles de la Tourette, Pierre Marie, and Paul Richer. Copy courtesy of Henri F. Ellenberger.

Hypnosis in the Relief of Pain

ERNEST R. HILGARD

JOSEPHINE R. HILGARD

WILLIAM KAUFMANN, INC.   Los Altos, California

Library of Congress Cataloging in Publication Data

Hilgard, Ernest Ropiequet, 1904-
    Hypnosis in the relief of pain.

    Bibliography: p.
    Includes index.
    1. Hypnotism--Therapeutic use. 2. Pain. I. Hil-
gard, Josephine Rohrs, joint author. II. Title.
[DNLM: 1. Hypnosis. 2. Pain--Therapy. WM415 H644h]
RC497.H54   615'.8512   75-19490
ISBN 0-913232-16-5

Printed in the United States of America

Contents

Preface

Hypnosis has had a cyclical history of acceptance and rejection since the time of Mesmer, two hundred years ago; it has now attained a significant place in medical and psychological science. This acceptance is based on the involvement of well-trained clinicians and investigators whose studies of hypnosis and its applications employ the same critical methods used in studying other medical procedures or topics within experimental psychology. Although not all people are equally hypnotizable, enough can profit from hypnosis to justify its wider use.

The study of pain provides an unusually fortunate intersection of the clinic and the laboratory; thus it is a useful testing ground for hypnosis. If hypnotic treatment can relieve human suffering as well as—or in some cases better than—other methods, its use is justified and its neglect unfortunate. If experimental research can explain how hypnotic pain relief comes about, for whom, and under what conditions it is effective, the experimental findings will undergird the work of the clinician. Basic science in a medical setting often performs this service for clinical practice. Examples abound in the study of drugs, dietary deficiencies, immune reactions, and the genetic basis of molecular disease. The clinical treatment of pain with the aid of hypnosis must rest on the same careful research required in all fields of clinical practice.

In substantiating the foregoing propositions, we have taken advantage of our differing backgrounds, which include the experiences of a practicing psychiatrist and clinical investigator (J. R. H.) and those of a laboratory worker in experimental psychology (E. R. H.). We came to hypnosis after our careers had been well established, so we had acquired the skills resulting from interviewing, therapy, and laboratory investigations unrelated to hypnosis. The subsequent twenty years of studying hypnotic manifestations have convinced us of the practical importance of hypnosis as well as of its theoretical interest. Our earlier books on hypnosis have dealt with its more general features, applying to hypnosis the quantitative techniques familiar in psychological investigation (E. R. Hilgard, 1965; 1968), and relating hypnotic phenomena to other aspects of personality through an extensive interview study (J. R. Hilgard, 1970). The studies of pain have taken form since the writing of those books, so the material reported here from our laboratory is new, although influenced by our familiarity with hypnosis in other contexts.

The first four chapters are designed to orient the reader to problems of hypnosis, pain, and hypnotic practices related to pain. These are followed by four chapters which deal with clinical pain—in cancer, in obstetrics, in surgery, and in dentistry. One of us (J. R. H.) has had experience in the clinical use of hypnotic methods in cancer. She has also had experience interviewing mothers who have used hypnosis in childbirth, with phantom limb pain, and in the treatment of other pains referred to in the course of our discussion. In the clinical areas, we have relied on the advice of recognized experts to supplement our review of the literature. It is hoped that the clinical material we present will give an unbiased account of clinical practice of hypnotic pain relief in the areas discussed.

We have deliberately selected and emphasized categories of pain in which the organic component is high, because pain reduction through hypnosis is especially convincing in those cases. We are well aware that pain experiences have many components; a career in treating patients by psychiatric methods assures an awareness of psychosomatic problems. Because our subject is pain—where clinic and experimental laboratory meet—we have emphasized clinical pains of known causes, comparable to pains of known causes in the laboratory. Hence we have paid primary attention to pain in which the diagnosis is not at issue.

The final chapters break new ground. The concept of a "hidden observer" is introduced as a metaphor, representing the part of the hypnotized person found to sense covert pain even when the person under hypnosis experiences no overt pain or distress whatever. This puzzling discovery leads to an attempted explanation according to theories of pain and hypnosis. The final chapter seeks to tie together the appropriate generalizations from the clinic and the laboratory as they bear on the future utilization of hypnosis.

We found it difficult to decide at what level to write, because we wanted the book to be readable both by those with specialized professional training and by those without it. We noted also that hypnotic phenomena are so inherently interesting that writers tend to make extensive claims for hypnosis. We felt that a cautious approach was essential, even though hypnotic phenomena might thus appear less dramatic. Our hope is that because we have preserved scientific integrity and caution, members of the medical and psychological professions—whether familiar with hypnosis or not—will find a considered statement of the role of hypnosis in relation to pain. In addition, research workers concerned with pain, whatever their disciplines, may find here an introduction to an aspect of pain often neglected in their journals and textbooks. As an aid to professional workers, extensive notes are provided for each chapter, adding critical details not required by the text, and exact citations to the literature. The separation of such specialized material frees the discussions in the text from digressions and from the potentially disturbing need for footnotes. The cited literature, compiled in a single reference list, serves also as an index to the pages on which a study is mentioned.

We respect the "intelligent layman" who would like to know what to expect from hypnosis; therefore we have tried to define specialized terms as necessary. We hope the nonprofessional will find this book informative.

In the course of preparing the book we have received valuable criticism and advice from others whose familiarity with pain, or with pain and hypnosis, supplements ours in important ways. We wish to express our gratitude to Ronald Melzack for his review of Chapter 2; to Richard G. Black for Chapter 3; to George L. Hoffman, Jr. for Chapter 6; to Ronald L. Katz for Chapter 7; and to Kay F. Thompson for Chapter 8. Reading of early versions of the whole book by Donald W. MacKinnon and by J. M. B. Edwards proved very helpful, and resulted in major changes. We, of course, must bear full responsibility for the final product. Our publisher, William Kaufmann, and his associates have been most helpful throughout. We are indebted also to the foundations, agencies, and individuals who have supported and participated in our researches on hypnosis and pain. The names of our collaborators appear in the citations of their work. Financial support has been received over the years from the Ford Foundation, and the U.S. Air Force Office of Research (Contract AF 49[638]-1436). The longest continued financial support has been that from the National Institute of Mental Health (Grant MH-03859). We wish to express our appreciation to all of these, to Stanford University, and to some private donors who have made possible our collaborative efforts.

E. R. H.

J. R. H.

Stanford, California
August, 1975

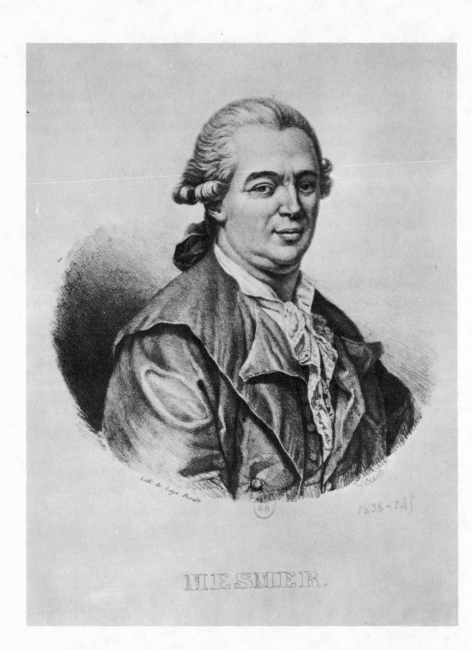

Franz Anton Mesmer (1734–1815). Although always a controversial figure, modern hypnosis began with him and his disciples, who called it animal magnetism. From the collection in the Institute for History of Medicine, Vienna. Copy courtesy of Henri F. Ellenberger.

PART I. *Pain and Hypnosis*

The scientific foundations upon which the understanding of hypnosis is based have become much firmer in the last two decades. In the course of research, much has been learned about the effectiveness of hypnotic procedures in the alleviation of pain.

To keep all in perspective, the account begins with an orientation to hypnosis, and then turns to pain—knowledge about it and theories to explain it. The more usual methods of controlling pain—drugs, surgery, physical medicine, and psychological procedures—are reviewed. The evidence for hypnotic relief of pain is then examined, in the light of experimental evidence gathered under well-developed methods of control and measurement.

1 Hypnosis

It is possible to discuss the relationship between hypnosis and pain with confidence because of the advances in the understanding of hypnosis that have occurred in the last two decades. With the establishment of research laboratories working continuously on problems of hypnosis, and of professional societies composed of those interested in a scientific basis for its clinical use, hypnosis must now be considered as a serious topic in psychology and in the healing arts.

Hypnotic-like behavior has been reported from the dawn of history, and such behavior can be observed today in the rites of cultures little influenced by modern civilization. The early origins are shrouded in mystery and magic; for our purposes we may begin two centuries ago, with Franz Anton Mesmer (1734–1815), an Austrian physician who came to prominence in Paris. His form of hypnosis under the name of *animal magnetism* was important enough to be known as *mesmerism* (with a small *m*), a name still heard occasionally as a synonym for hypnosis.

Disparaging remarks have been made about Mesmer because of the dramatic manner in which he conducted his therapeutic sessions in Paris in the late 1700s. The patients sat around a *baquet*—a tub filled with water and iron filings—holding onto iron rods through which the magnetic influence might reach their bodies. The master himself would appear in his elegant silk robe, assisting in the transfer to the patients of the marvelous animal magnetism exuding from him. The patients would eventually go into convulsions, and would then be taken to a recovery room where they became normal again, hopefully rid of their complaints. A committee of inquiry was set up in 1784 by the King of France, composed of leading scientists of the day, including Benjamin Franklin, ambassador from the young United States. Using good experimental designs, the committee showed that the "magnetic" influence could be transferred as well by wooden rods as by iron bars, and that the influence upon the patient, although present, was a result of the imagination. Hence Mesmer was discredited, although his methods and theories lived on.

Mesmer was obviously wrong in his theory, but two things may be said in his defense. In the first place, he was attempting to use modern physical science to replace some of the superstition of his day. It may be remembered that this was the Age of Enlightenment in France, the time when Diderot's famous *Encyclopedia* was appearing. Second, even though the results were produced by imagination, they were indeed being produced; we shall note later how important imagination has become in the interpretation of hypnosis.

The first point—that he was trying to use modern science, even if he did not use it well—can be documented by a controversy he had with Father Johann Joseph Gassner (1717–1799) an exorcist of the time. Father Gassner was a Catholic priest in a small village in Switzerland; through the Church's practices of exorcism, he got rid of "the Evil One" and cured himself of headaches, dizziness, and other disturbances that had been troubling him. He then began to exorcise others within his parish, and by 1774, patients began to come to him from miles around. He soon received invitations to practice elsewhere. There was much opposition to Gassner, for many of those participating in the enlightenment wished to be rid of practices that they considered irrational. The Prince-Elector Max Joseph of Bavaria appointed a commission of inquiry in 1775 and invited Mesmer to show, if he could, that the results of exorcism could be obtained as well by "naturalistic" methods. Mesmer was able to produce the same effects that Gassner had produced—causing convulsions to occur and then curing them. He declared that Gassner was an honest man, but that he was curing his patients by animal magnetism without being aware of it. Mesmer won the day, and Gassner was sent off as a priest to a small community. Pope Pius VI ordered his own investigation, from which he concluded that exorcism was to be performed with discretion.

Mesmer was not prepared to consider the role of imagination, the explanation which the Royal Commission had proposed, because psychology was not then far enough advanced for imagination to be taken seriously in relation to science. However, despite a temporary setback, mesmerism spread to other parts of the world. Among its adherents in the United States, one to be remembered is Phineas Parkhurst Quimby (1802–1866), who cured a bedridden invalid later to become famous as Mary Baker Eddy (1821–1910), the founder of Christian Science.

Undaunted by scientific objections to their explanations, later mesmerists were impressed by the results they could achieve, most dramatically in relieving pain in major surgery. An English surgeon, John Elliotson (1791–1868), reported in 1834 on numerous surgical operations performed painlessly under mesmeric sleep; in 1846 a Scottish doctor, James Esdaile (1808–1859), reported on 345 major operations performed in India with mesmerism as the sole anesthetic. General chemical anesthetics were not yet in use; ether was introduced in 1846, chloroform in 1847. The opposition to surgery under mesmerism was intense, and the practice died out rapidly after the chemical anesthetics became available.

Hypnosis was rescued from oblivion by another English physician, James Braid (ca. 1795–1860), who wrote in the 1840s. Braid divorced himself from the mesmerists, relating hypnosis to "nervous sleep;" he eventually gave it the modern name of "hypnotism." He never broke with the medical profession and was a far less controversial figure than Elliotson. In some sense, hypnosis as we know it began with Braid, who used it widely in his medical practice, even treating his own pains with self-hypnosis.

Despite the moderation of Braid's views, hypnosis declined again until another revival occurred in France. Here we find two schools of thought in disagreement about hypnosis—that of the Salpêtrière, headed by Jean-Martin Charcot (1835–1893), and the Nancy school, led by Auguste Ambrose Liébeault (1823–1904) and Hippolyte Bernheim (1840–1919). From them we are led to Sigmund Freud (1856–1939), a name more familiar today.

Charcot was the most distinguished neurologist of his day; the fact that he gave demonstrations of hypnotic phenomena in his clinic and explained hypnosis neurologically gave it scientific respectability. Charcot presented his findings on hypnosis in a paper read in 1882 before the French Academy of Sciences—the same academy that had assisted in the earlier rejection of mesmerism. Charcot believed that hypnosis was essentially hysterical and that its major manifestations were limited to those who suffered some abnormality of the nervous system. He was wrong in this, but because he linked hypnosis to disease, his findings became acceptable to his scientific colleagues. Freud spent some time with Charcot in 1885–1886, while Charcot remained interested in hypnosis. The Nancy school, on the other hand, regarded hypnosis as an entirely normal phenomenon and attributed it to the influence of suggestion. History has proven the Nancy school more nearly correct. Freud wished to learn from both sides and, in fact, translated the works of both Charcot and Bernheim into his native German.

Because both Charcot and Bernheim were medical men of sound reputation, their disputes were considered as part of normal scientific discussion; hypnosis now became a matter of scientific interest and investigation. This interest was soon so general that the First International Congress for Experimental and Therapeutic Hypnotism was held in Paris in 1889. The list of participants includes many distinguished names, such as the American psychologist William James, the Italian psychiatrist and criminologist Lombroso, and the psychiatrist Freud, who did not establish psychoanalysis until later.

At this peak of interest in hypnosis in the 1880s, academic psychologists took their places along with the clinicians. It was most natural for William James, in 1890, to include a chapter on hypnotism in his classic *Principles of Psychology*; Wilhelm Wundt, often called the father of modern experimental psychology, wrote a book on hypnotism; Wilhelm Preyer, important in the history of child development, had his book also; and there were many others in many languages. Several journals devoted to hypnosis appeared, and long bibliographies were assembled to help keep abreast of the flood of books and articles. By 1900, however, it was almost all over.

In Vienna, Freud, along with Joseph Breuer (1842–1925), had begun to use hypnosis successfully in psychotherapy with patients then classified as hysterical. The result was their classic book, *Studies in Hysteria*, published in 1895. By the time the book appeared, however, Freud had rejected hypnosis. He had already substituted his method of free association and psychoanalysis; only the couch remained from his hypnotic practice. This was another blow to hypnosis, for because of their psychological orientation, Freud's followers might have been sympathetic to the use of hypnosis had not a kind of taboo been set up against it.

Pierre Janet (1859–1947) was Charcot's successor, although too independent to be thought of as a disciple. He had a large share in developing the theory of dissociation of personality as an aspect of hypnosis, and had followers in the United States early in this century—particularly Morton Prince (1854–1919), founder of the Psychological Clinic at Harvard. Janet lived a long life and was aware of the fluctuations of interest in hypnosis. In one of his books, published in English in 1925, he remarked that hypnosis was quite dead—until it would come to life again.

The new life for hypnosis began at the end of World War I. Treatment of soldiers with "shell shock" from trench warfare by English psychologist William McDougall (1871–1944) and others brought hypnosis to the attention of scientists. An important milestone in the experimental study of hypnosis was reached when Clark Hull (1884–1952) began experimentation as a professor at the University of Wisconsin, and later at Yale University. Hull published a classic book on *Hypnosis and Suggestibility* in 1933. This work, meticulous in its use of scientific controls and statistical tests, stands even today as a model for scientific method as applied to hypnotic phenomena. Unfortunately Hull, like Freud, abandoned hypnosis once he had worked successfully with it; few of his students followed up this interest, despite his listing more than one hundred studies that needed doing but that he had not gotten around to. But enough work was done that when Weitzenhoffer reviewed the experimental literature twenty years later, he could cite 508 references, many of them, of course, preceding the date of Hull's book.

A resurgence of interest followed World War II and the Korean War. Psychiatry was more advanced by this time than it had been in World War I; many psychiatrists found advantages in hypnotherapy, in part because it could achieve results more quickly than the methods of psychotherapy in which they had been trained. Dentists, too, found that they were able to use hypnosis when their normal supplies of local anesthetics might not be available. Clinical psychologists, drawn into service, also found hypnosis useful. After the war years, societies related to clinical and experimental hypnosis were established, with journals to publish research findings and case material. Speciality boards were established so patients could be directed to hypnotic practitioners with adequate credentials. Both the British Medical Association and the American Medical Association passed resolutions stating that training in hypnosis might appropriately be given in medical schools. Research laboratories were established at some leading universities, with support from government agencies and private foundations. Hypnosis was now on firmer ground and could advance without the sharp fluctuations of interest that had occurred in the past.

We are now prepared to consider the knowledge about hypnosis that has accumulated through the research efforts of recent decades, following this awakened interest.

Hypnotic Responsiveness

It has long been known that , quite apart from the skill of the hypnotist, people differ in the degree to which they are responsive to hypnosis. Records kept on nearly 20,000 cases by various investigators in the nineteenth century showed that roughly 10 percent of the subjects were refractory or essentially nonsusceptible to hypnosis; about 30 percent reached only a drowsy-light state; another 30 percent reached a moderate state; and the rest reached a deep state, often called "somnambulistic" by analogy with sleepwalking. The figures differed widely from one investigator to another, however, because there were no standard measurements. Intensive efforts in recent years have been devoted to producing better tests of hypnotic responsiveness, and then to finding personality characteristics related to scores on these tests. As with nearly all human measurements, subjects would be expected to vary in their responsiveness from one end of the scale to the other, with more people achieving intermediate scores.

The construction of a hypnotic responsiveness scale is logically very simple. The person to be studied is first given a brief standard induction of hypnosis, of the kind that long experience has shown makes a person feel hypnotized if he is responsive to these induction procedures. Two favorite methods of induction are the eye closure method and the hand levitation method. In the eye closure method, the subject stares at a small target, such as a tack on the wall, while the hypnotist suggests relaxation, drowsiness, and eventually, eye-closure. The intent is that the subject should hold his eyes open as long as possible and have the feeling of involuntary action as the eyes "close of themselves." Once the subject's eyes are closed, the assumption is that he has become lightly hypnotized; further suggestions are given to make the involvement in hypnosis more profound. When the hand levitation method is employed, the subject is told to concentrate on a hand in his lap. He is then instructed to note that the hand is getting light and is beginning to lift, to move up toward his face. The subject becomes relaxed, his eyes close, and, when his hand touches his face, he is comfortably hypnotized and the hand descends slowly to his lap. There are many variations, but if a standardized test is desired, the suggestions follow a standard pattern and are given in a uniform manner.

Following such a routine induction, the subject's hypnotic responsiveness is tested by giving him suggestions to which hypnotized persons are known to respond. For example, the subject may be told to hold his arms out in front of him at shoulder height, with his hands about a foot apart, palms facing inward. Placing the hands in this position is merely a cooperative response, made as well by the less hypnotizable as by those more highly hypnotizable. Next the subject is given the suggestion that his hands are moving together involuntarily, as though an external force were acting upon them. For many people, the hands begin to move together; then they report that it does indeed feel as if the hands are being attracted toward each other, or being pushed together. If the hands move some specified amount—say to within 6 inches of each other—that item is "passed" as an indication of responsiveness. In a standardization test with college students, 70 percent passed this item, making it an "easy" item. Others are much harder. In one such item, the subject is told to place the palms of his hands together and to interlock his fingers. He is then given the suggestion that the hands will be so tightly locked together that he will be unable to open them when he is told to do so. He is then told, "Try to open your hands. Go ahead and try." Only one-third of the students tested in a standardization sample were unable to open their hands in the 10 seconds allowed—half as many as had their hands move together in the easier item above. By collecting together a dozen such tests of hypnotic responsiveness and observing varied performances, a larger sample of hypnotic responsiveness may be obtained. Age regression (return to childhood); hallucinating something not present; performing an act at a signal when out of hypnosis (posthypnotic suggestion); forgetting what was done in hypnosis until a release signal is given (posthypnotic amnesia)—these represent other kinds of performance that may be called for. A "score" is derived by counting up the number of items "passed;" the least re-

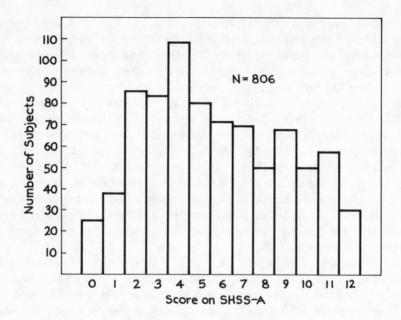

Figure 1. Hypnotic responsiveness scores of 806 college students. The scores were earned on individual tests with the Stanford Hypnotic Susceptibility Scale, Form A; the least responsive scored 0, the most responsive 12. Most scores lie between these extremes. Unpublished data, Stanford Laboratory.

sponsive subjects pass none of them, the most responsive all of them. In addition, some determination may be made of the reality of the experiences to the subject, and the "objective" scores may be modified according to these "subjective" reports. The scores obtained from standard testing of students show that hypnotic responsiveness is indeed widespread, few are totally unresponsive, most are in the medium range, and an appreciable number score high on these scales (Figure 1).

It is surprising to find how consistent scores obtained in this manner can be when the same subject is tested twice by different hypnotists, or tested again many years later with no hypnotic experience in the interim. Retest scores over a few days tend to correlate around .80 or .90; even after ten years, the correlation is still around .60, about as high as would be expected with adult intelligence test scores repeated over that interval.*

---

* For those who are not familiar with coefficients of correlation, it suffices to point out that they are not percents; they vary from 0 (no relationship) to 1.00 (perfect correspondence) between the two tests.

These hypnotic responsiveness tests have also been developed in forms that can be used with children; one of the by-products of responsiveness testing is an understanding of the change of hypnotic responsiveness with age. Tests of this kind become appropriate for use with children when they reach the age of 4 or 5 and have acquired the necessary language skills. Scores rise rapidly in the early years, reaching a maximum between the ages of 8 and 12, in the preadolescent years. Scores then tend to fall off gradually with age. These are, of course, average results; some individuals remain highly hypnotizable throughout life, and others are insusceptible all along.

The impression must not be given that, because these scores are relatively consistent, they are immutable. A few striking changes are commonly found on retests; these are often caused by factors in the test situation rather than a change in the person. For example, a person may resist hypnosis in the first experience out of fear that, if hypnotized, he may be asked to do something of which he disapproves. The next time he may not be so fearful, and so may achieve a higher score. Anyone can prevent himself from being hypnotized if he wishes, so a score is useful only if the subject is fully cooperative. At the other side of the spectrum is the person who so much wants to be hypnotized that he "helps out" by doing voluntarily what is supposed to occur involuntarily. Sometimes this does indeed work, and the person finds that involuntary processes "take over;" but he is more likely to be disappointed and to experience no genuine change in himself or in his responsiveness. Hence the next time, when he follows the suggestions as intended, his score is reduced. In practice there are not many such cases, or the correlations would not be so high.

What interests us more, however, is whether a person can *learn* to become hypnotized or can be *trained* to be a more responsive subject. Many practicing hypnotists assume that these results can be achieved, but laboratory studies show that they are much more difficult than might be supposed. Although small gains in responsiveness have been reported in a number of studies, the final scores after training tend to be positively correlated with the initial scores. Thus improvement is often greater for the subject who was moderately to highly responsive in the first place than for the initial nonresponder who most needs to improve. A second point must be made, however: *general* hypnotic responsiveness, as measured by the scale, is different from *specific* responsiveness, more appropriately described by a single item on the scale or by a special subscale designed to reflect a particular hypnotic ability. An analogy might be drawn here to efforts to increase scores on intelligence-type tests: general efforts, such as early education programs, are not usually very successful; improvement of reading, which is a more specific ability than general intelligence, is often a more successful approach. In hypnosis, a person who can, at first, have visual hallucinations with eyes closed but not with eyes open may perhaps be taught to have the hallucination with eyes open; that would be a change in a specific ability, which might not be reflected in general hypnotic responsiveness scores apart from the hallucination item.

The next step, after finding that hypnotic susceptibility was both measurable and relatively stable, was to see if the differences in that ability could be accounted for by personality characteristics of the subject. The old idea that hypnosis was related to hysteria was readily disposed of, because people with no evident personality problems proved fully as susceptible to hypnosis as those who were obviously neurotic or psychotic. It was not easy, however, to find personality characteristics that could predict hypnotic responsiveness. The standard personality inventories of the "troubles" type (such as the Minnesota Multiphasic Personality Inventory, MMPI), in which a person reports things that have bothered him, did not prove to be predictive; the freer tests, such as storytelling to pictures (Thematic Apperception Test, TAT) or describing what is seen in standard ink blots (the Rorschach test) did not fare any better. Some inventories of experiences similar to those of hypnosis but occurring outside hypnosis proved mildly related to hypnosis, but most of the correlations, even when positive, were quite low.

This disappointment in finding general personality correlates of hypnosis led to the possibility that hypnotic ability might be something very specific, which would be limited to the experiences in hypnosis. Were that the case, there might even be a hereditary component, as there often is with specific individual characteristics, such as colorblindness, taste blindness, and even diabetes. One way to test this was to do a twin study. If hypnotic responsiveness is hereditary, identical twins (homozygous or one-egg twins) should prove to be more similar in their hypnotic responsiveness than fraternal twins (dizygous or two-egg twins). In addition, of course, hypnotic ability ought to be inherited from parent to child. A careful study showed that this possibility cannot be ruled out, because there is a low but positive correlation between parent and child, and because identical twins were indeed more alike in their hypnotic responsiveness than either fraternal pairs or nontwin siblings. A study of this kind cannot be fully decisive because identical twins, who look alike and are always of the same sex, share a more common environment than fraternal twins. However, the results leave open the possibility of a hereditary component.

The hint of a hereditary aspect makes all the more plausible a search for some uniqueness in the personality of the hypnotizable. Some answers are now beginning to emerge more clearly than before, and they all point in the same direction: to something involving the life of imagination.

The evidence first began to mount in a large interview study conducted in our laboratory. To avoid the bias that enters into after-the-fact explanations, students were interviewed *before* they were hypnotized, in an attempt to predict how hypnotizable they would be. They were then hypnotized, and the actual scores were compared with the predicted ones. To improve such predictions, the interviewer must learn from both his successes and his failures. So, after they were hypnotized and their scores determined, the students were again interviewed. They were asked if they themselves saw in hypnosis any connection with what the interviewer had used as his basis of prediction, or why what he had thought relevant had nothing to do with it. This process of successive approximation led finally to an emphasis on *imaginative involvements,* usually developed in childhood and often acquired from parents who shared such involvements.

Imaginative involvements may be in reading, in dramatic viewing or acting, in music listening or performing, or in some forms of adventure. The person who becomes involved temporarily sets ordinary reality aside to become totally absorbed in the imaginative experience; he finds this absorption refreshing and wholly satisfying. The student listening to his favorite selection on the phonograph—and transformed by it—may literally beg it to go on when the record ends. But the departure from reality is temporary, and the person returns to his normal coping with external reality. Those who habitually had such experiences proved to be among the most hypnotizable, while those who could report none of them were among the least hypnotizable. The findings from the interview study were converted by other investigators into a self-report scale called an absorption scale that could be given to subjects along with items measuring introversion-extroversion and normalcy-neuroticism. The whole scale could then be studied in relation to measured hypnotic responsiveness. Hypnosis was found not to be related to introversion-extroversion or to normalcy-neurotism— a result consistent with the earlier negative findings. But hypnotic responsiveness was substantially related to the absorption scale, thus supporting the conclusions from the interview study.

Additional evidence consistent with the role of imaginative experience came from an unexpected source: the study of brain function. Efforts through the years to find physiological indicators distinguishing the hypnotic state from the waking state have not proved successful, but new evidence is accumulating to show some differences between the more and the less hypnotizable person in the normal, nonhypnotized state. Among the first signs to show up was a difference in the electrical activity of the brain in the relaxed waking state, as measured by the electroencephalograph. The electroenphalogram (EEG) that results when a subject sits quietly with his eyes closed in a semidarkened room shows some periods of regular waves known as EEG-Alpha, at a frequence of 8 to 13 cycles per second. The proportion of time that these EEG-Alpha rhythms appear on the record turns out to be correlated with hypnotic susceptibility: the more hypnotizable the subject, the higher the proportion of time in EEG-Alpha.

An extension of the EEG studies took off from another starting point. Sperry and his colleagues had done research on patients who, to counteract the effects of severe epilepsy, had had the fiber bundle between the cerebral hemispheres (the corpus callosum) severed surgically. This research revealed that the two halves of the brain are essentially two brains, almost identical but differing in what they can do. In right-handed people, the left hemisphere is primarily concerned with verbal behavior and analytic tasks, whereas the right hemisphere is concerned with more global and patterned tasks such as imagination, space perception, and music. To use two analogies, the left hemisphere acts like a digital computer, the right hemisphere like an analog computer; or, the left hemisphere acts like a stimulus-response brain, the right acts like a Gestalt brain. The relationships are usually reversed in left-handed people.

If electrodes are placed appropriately on the two sides of the head to detect which hemisphere is being more actively used, people with perfectly normal brains can be shown to use their half-brains differentially, as had been shown with the split-brain patients described above. If, for example, a right-handed person speaks the words to a song without singing them, he can be shown to use the left (verbal) hemisphere; if he hums the music without the words he uses the right (nonverbal, patterning) hemisphere; if he sings the song—words and music—both hemispheres are activated.

Other methods are also available for studying when the two hemi-spheres are activated preferentially. One of these makes use of the tendency to divert the eyes while solving mental problems. A questioner sits behind a strongly right-handed subject, who is looking ahead while being questioned. If the questioner asks a question of analytic type, such as mental arithmetic, the person tends to divert his eyes to the right while figuring out the answer. This indicates that he is activating his left hemisphere, the analytic one. If the question involves imagination ("imagine a child swinging in a rope swing out over a garden") the subject tends to move his eyes to the left, indicating that the right hemisphere has been activated. The degree to which eye move-ments correspond to the type of question indicates how "lateralized"—how completely right- or left-handed—the subject is.

Something else happens, however, when the questioner sits facing the subject. Now the subject's eye movements have other components; they are avoidance movements as well as being related to the nature of the question. For reasons that are not simple to explain, people in this situation differ in their *preference* for looking to the right or to the left, with the same set of questions. In the first case, with the questioner behind, the determining factor was how *lateralized* the person was. Now, however, something else has entered—a habitual preference for diverting the eyes one way or the other, or, in terms of brain function, a *preference* for using the right or the left hemisphere. This preference correlates with measured hypnotizability: right-handed persons who show hemispheric preference by looking more often to the left and are therefore activating the *right* hemisphere (that related to imagination) are the more hypnotizable. At present the relationship has been established primarily for right-handed males, but it is so striking as to be convincing.

We are still referring to hypnotic responsiveness—an ability or talent some people have for responding to hypnotic procedures—not to a change that takes place within hypnosis itself. As pointed out in Chapter 2, there is no single physiological indicator of pain, although under appropriate circumstances cardiovascular changes occur in orderly fashion as pain increases. The physiological situation in hypnosis is even more ambiguous, for there are no physiological signs whatever that indicate the degree of hypnotic involvement. The physiological signs we have, such as hemispheric preference and a greater proportion of EEG-alpha in the resting waking state, refer to the hypnotizable person as he presents himself before he has been hypnotized.

The State-Nonstate Issue

Those acquainted with the controversies among contemporary writers on hypnosis are sometimes confused by experts in hypnotic research who seem to conclude that there is no reality to hypnosis. That is not in fact their conclusion, for the data obtained in their studies are like those obtained by the majority of the researchers who accept the reality of hypnotic phenomena. How can this be?

The disagreements are not primarily over facts, but over conceptualizations. By stepping aside from hypnosis to consider another controversy in psychology, we may be able to clarify the differences in viewpoint by analogy. An old controversy, dating back to the 1920s, was over *instinct* as a concept in psychology. The facts of the matter were quite clear. Birds build nests corresponding to those of their species, even though they may be raised in isolation. The nests of some bird species are quite remarkable, such as that of the weaver bird, in which the cords holding the nest together are skillfully tied in knots. Some species of pigeons, released at a distance from their homes, will return promptly, but others will not. Salmon return to the rivulets in which they were spawned, despite spending their growing years at sea. These are all illustrations of instinctive behavior. Why, then, was instinct ruled out as a concept in psychology? As a classificatory label, the word was—and is—quite satisfactory; it is only because of the old controversy that the classificatory term has now been changed to "species-specific behavior." The objection was that the word *instinct* was often used in a circular manner in attempts at explanation. Why does the pigeon come home? Because it has a homing instinct. How do you know it has a homing instinct? Because it comes home. Nevertheless, the statement that the pigeon has a homing instinct is not an empty one, for races of pigeons can be classified into those which come home under specified circumstances and those which do not.

To return now to hypnosis: those who reject hypnosis as a concept do so for reasons like those used in the past for rejecting instinct. There is a danger in saying that an individual behaves in a certain way because he is hypnotized, when the only way one can tell that he is hypnotized is that he behaves in this way. Again, the reply is that some people respond to hypnotic procedures, and others do not; this corresponds in its way to the presence or absence of a given instinct in a given species. What we may learn from this controversy is that a basic conceptual issue may have very little to do with the observations made, but rather with the explanations offered. That is clearly the case with Barber and Sarbin, whose writings raise doubts about the conceptual usefulness of hypnosis.

Although the controversies do not, then, concern the reality of hypnotic phenomena, the differences in conceptualization have sharpened some empirical issues. Because we seem able to find out more about individual differences among those who can and cannot be hypnotized than about specific indices of the hypnotic state, the alternatives have become polarized over an issue between *trait* and *state*. The non-state theorists, among whom Barber and Sarbin would be included, object to hypnosis as a special *state* of consciousness. Accepting the *state* concept would imply that hypnosis is a change from normal, just as sleep differs from waking, or drunkenness differs from sobriety. However, both investigators are forced to recognize that the individual differences that characterize the more and the less hypnotizable represent an ability component, which we may call a *trait* of hypnotic responsiveness. It is possible to hold to a strictly *trait* theory, denying a state of hypnosis, or to hold to an extreme *state* theory, on the assumption that everyone can enter the state of hypnosis if circumstances are favorable. Of course, one can also hold at once to both *trait* and *state*. Those who accept both trait and state recognize differences in hypnotizability, but are aware that even the highly hypnotized person is not in the hypnotic state all of the time. Most workers do, in fact, accept this latter position.

One practical consequence of objecting to hypnosis as a state is to minimize the importance of hypnotic induction. If there is no state to enter, why go through a ceremony of entering it? This idea has led to a number of experiments comparing the results of the same suggestions given *with* a prior induction of hypnosis and *without* a prior induction. For example the standard hypnotic responsiveness scales can be given in both ways, to see what happens. It was known long before the question of state became a critical issue that most results could be obtained through what has traditionally been called "waking" hypnosis—that is, hypnotic-like suggestions given without a prior induction. Hence the question becomes whether or not induction *adds* something. This indeed it does: subjects are found to be more responsive after an induction than if given suggestions without an induction. The result, which favors a state theory, has been found by opponents of state theory as well. In order to explain this result, the non-state theorists have proposed other tests to deny state, such as substituting for no induction special exhortations known as "task-motivation instructions." After such instructions, to be sure, results more closely resembled those following an induction. However, the instructions given to substitute for an induction made such strong demands for compliance that critics pointed out a need to make a correction for the honesty of the performance. When such a correction was made, the task-motivation instructions were found to produce results superficially similar to those following an induction, but not exactly like them. This is still a matter of some ambiguity, and the state-nonstate issue is, therefore, not fully resolved. The nonstate supporters are correct in pointing out that for highly hypnotizable persons, the role of induction may be minimal. Hypnotists have known all along that after a person has been hypnotized once or twice, he can become hypnotized again quite rapidly at a signal implanted for the purpose. There is some uncertainty as to where to draw the line between such a brief induction and none at all. All this should not be surprising, for the induction itself must make use of waking suggestion; unless the subject responds to suggestion before he is hypnotized, his eyes would not close during the induction, nor would his arm rise when that induction method was being used.

One further aspect of hypnotic induction must be noted: a person can hypnotize himself. At first this seems very illogical; how can a person be both hypnotist and subject? A little thought reveals, however, that we commonly talk to ourselves, telling us what to do. "It's time you went home and got some sleep." "Don't eat any more of that rich dessert; remember that you're trying to reduce." What part of us does the talking? What part does the listening? These are puzzling questions, but the fact that such splits within ourselves are occurring all the time is familiar; self-hypnosis is merely another example. Once a person has been hypnotized, he can follow the same routines used by his hypnotist, both to enter hypnosis and to come out of it. Surprisingly, it has been found that an individual can do this even *before* he has been hypnotized by someone else and that how well he does it for himself is highly correlated to his responsiveness to an external hypnotist. There are some cautions to be exercised, and it is preferable to learn self-hypnosis under the guidance of someone who knows hypnosis, but self-hypnosis is more effective than it might be expected to be. Self-hypnosis or auto-hypnosis, a newcomer to the laboratory, was known for a long time in clinical practice. Braid used it on himself; Emile Coué, who had studied hypnosis under Liébeault, went around teaching autosuggestion many years later. Coué became widely known in the United States for teaching people to say, "Day by day, in every way, I am getting better and better." In Germany, Oskar Vogt taught methods of self-hypnosis as early as 1900; one of his followers, Johannes Schultz, developed a method called *autogenic training*, beginning in the 1920s. This method, a somewhat ritualized form of self-hypnosis, has many contemporary advocates.

In addition to increased scores on hypnotic responsiveness scales following induction, there are other ways of testing whether or not the hypnotic condition *adds something* to the behavior of the hypnotized person that distinguishes him from the nonhypnotizable. The hypnotist, through his suggestions, invites the subject to act in specific ways; other suggestions are implied in the expectations he creates, perhaps even unknowingly. Orne developed a special experimental design that seeks to test whether or not the hypnotic state adds something that is not demanded by the hypnotist, either openly or covertly. Orne recognized that hypnosis and suggestibility are closely related, although not necessarily the same, and that habitual social conformity might be mistaken for involuntary response to suggestion. He therefore sought a method to separate responsiveness to the demands made by the hypnotist upon the subject—whether obvious or subtle—from kinds of behavior clearly associated with the state of hypnosis. To make this separation, he proposed comparing a group of highly responsive hypnotic subjects ("reals") with a group of insusceptible subjects *instructed* to behave as they thought a highly hypnotized subject would ("instructed simulators"). The use of the word *simulator* may be misleading; Orne's purpose is not to find a method of detecting deliberate "faking," which is very rare and not important. What the experimental design does is to determine how well what a "real" subject does can be matched by an "instructed simulator." Even if no differences were detectable, this would not mean that the "real" is actually simulating. It would mean only that the experiment is not sensitive enough to show anything unique about the hypnotic state. If, however, the "reals" *add* to their behavior something associated with being hypnotized—and not the result of overt or implied demands of the hypnotist—then the experiment is indeed relevant to the state-nonstate controversy. Orne and his collaborators have been able to show differences between "reals" and "instructed simulators" in their experiences of pain from electric shock, in their responses to posthypnotic suggestion, when the suggestions are tested outside the experimental session; and in what happens when the hypnotist is called away, leaving the subject hypnotized. In brief, the "reals" show true pain reduction, which the "simulators" do not, they perform the posthypnotic act outside the experimental setting, whereas the "simulators" have forgotten their instructions by that time, and they come out of hypnosis more slowly than the "simulators" when the experimenter has disappeared. These results give evidence that, for the truly hypnotizable, real changes occur with hypnosis. Objections have been raised because this design compares responsive subjects with refractory ones, but that implies more personality differences between highs and lows than are usually found.

In summary, hypnotic phenomena appear to have a rather robust quality; they survive repeated attacks upon them and upon the manner in which they are conceptualized. Continuing controversy is valuable in that it demands ever better proof to replace conventional lore. The study of hypnosis is strengthened as it survives attacks by its critics and makes advances through critical, systematic research free from prior commitments to one or another position on controversial issues.

The Hypnotic Experience and the Relation to the Hypnotist

Despite the interest in making psychological science as objective and as much like other sciences as possible, the human mind and human experience are still better captured through what people tell us than in any other way. This has proved to be the case in measuring something as objectively real and as physiologically based as pain; it is equally true in attempting to find the essential characteristics of the hypnotic experience.

Regardless of the problem of "state," the hypnotized person has little doubt that he feels different when hypnotized; he senses a change when hypnosis is induced and when it is terminated. The following account is based on numerous interviews with subjects out of hypnosis, in an attempt to reconstruct what hypnosis was like to them. The quotes are verbatim remarks made in those interviews. Many subjects found it difficult to describe the experience in words, but that is equally true for many human experiences; the recurrent themes expressed in the descriptions of hypnosis were so prominent that it is possible to characterize certain experiences as typical.

One common theme is a sense of *relaxation*, both mental and physical. "It is a relaxation such as I have never experienced before: very deep, complete, with escape from all tension." To be sure, this feeling is engendered in part by the kinds of suggestions commonly given in hypnosis; a more alert hypnosis can also be induced. However, because relaxation is often an aim in the use of hypnosis, the finding that it is experienced so profoundly is itself important.

A second frequent comment is that *attention* has been narrowed. This may take various forms, and does not necessarily mean a highly concentrated attention. In fact, the mind in hypnosis may sometimes be almost blank, attending scarcely at all. At other times the attention is only on the hypnotist's voice and on what he is saying, with inattention to any distracting sounds. When the attention is directed to specific experiences, these are often so central that conflicting thoughts do not intrude. "It's like narrowing the thread of existence to a single strand, so that things that usually matter seem to drop away one by one. All that is left is the hypnotist and the hypnotist's voice." Or: "Psychologically, it was an easy way to detach myself from present problems." Shor, in his theoretical accounts, has emphasized this fading of reality orientation. The positive side of the singlemindedness can be utilized when hypnosis is directed toward reality in a therapeutic way. The patient can make plans—such as to eat fewer rich desserts—with the single idea before him of how fine it would feel to be strong enough to resist, and to have a body-image to be admired. The usual distractions—"How good cake and ice cream taste!"—need not intrude.

The future orientation implied in such suggestions is not characteristic of the usual hypnotic state, which is much more a here-and-now experience. "You don't have to worry about what you did yesterday or what you'll do tomorrow. . . . It's a respite from the uptightness of the day. I'm normally worrying about tomorrow—studies, roommate, job." This timeless, carefree quality of hypnosis is frequently expressed.

The prevalence of imaginative involvement outside hypnosis for those who can become hypnotized is reflected in the rich imaginative and fantasy experiences that are aroused in hypnosis itself. "Hypnosis was very much like a day-dream to me." Sarbin's characterization of hypnosis as "believed-in imagination" is an apt one. When age-regression is suggested, visual memories from childhood may take on the vivid quality of actual experience—being a child again. Anyone can imagine a puppy on the floor beside his chair, wagging its tail and begging to be picked up. In hypnosis, however, the imagination may be converted into a hallucination with the vividness of perception, so that the puppy appears actually to be there and may be picked up and petted as though real. Reality testing is set aside, so that the imagined experience is accepted as real. There are gradations to acceptance of these experiences within hypnosis, so that hallucinations may be accepted and acted upon with some reservations, just as in night dreams the sleeping person may have a genuine dream, and yet know that he is dreaming.

The reason for not mentioning *suggestibility* as a primary aspect of the hypnotic condition is that it is often overemphasized, largely because it is so easily seen by an observer. If the subject is asked about it, he usually notices his heightened suggestibility; subjects capable of self-hypnosis report being more suggestible in self-hypnosis as well as in heterohypnosis. This suggestibility may be an illustration of what James called ideo-motor action: if an idea of some action is before the mind, without any conflicting idea, then that idea will express itself in action. Subjects often report that they would not have to do what the hypnotist suggests but see no reason not to. The same is apparently true within self-hypnosis; if a person tells himself that an arm is stiff, it then feels stiff.

Consideration of suggestibility raises the important issue of control. Is the subject a passive person, an automaton doing what the hypnotist asks? Clearly not; but the matter is complex, and may depend in part on the nature of the rapport between the hypnotist and the subject. The modern hypnotist is not authoritarian, as the classical hypnotist was, and the general tone of professor-student and doctor-patient relationships has changed. The hypnotized person has at least two ego fractions operative at once: a hypnotized part, on the center of the stage, doing what the hypnotist suggests; and an observing part, in the wings, monitoring what is going on—and quite capable of interrupting if anything untoward is suggested. "If the hypnotist ever suggests things you don't want to do, you don't do them. . . . I have absolute control." "There is no situation where I feel I'm not in control. Suggestions are made, but it's me that's doing it, and I'm the one accepting or rejecting. . . . If I trust a hypnotist, I give up most of my controls, but a strong part of my mind knows what is going on."

One subject illustrated how she had resisted a suggestion. While under hypnosis she was told that she would be regressed back to the age of seven. She spoke up to the hypnotist: "No, I don't want to go back to seven, because when I was seven I had a dog I very much liked and the dog died. I don't want to go through losing that dog again."

One reason the practice of hypnosis requires experience and should remain in the hands of trained professional workers is that not all subjects conform to these generalizations. For an occasional subject, the observing ego recedes in hypnosis and does not function in the manner just described. One subject said: "Usually I can't bring myself out of hypnosis when someone else has put me in." She then gave an example. "I was supposed to waken myself and go home. I went home, but I was relaxed and rubbery, and couldn't remember about going home." This subject gradually regained normal functioning, but such an experience is potentially hazardous, and should and can be avoided.

Subjects may be asked within hypnosis to do tasks requiring a high order of hypnotic ability, such as eliminating the pain of normally aversive stimulation or being unaware of one task (such as automatic writing) while consciously doing another. They report that such tasks require great effort.

Subjects may come out of such hypnotic experiences tired instead of merely pleasantly relaxed. In other words, they have had to work to conform to the demands and are not merely passive.

The matter of control is illuminated by what subjects say about the hypnotist's role. We asked twenty-six highly hypnotically responsive subjects to tell us how the hypnotist appeared to them, and then had them choose the most appropriate description of the hypnotist from among the following:

Authoritarian person

Permissive person

Parental figure

Guide

Helper

Other

The hypnotist as guide was the predominant answer, given by twenty-five of the twenty-six subjects. Some insisted on adding their own supplements: "guide and helper;" "permissive guide, helper, and friend;" "permissive guide and teacher." The hypnotist as a parental figure was mentioned by only one: "combined guide with parental figure." Many were careful to deny any authoritarian aspect: "There's only a little authority, not much. I really don't enjoy authority figures. If the hypnotist were largely authoritarian, I don't think I could do well at all."

In describing what hypnosis is like to the person experiencing it, we must say something further about the intense personal experience the individual has when his hypnotic involvement is much more profound than that usually achieved. "Depth" of hypnosis is not a clear metaphor, but it is a familiar way of characterizing the profound and encompassing quality of an experience, just as sleep may be described as light or deep. Hypnotic responsiveness or susceptibility scales have occasionally been referred to as "depth" scales, on the assumption that the more responsive to the suggestions a subject is, the "deeper" into hypnosis he must be. To some extent this may be the case, for, with the same exposure to suggestions, the more hypnotizable person probably has a more profound experience of hypnosis. Depth is not the same thing as responsiveness to suggestions, however; a highly responsive subject can give many of the responses in the normal waking condition, but he does not go around hypnotized all the time. In other words, even if his responsiveness is relatively constant, his *depth* can vary. Analogous distinctions can be made in other areas: a person with a generally good appetite is not always hungry, and a finicky eater may be very hungry on occasion. His temporary state is not defined by his enduring characteristics.

The term *depth* should refer to momentary depth, which may fluctuate widely within a single hypnotic session; the best measure that has been devised is a verbal report by the subject on a numerical scale. After a little experience of hypnosis, a subject can indicate his degree of involvement on a scale with which he is familiar. For example, such a scale may use 0 for wide awake; 1 for drifting into a drowsy state; 2 for beginning to feel hypnotized; 3 for feeling that hypnosis has been entered; and so forth, with higher values going up perhaps to 10 for the condition in which most of the responses to suggestion can be given. The scale is open at the top, however, and with continued deepening, subjects may report depths well up toward 100 on this scale. For the scale to be useful, one subject need not agree with another. Despite the ambiguity of defining depth, subjects report no difficulty in assigning numbers to progressive changes they experience. In studies of hypnosis at greater depth, two findings are relevant. The first is that responsiveness to the standardized hypnotic scales takes place in the very low portion of the total scale of depth. Pain reduction, posthypnotic amnesia, and hallucinations do not require depths beyond 8 or 10 for most subjects; if a person does not succeed in pain reduction at, for example, a depth of 10, he is not likely to succeed at a depth of 20. The second finding is that at great depths responsiveness to suggestion falls off. In fact, without special arrangements, communication with the hypnotist may become essentially absent. Those rare cases in which a hypnotist has difficulty arousing a subject from hypnosis may be ones in which such depth was spontaneously achieved, when the hypnotist had not prepared for it. A simple preparation is to provide a nonverbal signal, such as placing the hypnotist's hand on the subject's arm, to reduce the hypnotic depth to a level at which the subject will again talk with the hypnotist.

What is hypnosis like at these greater depths of involvement? After the signal to return to a lighter depth, subjects can report how deep they were and what it felt like. A careful investigation by Tart of these deeper states shows the progressive changes occurring in one subject in the following order, as the hypnosis deepened. First relaxation of the body increased for a time, but he eventually no longer felt identified with his body. It was though it was just a "thing" left behind, so that it no longer made sense to ask him further about body relaxation. Relaxation of the body was succeeded by a peacefulness of the self, but beyond a certain depth this concept also became meaningless, because the self was no longer present. The environment also faded progressively, until finally a state was reached in which the only part of the environment that remained present was the hypnotist's voice. Time passed more and more slowly, finally reaching a point at which it ceased to be a meaningful concept. Spontaneous mental activity declined steadily until it finally reached zero.

In our experience, loss of contact with the hypnotist can occur if the deepening is a self-deepening process by the subject, not interrupted by continued talking by the hypnotist. What is found out can be expected to be in part a result of the arrangements under which the experiment is conducted; it may be expected to differ if, as in Tart's case, the hypnotist keeps on talking. Many subjects, when they deepen the experience themselves, report something akin to mystical experience; they feel that some kind of illumination has occurred, but of a kind that is not communicable.

These experiences are fascinating; they show that hypnosis is not completely defined by responsiveness to suggestion and indicate something about the limiting conditions. For therapy with hypnosis, these deeper states are not likely to prove practical because they leave behind some of the most useful features of hypnosis: a cooperative person who remains active and can eventually take responsibility for his own treatment. The successful patient not only experiences hypnosis, but directs it himself. In laboratory tests it was found that subjects who could not experience hypnotic analgesia at the ordinary levels could not experience it in the deeper stages either; thus the usefulness of responsiveness to suggestion occurs at the lighter levels of hypnotic involvement. The very profound levels may also present hazards, so that, except under appropriate conditions, it is probably wise to remain at more familiar levels.

The Laboratory and the Clinic

Because we shall present both experimental and clinical findings on pain and hypnosis, a word on the relation between laboratory and clinic may be worth adding in this largely laboratory-oriented chapter. The logical relationship between the researcher and the clinician is obvious: each needs to learn from the other. The social fact, however, is that those drawn to practice tend to have somewhat different motivations from those drawn to the laboratory; as a consequence there is often a gap between the clinical practitioner and the laboratory worker. This can readily be understood. The clinican must believe in what he is doing and communicate confidence to his patient; but the mark of the research scientist is skepticism. He sets up experiments to test his own favorite theories, and is obligated to relinquish his theories if they are disproved by the experiments. If the clinician has a long history of "training" his patients to become better hypnotic subjects, he will not accept very quickly the researcher's finding that such training is largely ineffective. Actually, both may be right. For the specific purposes of the clinician, the training may be effective; for changing the general responsiveness of the subject on a scale of hypnotic responsiveness, the training may not be effective. Resolving the difficulty calls for a collaboration in which the experimenter, by appropriate methods, determines what changes do in fact take place in the patient trained by the clinician. The research worker is not playing an irrelevant laboratory game; he is seeking appropriate generalizations based on the evidence, and should ultimately prove indispensable to the clinician who wishes his practice to be scientifically based. Our aim, then, is to bridge the gap between the clinic and the laboratory as best we can, as both of them deal with problems of hypnosis and pain.

Notes

The early history of hypnosis has been thoroughly covered in several books written near the turn of the century and later reprinted, such as Bramwell (1903; reissued 1956), and Moll (1890; reissued 1958). In their collection of basic writings, Shor and Orne (1965) include a number of pertinent early papers along with more recent ones. They also give a selected bibliography of historically important books, indicating the current editions of those which have been republished. A thorough book by Ellenberger (1970), although written primarily as a historical background for dynamic psychiatry, has a mine of information on early hypnosis.

The Mesmer-Gassner episode is fully recounted in Ellenberger (1970, pp. 53-57). An interesting account of Mrs. Eddy's cure by magnetiser Quimby is contained in Podmore (1902).

Esdaile's book on his surgical successes in India is available in reissued form (Esdaile, 1846 reissued, 1957). Braid's chief work is Braid (1843); an edited version appeared in 1889 and was reprinted in 1960. Freud's effort to resolve the conflict between Charcot and Bernheim is explained in his preface to the German edition of Bernheim's book (Freud, 1888). This is said to be Freud's first strictly psychological writing; his earlier writings can be classified as neurological. Freud's use of hypnosis in psychotherapy is in Breuer and Freud (1895).

The prominence of hypnosis in the 1880s, is evidenced by two long bibliographies by Dessoir (1887; 1890), listing 1182 works by 774 authors. Janet's remark that hypnosis would come back again appears in his two-volume English work (Janet, 1925), which had been written in French much earlier. McDougall included his World War I experiences with hypnosis in his *Abnormal Psychology* (McDougall, 1926).

The research program of Clark Hull led to his book, now considered a classic in the field (Hull, 1933; paperbound reprint, 1968). The papers in which he listed many topics left to be investigated are Hull (1929; 1930; 1931). His notebooks, published after his death (Hull, 1962), give interesting reflections on the courage it took to do research on hypnosis at the time. The next important research summary was by Weitzenhoffer (1953). The major research contributions during the decade 1955-1965 were reviewed by E. R. Hilgard (1965b); those of the next decade were summarized in E. R. Hilgard (1975b). Many research developments are given in the book edited by Fromm and Shor (1972). The general status of hypnosis around the world in the early 1960s is recounted in Marcuse (1964). The favorable actions by the British Medical Association and the American Medical Association are noted there.

Hypnotic Responsiveness

A summary of the estimates by nineteenth century writers as to how many people can be hypnotized may be found in E. R. Hilgard (1965a); modern hypnotic responsiveness scales are also described in detail, and evidence for the stability of scores on retest is given there. The follow-up over ten years is reported by Morgan, Johnson, and Hilgard (1974). For induction techniques, the most thorough source is still Weitzenhoffer (1957).

The best-known children's scale is that developed by London (1962), with normative data by London and Cooper (1969). We are now developing a new, short clinical scale in our laboratory for use with child patients. Scores according to age have been reported also by Barber and Calverley (1963b) through childhood, and throughout the lifespan by Morgan and Hilgard (1973).

Many active attempts to improve hypnotizability are covered in a thorough review by Diamond (1974); the reader must be warned, however, that the flavor of his conclusions is more favorable to change than the data on which they are based.

The personality correlates of hypnosis, leading to disappointing relationships, were reviewed by E. R. Hilgard (1965a). The twin study referred to is by Morgan (1973). The interview study was first reported in J. R. Hilgard (1965) and later in book form, J. R. Hilgard (1970). Further interviewing of those high and low in hypnotic responsiveness has confirmed the original findings of the importance of imaginative involvement (J. R. Hilgard, 1974a). The supporting study in which an absorption scale, developed by personality test methods, was found to correlate with hypnotizability is that of Tellegen and Atkinson (1974). It should be pointed out, however, that the best method of finding out whether an individual is hypnotizable is still to try a short hypnotic procedure with him. Correlations between hypnotic susceptibility and EEG-alpha are reviewed by E. R. Hilgard (1975a).

The work of Sperry and his associates on split brains is accessible in a book by one of the associates, Gazzaniga (1970). The study of normal subjects reciting, humming, and singing is by Schwartz and others (1973). The eye-divergence method was brought into hypnosis by Bakan (1969), working in our laboratory; the study of preference for right hemisphere function was also done here (Gur and Gur, 1974).

The State-Nonstate Issue

Barber and Sarbin have repeatedly attacked the usefulness of hypnosis as a concept, without thereby denying the phenomena of hypnosis, although Barber has frequently written the word *hypnosis* in quotation marks to show his dissatisfaction with it. Useful sources of their views are Barber (1969, 1972), and Sarbin and Coe (1972). The instinct controversy, used as an analogue, came up again after the ethologists (who have since won Nobel prizes for their work) used the word *instinct* in describing their naturalistic observations of birds and fishes (for example, Tinbergen, 1951). Rather than fighting, they were satisfied to speak later about species-specific behavior, which is simply instinct under another name. Some former hypnotic practitioners, particularly in Spain and South America have substituted the word *soph-rology* for hypnosis, thinking thereby to avoid some of the ancient stigma. The sophrologists have an arrangement whereby they publish their articles in English in an American hypnosis journal.

That hypnotic induction increases scores over ordinary noninduction procedures of testing susceptibility was first systematically pointed out by Weitzenhoffer and Sjoberg (1961). The result was immediately confirmed by Barber and Glass (1962), and more recently by Ruch, Morgan, and Hilgard (1973). Barber and Calverley (1963a) introduced the task motivation method in an attempt to show that it was not hypnotic induction that produced the increase; the technique was used in numerous subsequent studies. Eventually Bowers (1967) showed that statements such as "Everyone passed these tests when they tried" led to a falsification of what the subject did and reported. Bowers found this out by having subjects interviewed afterward by someone other than the experimenter, under instructions for absolute honesty. In a test of Bowers' conjectures, Spanos and Barber (1968) supported his conclusions for at least one of their hallucinatory tasks; the result for the other was a little ambiguous. Hence the strongest argument against induction doing anything turns out to be a weak one. For this and other reasons there are some signs of a growing theoretical convergence (Spanos and Barber, 1974).

The increasing ease with which eye closure could be achieved in repeated hypnotic inductions led Hull (1933) to propose a learning theory of hypnosis. He was misled in this, because the learned rapidity of eye closure did not mean necessarily that the subject had learned to go more deeply into hypnosis.

That self-hypnosis is effective with minimal instructions, even for someone not previously hypnotized, has been shown in a doctoral dissertation by Ruch (1972). Coué's variety of self-hypnosis is described in his book, (Coué, 1923) and in Brooks (1922).

Orne's paradigm for the experiment comparing instructed simulators with reals is presented in detail in Orne (1972). Orne gives a number of illustrations in which a difference was found between the "real" and the "instructed simulator" supporting the interpretation that hypnosis adds something beyond the experimenter's demands. Some failures to find differences are also given.

The Hypnotic Experience and the Relation to the Hypnotist

Some of the phenomenal differences that subjects report when hypnotized, and some of the differences observed by experimenters, are summarized by E. R. Hilgard (1965a, pp. 5–14) and by Barber (1969, pp. 105–122). Although the observations made are quite consonant, they are differently evaluated with respect to the nature of the hypnotic condition. The observations themselves agree essentially with the later interview material reported in this chapter. Shor's characterization of the hypnotic experience can be found in Shor (1959b; 1962a; 1970).

The material on how the subject perceives the hypnotist has been drawn largely from J. R. Hilgard (1971).

The discussion of more profound hypnotic states, coordinated with subjective scales of depth, depends heavily upon Tart (1970; 1972). In one of his scales, Tart assumed that certain kinds of hypnotic behavior in response to suggestion could be used to define depth. Subsequent work has shown that a simple numerical scale without an upper limit is preferable. An unpublished doctoral dissertation following up some of Tart's earlier observations also contains relevant observations on great depth (Sherman, 1971).

The Laboratory and the Clinic

It is common for clinical practitioners to express impatience with experimenters and to fall back on their experiences with patients as "proof." Because a few patients who were at first resistant to hypnosis later became sufficiently cooperative to accept hypnotherapy (as in Dorcus, 1963), is hardly a sufficient answer to the laboratory studies that find hypnotic talent difficult to modify. It is quite possible for patients with only slight hypnotic responsiveness to profit from suggestive therapy. If the patient is cooperative enough merely to sit with his eyes closed and listen to the therapist, he can be treated by a method known in Russia as the Bekhterev-Bernheim method of direct suggestion, named for two famous older users of hypnosis (Platonov, 1959, p. 426). If, therefore, we ask for critical cooperation between experimenter and clinician, it is only to base hypnosis on as firm scientific ground as possible.

2 Pain

A thumb pounded by a hammer throbs with pain. There is no question what caused the pain; the victim's immediate concern is how to relieve it. Pain is all too familiar to each of us. We take for granted that we must live with it some of the time, and most of us manage to do so successfully. Our familiarity with pain does not, however, lessen the importance of understanding it better. Pain reduction is a primary task of the physician, second only to the preservation of health against life-threatening disease. The prevalence of pain is evident from the attention pain-killers receive in advertising and from the millions of dollars that the public spends on them. Hypnosis has played some part in pain reduction for over a century in modern medical practice; at the same time, hypnosis has been confused with the mystical, the occult, and with faith healing—confusions creating obstacles to its acceptance in science and in the healing arts.

To remove the barriers against wider use of hypnosis, a sober critical appraisal is required, reviewing historical and contemporary clinical and experimental evidence as to the proper place of hypnosis in the control of pain. This book aims to fill the need for such an appraisal; it is also addressed, through what hypnosis has taught us, to some of the larger problems of understanding pain.

Pain and Suffering

A fundamental paradox involving pain is that it is at once beneficial and harmful. If a thorn scratches the skin or a splinter pierces it, the resulting pain is a sign that there is something to be avoided or some damage to be repaired. The information the pain conveys is useful because the site of the damage can be located and something can be done about it: the splinter can be removed, a bleeding wound can be bandaged, or a dressing can be placed on a burn. If an ankle is sprained or a bone broken, pain increases when that member is used in its ordinary way; the pain thus protects from further injury until the condition has been improved. Abdominal pain may be a warning signal that the appendix is inflamed and may burst. A toothache gives information that a tooth is infected. We can certainly say that some of the body's sensitivities have evolved to protect it against danger.

The beneficial results of pain are dramatized by careful studies of a few persons whose pain mechanisms are so defective that they are insensitive to usually painful stimuli. Such a deficiency is often first noted in childhood, after a child has suffered more than the usual number of injuries without complaint. These otherwise normal children show no known physical basis for their pain deficiency. Without feeling pain, they may damage their nostrils by picking away at them, bite off parts of the tongue or fingers, or back into hot stoves or radiators without knowing that they are burning their skin. Careful examination of the children will show many scars and other signs of damage, such as deformed joints, caused by accidents and injuries. These children are evidence of the usefulness to other children of the warning that pain brings. The consequences of feeling no pain may be lethal, as in known cases of patients who died of rupture of the appendix accompanied by painless peritonitis.

The other side of the paradox—pain that is not useful—is pain that comes too late. Many of the gravest diseases strike without prior warning of pain. The famous French surgeon Leriche said that an illness is a drama in two acts, of which the first goes on in the silence of the tissues, without a warning sign of pain. The second act is then a *denouement* in which pain announces a disease condition already far advanced, perhaps beyond remediation. The tumors of cancer do not announce themselves in the early stages of their growth; heart illness may reach the stage of a coronary accident before pain is felt; and ulcers may cause no pain until perforation has occurred.

Chronic pain serving no useful purpose may go beyond being unpleasant; it may indeed be destructive and incapacitating. Disregarding for the moment the source of the pain, what can the prolonged *experience* of pain do to the sufferer? It may produce severe depression, have deleterious effects on heart and kidneys, disturb gastric and colonic processes, and upset heart regularity and blood pressure. The price of such pain, in reduced efficiency at work and in lessened enjoyment of life, is hard to measure; most people can find illustrations from their own lives or those of their acquaintances of the damage that continuous pain can do.

Those who ponder man's basic problems are soon led by the inevitability of pain to reflect upon it—along with death—as a basic fact of human existence. Religious literature dwells on the subject. Pains associated with childbirth are attributed in the Book of Genesis to Eve's punishment because she ate of the fruit of knowledge. Even the symbol of the Cross links pain to the understanding of human destiny; the word *excruciating*, applied to pain, is derived from the word *crucifixion*.

Because pain hurts and is so universally distasteful, it might be supposed that defining it would present no problem. Not so, however, for there are many discussions in the scientific literature about the problem of defining pain. By an *ostensive definition*, or definition by example, pain consists of such things as headaches, stomachaches, and the corresponding consequences of burns, cuts, bites, and broken bones. This "definition" does locate the general area of what we mean by pain, but borderline cases soon arise. Most of our examples point to some sort of injury, but we know that there are painless injuries and that there are ,pains caused by no known source of injury or irritation. Furthermore, although most pains have a sensory component, this does not completely describe the experience of pain. There is a triad of distress, incompletely described by sense perception, that includes *sensory pain, suffering,* and *mental anguish.* These concepts are familiar to lawyers who become engaged in controversies over personal injuries. It is no wonder that problems of definition arise.

In his book on pain, Sternbach said that after almost despairing in his attempt to define pain, he had finally settled on a definition that recognized three components in it: a component pointing to the pain source as a harmful stimulus signaling possible damage; a pattern of responses permitting the pain to be recognized by an external observer; and, finally, the subjective or private feeling of hurt. By pointing out that investigators from different perspectives choose to examine one or another of these components, he tried to bring a little order into the ostensive definition of pain. But, like those before him, Sternbach was unable to come up with a definition that caught the single "essence" of pain, beyond the common-sense notion that we are dealing with what hurts. We shall find repeatedly that the subjective aspects of pain are paramount in understanding it.

These problems of defining pain have a long history. When Aristotle settled on the five senses, he omitted pain; it was not until the nineteenth century that the sensory component of pain became a normal part of physiological and psychological science. The ancient pairing of pleasure and pain as opposites led to classification of both as "passions of the soul" rather than as senses. The scientific study of pain has improved on the common-sense, ostensive definition by sharpening the distinction between two components of pain, the *sensory* component and the *suffering* component. In considering pain as one of the senses, the nineteenth-century investigators tended to pay less attention to pain as a "passion." The distinction came back to prominence a few years ago, however, in a study of patients who received prefrontal lobotomies for relief of intractable pain. These patients commonly reported that the pain was there as before, but it no longer bothered them. The pain that remained was the sensory pain; the suffering had been relieved. Some lesions in the medial thalamus, created by surgeons to alleviate intractable pain, have also been reported to relieve distress without interfering with sensory functions. These areas of the brain are, interestingly enough, the same ones that are very sensitive to morphine.

The separate experiences of pain and suffering can be characterized in two ways. One way is to assume that *sensory pain* is like any other perceptual response to irritation or injury; it is informative about the location and intensity of whatever may be its source. If that is the primary experience, there is a secondary experience in reaction to it—an experience of distress, expressed by crying out, by movement, by facial expression, by autonomic responses. This is the *suffering* component, a reaction that follows upon the pain. Such a distinction, by now familiar in the literature of pain, corresponds in some respects to a classical interpretation of emotion and its expression: first an informative message comes, such as a letter telling of the death of a loved one. Then the expression of grief follows as a reaction, just as suffering follows upon the information brought by pain.

A second possibility is that the two components arise simultaneously rather than successively. Sensory pain and suffering might be two ways of reacting to a common source of irritation or stress, with separate parts of the nervous system responsible for activating the two systems. According to this view, it would not be correct to consider the suffering component merely as a reaction to the felt pain; both may be interacting components of the total pain experience from the start.

One might suppose that the issue would soon be resolved by scientific tests. Unfortunately, decisive experiments are difficult to perform, and there are puzzling issues to be resolved, as we shall note in reviewing the physiological aspects of pain. Whatever the conclusions about sensory pain and suffering, the distinction between them is here to stay because they are rooted in personal experience. Separate consideration of the two components is important practically as well as theoretically. It appears, for example, that morphine may indeed reduce suffering more than sensory pain; corresponding issues arise in pain reduction through hypnosis. Of course there are also situations in which there is discomfort without sensory pain. Consider a person attempting to sleep in a room that is too hot or humid: his discomfort may rise to a high level without his feeling pain. Similarly, if the room is too cold, he may be uncomfortable without "hurting." Such discomfort can be subjected to quantitative measurement; orderly changes of discomfort are found as the temperature moves in either direction from the comfortable range.

There may very well be more than two components to the pain experience. The psychologists Melzack, a student of pain, and Torgerson, a specialist in psychological measurement, selected 102 words used to characterize pain. They then proceeded to arrange these words into appropriate classes by a two-step process. In the first step, student judges grouped together those words that seemed to belong together in describing pain. They found that the words fell into three main classes: those describing sensory qualities; those describing affective, or emotional, qualities; and those that were evaluative of the total experience. The latter two classes comprise the reactive or suffering component of pain. In the second step in classification, patients, doctors, and students assigned numbers to the words that belonged together, in a scale of increasing intensity from 1 (mild) to 5 (excruciating). An idea of the words used can be gained from a few representative sequences, here arranged within each class in order of increasing intensity of the pain experience:

Sensory pain, temporal aspects: flickering, quivering, pulsing, throbbing, beating, pounding.

Sensory pain, constrictive pressure: pinching, pressing, gnawing, cramping, crushing.

Affective, fear: fearful, frightful, terrifying.

Evaluative: annoying, troublesome, miserable, intense, unbearable.

Melzack and Torgerson found enough agreement among their raters to encourage them to develop a questionnaire that may prove useful in experimental investigation of the pains that patients feel. It may also help in finding out how the dimensions of pain are modified by various methods of pain management.

Many pains are described as *intractable*, which means only that they are obstinate and resistant to treatment. In most cases, however, the tissue source of such pain is vague or absent. There are many pains that give us no information—or false information—about the source of irritation or injury. Three of these may serve for purposes of illustration: phantom limb pains, referred pains, and psychosomatic pains.

It is very common for a person who has had an arm or leg amputated to have the perception that the absent limb is still present. Such an absent but perceived member is known as a *phantom limb*. In some instances, the patient feels *pain* in the phantom limb; these are the cases that interest us. The possibility readily suggests itself that the phantom pain arises because of stimulation of the cut ends of the nerves that formerly led to the amputated member. Sometimes, in fact, phantom limb pain can be controlled, at least temporarily, by anesthetizing or surgically removing the growths (neuromas) that develop in the stump at the ends of cut nerves. However, this explanation is not sufficient, for even anesthetizing the whole stump may not eliminate the phantom. Even more striking is the fact that the pain as felt in the phantom limb is likely to reproduce a pain felt in the limb prior to amputation; hence the phantom pain appears to be based on some kind of memory. A striking case is mentioned by Melzack of a man who was being taken for treatment of a wood sliver jammed under a fingernail; he met with an accident and the arm had to be removed. When a phantom developed, he felt pain under the fingernail of his phantom hand.

Referred pains are those felt in one place although the source of irritation is somewhere else; one may feel shoulder and arm pain, for example, when having a heart attack. Sometimes stimulation of an analgesic leg may produce a pain in the upper abdomen on the opposite side of the body. A specialist trained to do appropriate testing can find the source of the pain on the basis of where it is felt in some cases; in others, however, there may be enough idiosyncrasy to baffle him.

Psychosomatic pains are so described because their origins are complexly related to the life of the patient with pain, the emotional meaning of the pain to him, and the subtle purposes it may serve. A headache which is felt while studying for an examination, but which disappears when going to the movies can serve as an illustration. Such a pain is real; its psychological origin does not mean that it hurts less than pain of somatic origin.

These three kinds of pain—phantom limb, referred, and psychosomatic—point out the uncertainties about the source of stimulation when pain is felt in a particular place. In addition, they call to our attention the possible importance of psychological factors, which must be taken into account if our knowledge is to move forward.

Another question is why individuals react so differently to the same pain-producing stress. People appear to differ not only in the openness of their expression of pain through complaints or overt signs, but also in their reports of sensory pain under identical conditions of stimulation. Of course, some differences may be present from birth, as in the extreme case of insensitivity to pain; perhaps other individuals not so extremely deficient may also have reduced sensitivity. There are undoubtedly life experiences that modify the individual's responsiveness to pain, such as the manner in which pain is treated in his childhood. Detectable differences in reactions to pain appear among various ethnic groups composing subcultures within America. Local circumstances, such as those found on the battlefield, also affect responses to pain. It has been reported that some wounded soldiers experienced no pain from severe wounds, although they were still sensitive to painful stimulation, as shown by their wincing at the puncture by a hypodermic needle. Laboratory studies have shown that motivational factors characteristic of a given setting can influence not only pain reports but galvanic indicators of pain. We shall review some of the evidence bearing on these statements.

We know little about the specific effects of childhood experiences, although some dramatic experiments have been performed with animals. Scottie dogs reared in a restricted environment did not develop normal pain sensitivity. Later, when exposed to a lighted match, they would explore the match until it burned their noses, without withdrawing from it as a normal dog would. A normal dog would not again face this experience, whereas these dogs would explore a second lighted match as though nothing had happened previously. A somewhat similar finding was reported with a young chimpanzee raised with restricted movement, but otherwise normally healthy. Hence it appears that something about reacting to pain in the process of growing up determines the way in which the aversive quality of pain is experienced.

Indirectly, the effects of learning are shown by differences in reactions to pain among ethnic groups and among members of families of different size. Children from larger families complain of pain more than children from small families, as though more complaint may be required to get attention in larger families. Ethnic differences have been found in reactions to pain, based in part on the tradition of giving overt expression, which is more pronounced in some groups than in others. Investigations have been done with veterans who were surgical patients and their families, with college student women, and with housewives; ethnic groupings commonly used in those studies were Yankee (or "Old American"), Irish, Jewish, and Italian. The Yankee groups tend to have a phlegmatic, matter-of-fact attitude toward pain, reflected in physiological measures such as rapid adaptation of galvanic responses to repeated shocks. The Italian women showed the least tolerance to pain, in view of their cultural approval of public suffering. Jews also seemed to feel free to cry out, believing that expression did some good; they were likely to try to understand the meaning of pain and to avoid using drugs to reduce the pain.

The experience of pain at any given time and place may be influenced by situational factors closely related to motivation. A common story is that of the injured athlete who is not aware of his pain until the play is over. Laboratory studies in much less exciting circumstances have shown ways in which pain can be modified by motivation. There is a strong tendency for a person to view his behavior as rational, and to perceive his actions as consistent with his beliefs. If, for example, a person wishes to continue smoking cigarettes, he is less likely to believe the surgeon general's report that smoking is harmful than if he is prepared to give up smoking. In experiments with laboratory pain, the curious effect has been found that the amount of pain felt may be related to the amount of pay received for enduring it. It is as though the subject, to be consistent, must give value received for his pay. In one study, for example, subjects drew lots to determine whether they would be paid nothing at all, or $1, $2, $4, or $8. By drawing lots, each subject's need for money did not enter into the determination of how much he would be paid. The outcome was that those who happened to be promised more money felt more pain in the experiment. In another study the subject, after having been required to undergo a pain experience, was invited to volunteer for doing it again. When the subject volunteered, he rationalized that it was not such a severely painful experiment after all, in order not to seem foolish to himself for doing so. In fact, he showed both behavioral and physiological signs of suffering less pain.

It is evident that to understand pain fully we must enter the area of social psychology, and go beyond the sensitivity of receptor mechanisms and the functioning of pain processing mechanisms in the nervous system.

Physiology of Pain and Suffering

Modern efforts to understand the physiology and psychology of pain began in the nineteenth century, when interest was high in all aspects of sense perception. Pain came into its own with the discovery that exploration of small areas of the skin with appropriate instruments revealed some spots sensitive to touch, some sensitive to warmth, some to cold, and some to pain. These spots were spatially separated; their discovery led to a search for appropriate receptors beneath the skin which would serve as transducers between stimulation and the transmission of nervous impulses. The tactual sense was thus divided into several; pain thereafter had its place as a sensory modality. Von Frey, who was prominent in this experimentation, claimed in 1896 that free nerve endings are specialized pain receptors. This led to his *specificity theory* of pain, according to which cutaneous pain (and probably other pains as well) were said to result from stimulation of free nerve endings, just as sight comes from stimulation of rods and cones in the retina. The specificity theory was widely accepted and remains influential today, although it has now come under attack as being too limited to cover all aspects of pain.

Contemporary with Von Frey's theory, Goldscheider's *pattern theory* emerged as a rival. The pattern theory, or summation theory, proposes that pain depends upon a summation of neural inputs that must reach a critical level for pain to be felt. Peripheral stimulation is not enough, because central systems are important in this summation. Modern pattern theories include both peripheral and central summation. The several pattern theories have in common an attempt to explain why pain may endure beyond the time of focal stimulation.

Dissatisfied with both the specificity and pattern theories as complete accounts of pain, Melzack and Wall in 1965 proposed a new two-component theory. Known as the *gate control theory*, it has been widely influential in recent discussions of pain. Actually, it is the latest in a series of two-component theories; some earlier two-component theories identified the components as fine discrimination (epicritic) and diffuse sensitivity (protopathic); as fast and slow fiber conduction; or as differentiated fiber systems, with small fibers carrying pain in a network while large fibers served an inhibitory function. The gate control theory has probably drawn from these earlier formulations, but it is clearly a new integration of knowledge about pain.

The gate control theory begins with an acceptance of the anatomical distinctiveness between two neural conducting systems from the spinal cord to the higher centers of the brain, after impulses have entered the cord as a consequence of peripheral stimulation. One of these systems is primarily informative; it carries data about the location and intensity of stimulation, with little relation to its noxious or aversive quality. This is called the *sensory-discriminative* system. The other system, closely related to the structures near the center of the brain that involve motivation and emotion, is called the *motivational-affective* system. It is more concerned with the suffering that pain causes. It may be noted that the gate control theory accepts the second of the options previously discussed for the sensory and suffering components (page 30), because both components are initiated at once and have separate processing systems. We shall not enter here into the evidence for the two systems, except to state that they are reasonably well established, both neuroanatomically and psychophysiologically. Once pain and distress are repeated or long-lasting, the priority of sensory pain or of suffering is no longer a central issue.

The gate theory rests on a further hypothesis about the modulation of pain as it is affected by impulses transmitted by the two systems. The hypothesis is that the large and small fibers that enter the spinal cord interact in such a manner as to affect the pain information that gets transmitted to the higher centers. This interaction is shown schematically in Figure 2. Both large and small fibers are shown entering the gate control system, where their interaction affects the discharges of the first transmission cells (T-cells) of the two systems, which then send the pain impulses on their way. A central control mechanism is also imposed upon this local mechanism at the cord level. A practical consequence of the gate theory has been to accelerate the use of electrical stimulation for pain management, either directly to the nerve trunks that carry large fibers or to the skin surface over the nerve trunks without penetrating the skin. The purpose of such treatment has been to counteract deep, persistent pains being carried by small fibers by stimulating large ones. According to the theory, this should succeed in closing the gate and reducing the pain. The practical successes of electrical stimulation have been great enough to give some support to the theory.

The central control mechanisms act as another set of pain modifiers. There are many possible pathways by which impulses from higher centers can descend to modify activity in the spinal cord. One such pathway starts

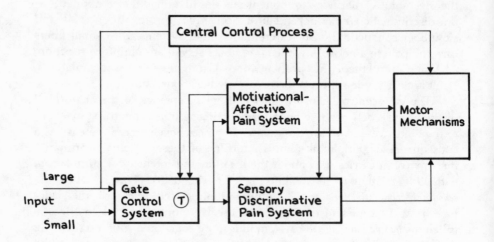

Figure 2. Gate control theory of pain. Large and small fibers deliver pain information to the gate control system in the spinal cord (lower left of diagram). There, the impulses from the two sources interact to modulate the impulses to be transmitted by way of transmission cells ⓣ. The transmitted impulses activate both the sensory-discriminative system and the motivational-affective system, leading eventually to responses to the pain (Motor Mechanisms).

The central control processes react on the basis of three sources of incoming information (shown by arrows pointing upward): direct, nonnoxious information from the large fibers about the location and nature of the stimulation (e.g., something hot on the left hand), shown by the vertical line at the left outside the gate control system; and separate information from each of the two pain systems. Descending control by way of central processes is indicated by arrows pointing downward, including one to the motor mechanisms. Modified from Melzack and Casey (1968), p. 427.

from the ventral posterior lateral nucleus, a center in the thalamus at which information about nonnoxious properties of stimulation arrives rapidly via the large fiber system. Because this information arrives before the motivational and affective processing has taken place, the higher center can modify the impulses at the gate while they are still being interpreted. Experimental evidence from several sources indicates that stimulation at these higher levels can affect pain impulses originating in the cord. Abdominal surgery in rats has been performed without chemical anesthetics by electrically stimulating the central gray matter of the midbrain. There was no evidence of responsiveness to aversive stimuli as long as the electrical stimulation continued; once it was discontinued, responses reappeared. Further experiments have shown that reactions to pain in cats can be abolished through electrical stimulation of electrodes implanted near the central aqueduct in the core of the brain. Again, reactions to pain reappear when the electrical stimulation is discontinued.

The gate control theory has gained clinical and experimental support for a number of its features, but not for all. Three difficulties with the theory have been listed by Casey, one of its supporters. (1) The complexity of interconnections in the dorsal spinal gray matter makes critical anatomical specification of the gate control mechanism extremely difficult. (2) Interneurons with all the necessary properties have not been located. (3) Some of the required interactions at the neuronal and synaptic level have not supported details of the theory. To these difficulties might be added the vagueness of the theory with respect to the central monitoring system. Another problem is that supplementary conjectures are required to explain why electrical stimulation and similar procedures, which supposedly close the gate, reduce pain not only while the stimulation is occurring but often for hours afterward. What does seem to be firmly established about the theory can be stated in three propositions.

1. Two distinctive mechanisms—one informative, the other motivational-affective—appear to be involved in the total pattern of pain perception. This distinction is supported by neuroanatomical considerations.

2. Deep, persistent pain can be modified by concurrent stimulation of large fibers. The pain reduction outlasts the counterirritant, so that some process enduring in time must be present to moderate responses to a pain source.

3. Central control processes, exemplified by psychologically recognized kinds or by brain stimulation, can clearly affect the perception of noxious stimulation.

These three features must be included in any satisfactory pain theory; the popularity of the gate control theory rests partly on its clear recognition of this total obligation. Even when a theory starts from a neuroanatomical and physiological base, psychological factors intrude themselves prominently —in motivation and emotion, in memory, and in "central" control that commonly means "cognitive" or "ideational" control.

A great deal more might be said about pain, the agents that produce it, and the action of the analgesics that reduce it. Lim and his collaborators demonstrated that the adequate stimulus for pain is often a chemical substance to which the viscera, the muscles, and other structures of the body are sensitive. Many of these substances are amines or peptides. Probably the most familiar is a peptide known as *bradykinin* that develops in the blisters formed when the skin is burned; it is responsible for the continuing pain. If bradykinin is injected into an artery, pain is felt. The analgesic action of aspirin is related to these substances; its action is primarily peripheral, not central as with morphine. It has been shown that aspirin acts on chemical receptors sensitive to bradykinin and related substances, hence reducing the pain their presence causes.

The laboratory pains used in our studies of pain and pain reduction probably involve some of these chemical mediators. Ischemic-exercise pain, for example, requires first that blood flow to the muscles of a forearm be reduced, so that the muscle tissue becomes blood-free, or ischemic. It has been shown experimentally that ischemia alone does not cause pain in muscle; the pain arises only following exercise of the muscle. Apparently exercise of the occluded muscle releases the pain-producing chemicals, which are normally washed away by the blood. Ischemic pain is, in fact, quickly recovered from when the circulation is restored.

Experimentally Produced Pains and Pain Measurement

The complexity of the pain experience must be noted again before we turn to the particular methods we have used in our own studies of pain. Alternative methods of measurement choose very different aspects of the total experience. The expression "pain sensitivity" is commonly used to describe threshold pain—the minimum amount of stimulation that can be detected as pain. There are well-developed laboratory devices for producing such pains, such as an instrument for painfully stimulating a spot on the forehead by radiant heat; a device for painfully stimulating a tooth by an electric current; and a concentric electrode for stimulation on a skin surface. Appropriate signal detection methods are available for treating the obtained data. We have chosen not to discuss such methods, because the problem facing the person suffering pain is not how little he can detect; rather, it is how to cope with enduring pains that are well above threshold levels. At the other extreme from the threshold we find the expression "pain tolerance." This is defined either by the maximum pain a person is willing to endure as the intensity of stimulation is gradually increased, or by the amount of time he is willing to continue accepting a pain at a given high level of stimulus intensity. We have also rejected the use of tolerance level in our studies, because it is a measure of heroism rather than of experienced pain. Two people, stimulated in the same way and experiencing the noxious stimulus as equally painful—both as sensory pain and as a distressing experience—may tolerate the pain very differently; one may grit his teeth and accept it longer than the other.

As already noted, other complexities are added to the pain experience by fears, anxieties, and expectations. We do not mean to minimize the importance of these factors, but at the same time we wish to emphasize the possibility of narrowing the study at first to pain reports correlated more specifically with circumstances of stimulation. For example, it is quite possible that some patients suffering from pain need tranquilizers or sedatives instead of analgesics. It would be a mistake, however, to believe that a tranquilizer reduces felt pain merely because it succeeds in quieting a patient; it might affect his tolerance rather than his pain. We shall meet such questions later on, but for the present we wish to concern ourselves with the narrower aspects of pain—both the sensory experience and the suffering viewed as functions of the intensity or duration of stimulation.

Our choice of direct magnitude estimates of pain and suffering instead of threshold sensitivity or tolerance limits left us free to choose ways of producing continuing suprathreshold laboratory-induced pains. Others have used enduring electrical shocks; pressures against bony structures, such as wedges against a finger or cleats against a shin-bone; tight headbands; and many others. Because we have used primarily two kinds of stimulation which are familiar also in other laboratories, our descriptions of procedures will be limited to them. What we have done is to induce physical pains similar to clinical pains, in order to show that such pains can be measured and then subjected to psychological reduction.

The first type of stimulation, which depends upon circulating ice water, is known as *cold pressor pain*. If a hand and forearm are placed in circulating ice water, the sensation of cold quickly becomes painful; the pain mounts very rapidly, reaching a maximum within a minute. After a minute, some complex things happen because of numbing, but for pain measurement, an immersion time of a minute or less is quite satisfactory. We have adopted the practice of asking for a report of pain every 5 seconds on a simple numerical scale, beginning with no pain at 0 and increasing to 10 as a critical or anchoring value, at which the subject would very much like to remove the hand from the water. We prefer not to call this a tolerance level, because subjects can tolerate much more pain than this; when we ask a subject to keep his hand and arm in the water beyond his report of 10, he continues to count. These pain reports are quite orderly; they can be repeated on successive occasions with little change. There are many evidences that reports on the simple numerical scale give a dependable measure of the pain that is felt. One kind of evidence is that the pain reported shows a very orderly relationship to the temperature of the water: the colder the water, the greater the pain reported. This relationship is shown in Figure 3.

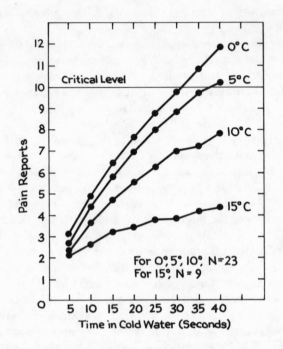

Figure 3. Reports of cold pressor pain corresponding to water temperature. The subject placed one hand and forearm in circulating ice water and gave a pain report every 5 seconds. The colder the water the greater the pain, as expected; water at 0°C and 5°C produced a maximum pain in 40 seconds that rose above the critical level of 10. The upper three curves represent the averages of twenty-three student subjects who experienced the temperatures in various orders; the lowest curve is for nine who were tested later. From Hilgard (1969).

The general orderliness of the pain reports over time in the cold water reflects a complex underlying process. When the hand and arm are being cooled in the water, the exact increase in the physical stimulus to pain is hard to specify, because the deeper layers of the skin are cooled less rapidly than the superficial layers, and because changes in blood circulation occur in response to the cold. As an empirical matter, however, time in the cold water can be used as though intensity of stimulation were increasing at a uniform rate.

Because of the many different qualities of pain, it is often well not to limit experimentation to pain produced in a single way. The cold pressor pain

has some disadvantages for study of the physiological aspects of pain, because of the cardiovascular responses that occur reflexively to the cold and
because the subject must discriminate between the sensory aspects of pain
and the sensory aspects of increasing cold. Hence we have used another
method, known as the tourniquet-exercise method, to which reference has
already been made (page 38). We call the pain produced by this method
ischemic pain to distinguish it from cold pressor pain, although there is some
ischemia in cold pressor pain also.

Ideally, a laboratory pain should approximate the postoperative pain of
surgical patients and respond as clinical pains do to chemical analgesics. It
has long been known that ischemic (blood-deprived) muscle, when exercised, gives rise to pain. The problem has been to develop the most appropriate way to produce and measure this pain in the laboratory. We have
adopted the method developed by Smith, working in Beecher's laboratory at
Harvard; they named it the submaximum effort tourniquet technique. In our
procedure, the subject's arm is first deprived of blood by raising it and
wrapping it to the elbow in an elastic bandage. Then the tourniquet—a
standard sphygmomanometer cuff—is inflated to 250 mm, and the bandage
is removed. Now the subject squeezes a dynamometer at a controlled rate
against a constant load of 10 kg for twenty squeezes, and waits; the pain
mounts very slowly at first, but eventually becomes unbearable. The time
required for pain to become unbearable is much longer than in the ice water,
a matter of minutes instead of seconds, and varies widely from person to
person. An important feature of ischemic pain is that it is sensitive to morphine, as postsurgical pains are; the amount by which the reported pain is
reduced depends upon how much morphine has been administered.

We have used the same numerical pain scale with ischemic pain that we
used with cold pressor pain, with comparable results. The reports of pain for
a given subject are quite consistent from one repetition of the pain experience
to another; a plot of increasing pain over time, as reported by the same
subjects in ischemia, shows little difference between one day and the next.

Although the distinction was not made in a number of earlier experiments,
we later introduced a rating for suffering, separate from that for sensory pain.
Suffering was defined for the subject as something other than the localized
effect of painful stimulation, having to do with general annoyance, disturbance, or distress as a consequence or accompaniment of the pain. It was
pointed out that people can have pain without distress, and that they can have
distress without pain. Although subjects gave their own interpretations to the
distinction, they did not find it difficult to make a distinction. Characteristi-
cally, subjects reported suffering as less intense than sensory pain; this
finding was sufficiently common for us to suppose that all were making the
distinction on a somewhat similar basis. A typical result for a mean of eight
student subjects is shown in Figure 4.

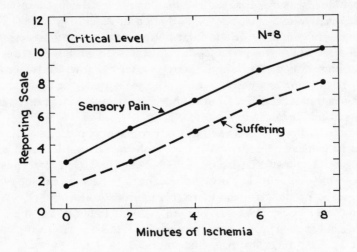

Figure 4. Reports of sensory pain and suffering in ischemic pain. The pain was produced by application of a tourniquet, followed by exercise. The rising curves indicate the pain and suffering as reported at 2-minute intervals; values are the means from eight student subjects. The reports of suffering tended to be less than those of sensory pain throughout. After Knox, Morgan, and Hilgard (1974).

With these satisfactory methods of measuring pain and suffering, we had a basis for experiments on pain control through hypnosis, which are described later.

We did not, of course, limit ourselves in these studies to verbal reports of pain and suffering, but measured some physiological accompaniments of the imposed laboratory stress, primarily changes in heart rate and in systolic blood pressure. Heart rates tend to accelerate as pain increases, and blood pressure tends to rise. An illustration of the relationship of blood pressure rise to time in water at different temperatures is given in Figure 5. This shows that the rise in blood pressure corresponds approximately to the rise in reported pain shown in Figure 3, but the blood pressure curves are not so smooth nor so distinct from each other as those for verbally reported pain. Thus physiological measures, which seem more objective and less subject to individual whim than verbal reports, turn out to be less satisfactory than what the subject says about his pain. This is partly because of individual differences in the responsiveness of the autonomic nervous system, and partly because the physiological indicators are affected indiscriminately by so many influences other than pain. Verbal responses are also influenced by more than one causal factor, but the instructed subject can attend selectively and give separate reports, for example, of sensory pain and of distress. Such separation for physiological indicators is almost impossible. As a consequence, no single physiological measure provides an infallible indicator of felt pain.

This survey of the manifestations of pain and suffering, ways of understanding pain physiologically and psychologically, and means of measuring pain and suffering prepares us to examine, in the next chapters, how pain is alleviated. We are prepared for the fact that the psychological component in pain is so important that modification of pain through psychological techniques, of which hypnosis is but one, is to be expected.

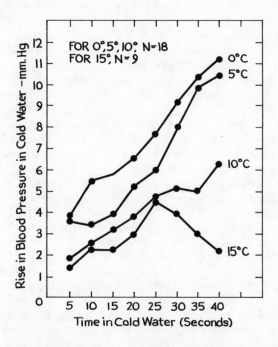

Figure 5. Rise in blood pressure corresponding to water temperature. The rise in systolic blood pressure at 5-second intervals when the hand and forearm were placed in circulating ice water corresponded to the rise in reported pain (see Figure 3); the greatest rise occurred with the coldest temperature. Blood pressure measures, however, discriminated between temperatures less well than verbal reports. From Hilgard (1969).

Notes

Useful sources on the general problems of pain, especially for those with a psychophysiological background or interest, are the books by Sternbach (1968) and by Melzack (1973), both of which contain extensive lists of references. The scientific reader desiring a very detailed and thorough review may find it in a large book of the papers presented at an international symposium on pain, edited by Bonica (1974).

Pain and Suffering

On congenital insensitivity to pain, there are useful reviews by Critchley (1956) and Sternbach (1963). The most extensively studied case of an individual who was congenitally insensitive to pain is that of a young woman reported by McMurray (1950). Her story, well summarized by Sternbach (1968), illustrates the point that pain is useful in that she underwent, without pain, extensive skin and bone accidents that contributed to her death.

The idea that illness comes in two acts, with pain associated with the second act and tending to come too late, may be found in a quotation from Leriche in Soulairac (1968). Buytendijk (1962) joins with those who believe that pain commonly causes needless suffering, and is more an enemy than a friend. The incapacitating consequences of long-continued experiences of pain are described by Wolff and Wolf (1958).

Bakan (1968) discusses the meaning of pain in the philosophical mode, partly in relation to sacrifice. The book by Buytendijk (1962) contains philosophical reflections on pain. The distress triad—pain, suffering, and mental anguish—is shown to have medicolegal implications by Smith (1970).

Many pain discussions (such as Beecher, 1959) begin with a despairing statement about trying to define pain; the multifaceted definition attributed to Sternbach is from his book (Sternbach, 1968).

Patients given frontal lobotomies who reported that they felt the pain as before but it no longer bothered them were described by Freeman and Watts (1950). The operation is no longer favored for treating pain, but the observations called attention to the difference between sensory pain and suffering. The related findings for patients with operations in the medial thalamus were reported by Mark, Ervin, and Yakovlev (1963).

The distinction between two major components of pain, here called *sensory pain* and *suffering*, has been made frequently. The second component is often called a *reaction* component (as by Wolff and Wolf, 1958), but this assumes that the pain perception comes first. The possibility of simultaneous activation through separate pathways arises in discussions of the gate control theory, for which references are given later in these notes. Those familiar with the history of psychology may recognize an analogy to the history of theories of felt emotion and emotional expression. William James argued, in the James-Lange theory, that bodily movements came first and that felt emotion was a repercussion from them ("I am angry because I strike"). The James-Lange theory has been the subject of periodic review and discussion ever since its announcement in the 1880s; Cannon and Bard later took the position that both components of emotion are released at once through a process of cortico-thalamic interaction. As with pain and suffering, the issue loses its importance for enduring emotional states such as moods, in which overt behavior and subjective experience have become inextricably combined.

The possibility that discomfort, in the absence of pain, can be studied quantitatively has been confirmed by Gagge and Stevens (1968), who changed the "comfort level" of an experimental room by increasing or decreasing its temperature.

The investigation designed to organize the language of pain empirically into a series of graded classes is that of Melzack and Torgerson (1971). They have developed a pain questionnaire based on their study; as an illustration of its use, see Melzack and Perry (1975).

Phantom limb pain has been well reviewed by Melzack (1971); much of what he found is summarized in his book (Melzack, 1973). Referred pains are also discussed in the book. Of special interest are "trigger points," pressure on which causes pain because of difficulties remote from where the pain is felt. For example, trigger points in the chest or back may be sensitive in cardiac cases.

A pictorial atlas of these relationships was published by Travell and Rinzler (1952). Pain in the chest or abdomen may result from stimulating an analgesic leg following hemisection of the spinal cord (Nathan, 1956). The problem of psychosomatic pain and other psychological and psychiatric aspects of pain are treated by Merskey (1965) and, at book length, by Merskey and Spear (1967).

The report of wounded soldiers feeling no pain is by Beecher (1956). The animal experiments on the acquired basis for pain responses are those with dogs by Melzack and Scott (1957) and one with a young chimpanzee by Nissen, Chow, and Semmes (1951).

The study of family size in relation to pain is that of Gonda (1962). The ethnic studies have been reviewed by Sternbach (1968). An earlier study by Zborowski (1952) also appeared in book form (Zborowski, 1969). The laboratory study of pain in which the amount of remuneration was determined by lot was that of Lewin (1965). Zimbardo and others (1966) were responsible for the study in which volunteering to experience pain reduced the pain.

Physiology of Pain and Suffering

Conceptions of pain and suffering through the ages were reviewed by Dallenbach (1939). He pointed out that because of Aristotle's influence, pain was not conceived formally as a sensory experience until the nineteenth century. Because of the assumed opposition between pleasure and pain, pain remained one of the "passions." Later, the pendulum began to swing the other way, until pain was conceived almost solely in sensory terms. Finally the two components, sensory pain and suffering, began to be distinguished and to be given neurophysiological explanation. The basic work on the specificity theory is that of Von Frey (1896). The pattern or summation theory was summarized by Goldscheider (1894). Von Frey's views have been widely held since, although attacked by those favoring the summation theory (such as Weddell, 1955). The matter has been reviewed by Melzack and Wall (1965) and Melzack (1973), to whom we are indebted for giving order to this complex material.

The gate control theory of pain, announced by Melzack and Wall (1965), has been amplified by them and their collaborators in the light of new evidence: Melzack and Wall (1968; 1970); Melzack and Casey (1968; 1970); Casey (1973); and Melzack (1973). Support for the implication that large-fiber stimulation can reduce clinical pain came first from a study by Wall and Sweet (1967); laboratory support has been found in experiments such as those by Higgins, Tursky, and Schwartz (1971), and Satran and Goldstein (1973), in which concurrent tactile stimulation reduced the pain of electric shock. Additional clinical evidence will be cited in a later chapter.

The evidence for pain control at the spinal level resulting from electrical stimulation near the center of the brain is that of Reynolds (1969) and Liebeskind, Mayer, and Akil (1974).

Some of the difficulties of the gate control theory have been listed by Casey (1970; 1973). Wall (1974) has written an essay on what needs to be done in the future of pain research; he selects descending controls as offering the most powerful chance of improving both understanding and therapy.

Lim (1970), in an excellent review of the physiology of pain prepared just before his death, gave primary attention to the role of chemical mediation and chemoreception, an area of great importance in understanding not only the nature of pain but also the action of chemical analgesics, and possibly the body's own defenses against pain.

Exercise of the occluded muscle rather than ischemia alone causes the pain in ischemia, as noted early by MacWilliam and Webster (1923) and since confirmed experimentally by others, such as Rodbard (1970). It appears likely that the muscles release some of the substances referred to by Lim.

Experimentally Produced Pains and Pain Measurement

The production of laboratory pains by various methods, including methods of estimating the pain, is discussed in review chapters by Tursky (1976) and by Hilgard (1976b). These sources may prove useful for the specialist. The psychophysical aspects of cold pressor pain, as measured in our laboratory, are given detailed consideration in Hilgard, Ruch, and others (1974). Other accounts of the pain measurement procedures from our laboratory, for a professional but nonspecialized audience, may be found in Hilgard (1967; 1969; 1971; 1975b).

The most important early source on cold pressor pain is Wolf and Hardy (1941). The tourniquet-exercise method for producing ischemic pain was developed, on the basis of earlier work, by Smith and others (1966); some follow-up data was given by Beecher (1968). The tourniquet method has been used conjointly with clinical methods to estimate the severity of clinical pain, with encouraging results, by Sternbach and others (1974).

The first published investigation from our laboratory in which a suffering scale was used along with a sensory pain scale was that of Knox, Morgan, and Hilgard (1974), with ischemic pain. A related study with cold pressor pain is reported in Hilgard, Morgan, and Macdonald (1975) and in Hilgard and Morgan (1975).

3 Controlling Pain

Before turning to the role of hypnosis in the control of pain, we wish to make note of methods used to alleviate pain through the ages and at the present time—drugs, surgery, and nondrug and nonsurgical methods, some of which are physical, some psychological. Hypnosis must eventually be assigned its appropriate place among other methods available, because it will occasionally be used alone but often in combination with these other methods.

A complete history of pain would consider the role of pain as an instrument of social control, through punishment for violation of the rules of the family in which a child is reared, or of the society to which an individual belongs. It is no wonder that the person who suffers pain often believes himself to be guilty of some transgression; this has been true through the ages. The infliction of pain is a feature common to many initiation ceremonies, in which accepting mutilation without complaint is a sign of fitness for adult status. One difficulty in interpreting these ceremonies as demanding stoical acceptance of pain is that we assume we are dealing with courage rather than with pain reduction. We have no way of knowing how much the pain may actually be reduced or even absent. In remote parts of India, at least until recent times, an individual chosen to represent the power of the gods had steel hooks inserted under the muscles of his back. In part of the ceremony, he would swing on ropes attached to these hooks as he blessed the children and the crops. Observers described him as being in a "state of exaltation;" he appeared to suffer no pain.

In addition to ceremonies involving pain or pain-tolerance, people all over the world have evolved forms of primitive medicine for dealing with pain. Alcohol has been familiar for many years and in many places; it is not surprising that alcoholic intoxication has often been noted as a pain reliever.

Many illustrations could be cited; one is the treatment of children in a nonliterate culture of South America known as the Caingang. A mutilation ceremony connected with initiation requires perforation of the child's lip. Before the initiation ceremony takes place, however, the children are intoxicated with beer. They are shaken until nearly unconscious, and then the lip is perforated with a sharp stick, apparently producing little pain.

A widespread surgical practice for the relief of head pain, still practiced in parts of Africa, is known as trephining the skull. A hole is cut into the skull, and the bleeding through the opening presumably relieves pressure and produces the cure. The practice has ancient roots; skulls with holes from trephining have been found in many archeological sites.

Physical methods of various kinds have been used for ages. Counterirritant methods include hot or cold packs, mustard or other skin irritants, and the method known as cupping. In cupping, a candle is burned beneath a cup inverted on the skin, driving out the air so that a vacuum is created when the cup cools. This vacuum sucks upon the skin, producing a painful irritation that is thought to be curative. This method probably works also through counterirritation. Acupuncture, in which needles are inserted at various points and twisted—in modern times, often electrified—belongs at least in part to these counterirritant methods.

These early methods, drugs, surgery, and counterirritants, all have their counterparts in modern medicine. In addition, there is a long history of treatment by methods that are called psychological today, but which in the past were magical or religious. Hanging around the neck a bag of some substance thought to be curative is an illustration of a magical cure; faith healing is a religious cure.

Modern medicine has not put an end to the practice of magical and religious cures; witness the copper bracelets recently worn in the United States for relief of arthritis, and the prevalence here of many religious groups with healing claims, such as Christian Science and Scientology. Because these practices are nonscientific does not mean they are never effective; they would not survive if they did not have a satisfied clientele. The point is not, however, that anything that works is to be recommended; a better way of putting it is that *the fact that some method occasionally relieves pain does not mean that the theory behind the method is correct*. A scientific approach asks for better evidence than some satisfied customers. The crutches discarded at a curative shrine do not tell us how long the cure lasted nor how many limped away on the crutches they came on.

If we accept the position that modern science seeks to provide tested truths based on evidence that any reasonable and competent person can accept, we will find that our knowledge of pain relief is, at best, on the borderlines of firm scientific knowledge. Science, however, is also an approach to evidence; scientific knowledge is not final but evolving. A great deal has been learned about the control of pain, and, fortunately, that knowledge is advancing.

Drugs and Surgery

The medical aspects of pain reduction center upon two large classes of pains: those brought to the physician by the patient who is already in pain, and those caused by the doctor in the course of treatment as in the process of surgery and in the postsurgical period. The two classes are not always separable: appendicitis, which is painful, is relieved by surgery, which is also potentially painful. We shall not here be concerned with the alleviation of pain by the removal of a tumor or a source of infection; important as these steps are, they belong to the ordinary practice of surgery and do not call for psychological methods of treatment.

Anesthesia in surgery to prevent pains caused by the surgeon's intervention is of interest, however, because the anticipation of surgery has an influence on the drugs that may be required and on the postsurgical recovery. General anesthetics have been a great boon because of their ability to relieve pain in major operations. Their history began only 150 years ago, when ether and chloroform were introduced. These have been supplemented by many other chemical anesthetics, along with local anesthetics that reduce pain but do not produce unconsciousness.

For the relief of nonsurgical pain, and for pains that persist after surgery, the most successful pain-killers have been morphine and other narcotics derived from opium. The success of morphine is blemished by its addictive potential and the severity of withdrawal symptoms following addiction. Just how successful is morphine? The individual differences in pain responses noted in Chapter 2 apply also to the effects of morphine. Investigations with hospitalized patients have shown that, in the relief of postsurgical pain by morphine in doses considered safe to use, the effects are roughly as follows: about one-third of the patients gain relief from morphine beyond that received from a placebo (a nonactive substance, such as saline solution thought to be morphine); another one-third gain the same relief from the placebo as from morphine; and the final one-third get little relief from this dose of morphine or from the placebo.

A further word about placebos may be in order. To study the effectiveness of drugs, experiments are commonly performed by the double-blind method; that is, neither the physician nor the patient knows whether the drug or the placebo is being administered. This guards against psychological influence upon the patient's pain attributable not to the effectiveness of the drug, but rather to the physician's manner or the patient's expectations.

Review of a large number of double-blind studies shows that the placebo tends to have about half the effectiveness of the drug, if the drug is a genuine pain reliever. This is a curious finding, because it shows that the placebo has a stronger effect when it is thought to be a strong drug than when it is thought to be a mild drug. This expectation must somehow be communicated to the patient by the physician administering the drug.

The necessity to control for the placebo effect tells us a great deal about psychological influences upon pain. It tells us that even drugs such as morphine that have clear organic effects in relation to pain also act through learned components. Pavlov, the distinguished Russian physiologist and Nobel prize winner, showed a learning effect upon injecting morphine in dogs. When morphine is injected hypodermically into a dog, the result is nausea, followed by vomiting, and then profound sleep. Pavlov found that, after receiving a few repeated injections, a dog would react with all those symptoms to the preliminaries of injection. Even seeing the experimenter come into the laboratory and open the box in which the syringe was kept could be enough to produce all the symptoms—nausea, secretion of saliva, vomiting, and sleep. The fact that these responses can be produced without morphine does not, however, mean that morphine was ineffective in producing them. This is one of the lessons that will have to be learned in connection with hypnosis and other psychological treatments: they work in complex interactions with the anxieties, expectations, and prior experiences of the experimental subject or patient. Because there is a psychological component to the responsiveness of the person does not deny very genuine organic components.

What applies to morphine applies equally well to the milder analgesics such as aspirin, which—although an organic pain reducer whose action is fairly well understood—also has a placebo component. A person who takes aspirin for a headache may find the pain diminishing almost immediately, far too soon for the aspirin to be absorbed into the blood stream. A placebo effect may enhance the drug itself; it need not depend upon a neutral substance substituting for the active agent.

In addition to the general relief that pain-killing drugs can produce, local anesthetics and other chemical agents may be used in more specific ways to relieve pain in local areas of the body or to assist in diagnosis of sources of irritation. A procedure known as a *nerve block* combines the use of anesthetic agents with neuroanatomical knowledge, and may serve as a guide to surgery. Bonica, director of the Pain Clinic at the University of Washington and one of the leaders in the use of nerve blocks, reports on many persons for whom appropriate nerves have been blocked successfully by injecting a local anesthetic or alcohol. With the local anesthetic, the beneficial effect may outlast the transient effect of the drug for hours, days, or even weeks. In some manner, then, the drug must interrupt a self-sustaining activity responsible for the pain.

In addition to therapeutic use, the nerve block procedure can be used in diagnosis. A chest pain, for example, may originate close to the painful area or in another part of the body. If injection of a specific spinal nerve shows where the pain is interrupted, the diagnosis can be made with more assurance. If the pain disappears only while the anesthetic is active, the assumption is more plausible that the pain has some contemporary stimulus, such as pressure on a nerve. If the effect outlasts the anesthetic, something may be involved in the way of self-sustaining activity with origins in the past.

Occasionally when the nerve block indicates a present source of painful irritation, a choice must be made between an alcohol block (which outlasts a block by a local anesthetic) and surgical cutting of spinal roots in the hope of more permanent alleviation. The local anesthetic may show the patient what he would feel like if the surgery were performed and proved successful. Because spinal roots are involved he might, along with the relief of his pain, have an objectionable area of numbness over some part of his body. Because cutting spinal roots does not always have the same effect as a transient block by a local anesthetic, Bonica may recommend an alcohol block that, though temporary, may last longer than the anesthetic block—perhaps for a year or a year and a half. After such continued pain reduction, cutting of the nerve roots (rhizotomy) is more likely to be recommended and more likely to bring permanent relief.

Surgical relief of pain depends upon well-known characteristics of the nervous system. Usually there is a definite afferent sensory pathway that conducts information to the brain from a source in the interior or periphery of the body. When the information is processed in the brain, the pain is felt. The logic of surgical intervention is as follows: if the pathway can be cut between the level at which the pain information enters it and the processing center in the brain, the pain should no longer be felt. There are also switching centers in the brain in which integration of impulses takes place; perhaps destroying such a center can also interrupt pain. An analogy with military operations attempting to interrupt the flow of railroad traffic is useful: if the main track can be bombed out, the flow will be interrupted; or, if the marshaling yards are destroyed, the freight cannot be properly deployed.

Surgeons have shown great ingenuity in designing operations to relieve intractable pain according to these principles, and they have shown great skill in carrying out the appropriate procedures. The sites are many, of which sixteen representative ones are listed in Table 1 to show the range of possibilities.

Unfortunately, an operation of this kind may succeed as a surgical procedure—with the appropriate incision made and the wound

Table 1

Sixteen Illustrative Surgical Procedures Designed to Alleviate Intractable Pain

---

1. Gyrectomy (cutting parts of the sensory contex)

2. Prefrontal lobotomy (cutting parts of the frontal lobes

3. Thalamotomy (cutting parts of the thalamus)

4. Mesencephalic tractotomy (cutting a fiber bundle in the midbrain)

5. Hypophysectomy (removing the hypophysis or pituitary gland)

6. Fifth nerve rhizotomy (cutting the sensory root of the trigeminal cranial nerve)

7. Ninth nerve neurectomy (removing a segment of the glossopharyngeal cranial nerve)

8. Medullary tractotomy (cutting a tract in the medulla)

9. Trigeminal tractotomy (cutting the trigeminal tract in the neck region)

10. Cervical chordotomy (cutting part of the spinal cord in the neck region)

11. Thoracic chordotomy (cutting part of the cord in the thoracic region)

12. Sympathectomy (cutting of connections to the sympathetic nervous system)

13. Myelotomy (cutting fibers in the central-dorsal part of the cord)

14. Lissauer tractotomy (cutting the transmission system in the dorso-lateral columns of the cord)

15. Posterior rhizotomy (cutting the sensory roots entering the cord at various segments)

16. Neurectomy (removing segments of sensory nerves in the periphery)

Modified from MacCarty and Drake (1956).

appropriately healed as the patient recovers from the surgery—without reducing the pain as intended. A baffling result is that an operation may reduce pain for one patient and not for another whose source of pain is similarly diagnosed by X-rays and other test methods. Furthermore, the pain may be temporarily reduced, only to return later at its original value. As White, the distinguished neurosurgeon, stated: "Given time, nature has a way of sooner or later frustrating the efforts of the most experienced neurosurgeon."

Surgery is, of course, effective in treating primary sources of pain—removing tumors, excising sources of infection, and correcting bone injuries. The operations listed in Table 1 are primarily for pain that persists after all the primary problems have been dealt with. For intractable pains such as neuralgias, phantom limb pains, and neck and back pains, surgery must be used very cautiously, with full knowledge of the many failures.

Physical Methods

For our purposes we have grouped together as "physical" a number of methods that treat pain by manipulating the patient largely from the surface of the body: massage, hot and cold treatment, counterirritants, electrical stimulation, acupuncture, and audioanalgesia. These methods have in common that they use neither drugs nor surgery. Furthermore, they do not claim to be psychological in their effects, whatever psychological components there may be in their effectiveness.

We shall not attempt to discuss the various palliative methods that rely on hot and cold applications, traction, massage, or exercise. Although some of these methods originated in folk medicine, there is increasing scientific knowledge supporting their use. In methods that have their origins in folk medicine, a measure of self-suggestion may well be involved. Practices outside established physical medicine may readily take on a cultish character, as recently with a deep pressure massage that is quite painful while it is being done, but is supposed to bring relief. Named "rolfing" for its originator Ida Rolf, it was apparently attracting a following in early 1975.

Superficial electrical stimulation of the skin over a painful area has become widely adopted as a method of pain relief. A rationale for it was provided by the gate control theory of pain described in Chapter 2. The gate control theory was first tested clinically by Wall, one of its originators, in cooperation with Sweet, a neurosurgeon. They temporarily abolished deep pain by directly stimulating nerves carrying large fibers which entered the spinal cord at the same level as the nerves conveying deep pain information over small fibers. It was soon found that it was not necessary to stimulate the nerve trunks directly, but that stimulation through the unbroken skin could serve the same purpose. Clinical applications became widespread, with favorable results. However, all new methods seem to work better during the period of initial enthusiasm, when the placebo effect is at its maximum; those now using the method find that the rate of success is much less than at first believed. If, however, some 10 to 30 percent of those suffering from chronic pain find relief through the use of electrical stimulators, they are worthwhile. Small portable devices are now available that can be used at home.

Needle stimulation in relation to pain has come to the fore with acupuncture, after this ancient method was newly sanctioned by the People's Republic of China. It shortly spread around the world—to Japan in 1950, to France the following year, and to the United States after a popular columnist, James Reston, had his appendix removed with acupuncture anesthesia in China in 1971. As scientists began to search the literature, they found that acupuncture had been known and tried many times before in the West. However, the modern surge of interest is so recent that established facts based on adequate research are still few. Some excessive claims are inevitable in a period of initial enthusiasm; this should lead to caution but not to a cynical attitude about the ultimate value of the method.

As an illustration of an implausible claim, we may point to the introduction of auriculotherapy in France. This is a form of acupuncture in which all the needles are placed in the external ear, with the rationale that points in the ear are homologous to portions of the human body. If the human body in the fetal position is superimposed upon the ear, it can be arranged so that the head is over the lobe of the ear and the rest of the body is draped around the ear canal (Figure 6). The procedure requires the appropriate use of gold, silver, or stainless steel needles, depending on circumstances. A leading French text on acupuncture notes that this method, invented in France, has been introduced into China. It is asserted that in one hospital in Nanking, 3,379 surgical operations were performed between 1965 and 1972 with auricular acupuncture as the only anesthetic. If this is so effective, what happens to all the famous meridians (needle locations) of classical acupuncture? There is obviously a body of unscientific lore associated with acupuncture; whether research will find a substantial basis for its successes remains to be seen. It is true that there are some successes; however, more than one explanation is possible, because successes in pain reduction are reported with therapies of many kinds. Some of these correspond in superficial respects to acupuncture without accepting its theories. For example, the success of acupuncture has been related by Melzack to surface electrical stimulation. Twirling or electrifying acupuncture needles may feel very much like the electrical stimulator, and can perhaps be given the same explanation when successful.

Another physical method is audioanalgesia, introduced a few years ago primarily to reduce the pain of dental patients. A machine was designed to play noise, along with music, to the patient. The patient could raise the intensity of the sound to a level at which he no longer felt pain; it then substituted for a local anesthetic. The method died out after a short vogue, in part because of danger of damaging the ears, in part because of uncertain effectiveness. A careful study was made of the effectiveness of this method and of suggestions of pain reduction. We have noted that physical effects often interact with psychological ones, and that is what was found. The measure of pain relief the investigators used, called pain-tolerance-duration, was influenced by joint auditory stimulation and suggestion. If auditory stimulation was combined with suggestions of reduced pain, the pain-tolerance-duration increased substantially; if, however, auditory stimulation was used alone, without suggestion, no effect could be detected. Correspondingly, if the auditory stimulation was kept at a low intensity, but the same suggestions were given, there was no appreciable effect.

These, then, are a representative sample of physical methods for alleviating pain: physical medicine, superficial electrical stimulation, acupunc-

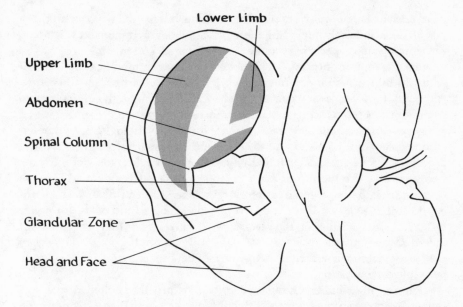

Figure 6. Diagram of the ear for the purposes of auriculo-therapy. The points are those in which needles are to be inserted to be effective in different regions of the body, according to the correlation between the shape of the ear and the fetal position superimposed on it. After Nogier (1972).

ture, and audioanalgesia. They are all doubtless effective to some extent, particularly if the psychological setting is favorable.

Psychological Methods

Psychological methods of dealing with pain can be classified into three major groups: first, those based on principles of learning, which treat pain as a response that can be learned and hence unlearned; second, those using principles of suggestion and hypnosis, which are considered in the next chapter; and third, those that attempt to deal with pain according to its personal significance to the person based on dynamic principles. An individual dealing with pain need not limit his approach to one or another of these, but for expository purposes there is some advantage in discussing them one at a time. In this discussion, we shall consider only those methods based on principles of learning. The dynamic aspects involve a great deal besides pain; they will be discussed in Chapter 10.

Behavior modification has come to be a term for the application of learning principles to changing behavior in desirable directions. For this purpose the word *behavior* is not limited to overt movements but is used to cover all that a person does and feels, including thoughts, anxieties, and pains. It was noted earlier that some aspects of pain are clearly learned, and that memory has an influence upon present pain. The rationale of behavior modification is that if pain can be learned and remembered, it can be unlearned and forgotten. Although there are several competing theories of learning, the easiest one to communicate and to incorporate into a practical program of treatment is that known as *operant conditioning*, based on the work of psychologist B. F. Skinner. Although operant conditioning differs in many respects from the classical conditioned reflex methods of the Russian scientist Pavlov, some of the same terms are used. To the extent that a given response is strengthened by what comes after it, perhaps in the form of a reward for successful performance, it is said to be *reinforced*. If it is desired to reduce some kind of performance instead of strengthening it, the reward, or *reinforcer*, is omitted. The behavior then decreases, that is, undergoes *extinction*. By an appropriate balancing of reinforcement and extinction, behavior can be *shaped*, or made to move in desirable directions.

These rather easily understood principles can be applied to pain, as though pain were itself a conditioned response. Pain may be reinforced because it gets attention, or it may be reinforced by the very act of reducing it. If, for example, a person in mild discomfort gets a pain-reducing drug only when the pain becomes more severe, the subsequent pain reduction, rest, and comfort may reinforce the very increase in pain that the pill is designed to relieve. These are subtle matters and not something for which the sufferer should feel responsible; such "conditionings" are occurring all the time, out of awareness.

Skinner speaks of the repeated association of a reinforcer with a specific state of affairs as a *contingency* established between them: sympathy may be contingent on signs of distress, administration of a pain-relieving drug may be contingent on mounting pain, and so on. If habitual pain is to be reduced, these contingencies must be interrupted so extinction can occur.

How are these abstract principles put into operation? Some concrete illustrations will help. A person debilitated with pain may have taken to his bed for so long that he now finds it hard to walk without feeling pain, and therefore has to lie down and rest after a short walk. The sequence walking–pain–rest is one of the subtle ways in which the pain is reinforced by the comfort of the rest afterwards. To break this contingency, the person may be taught to calibrate the amount of walking he does so that he stops short of pain; then he no longer needs pain relief, and walking loses its association with pain. At first, of course, he can walk only a short distance. However, with daily walks, each a little longer than the preceding one, he soon walks beyond the distance at which he formerly began to feel pain.

Or consider pain medication. If an individual is told to restrict his medication to relieving severe pain lest he become addicted to it, his pain begins to mount. When the pain becomes severe enough, he is permitted the relief that the medication brings. This is a pleasurable outcome based on contingent reinforcement between mounting pain and relief through a pill. How can this be broken? Suppose that the amount of medication the person is accustomed to taking—or at first, even somewhat more—is given him in a disguised form, such as a pleasant fruit drink, or "pain cocktail." If this dosage is divided so as to be taken at regular hours during the day, then the contingency is broken. The individual gets relief on an average basis throughout the day, whether his pain is high or low at the moment, and the pain does not signal its own relief. On successive days he receives the "cocktail" as before, but the medication is gradually reduced (with his full knowledge). After a while he may no longer need any medication at all. It should be pointed out that ingenious methods of doing these practical things have to be invented; they do not follow automatically from the learning principles, although these principles do explain why the invented methods are effective.

A recent addition to psychological methods is a technique known as *biofeedback*. Biofeedback consists in amplifying some of the body's usually involuntary processes so the person becomes more aware of them. When he is more aware of them he learns to achieve control over them, often to his benefit. For example, heartbeats can be converted to audible sounds or to displayed numbers describing the momentary rate. The person who wishes to slow or speed his heart may learn to do so with these indicators before him. Biofeedback has been applied to pain alleviation in the control of some forms of headache in which pain can be lessened by reducing pressure in the enlarged blood vessels of the scalp. One way of doing this is to dilate the blood vessels of the hands by warming the hands. This hand-warming can be taught by biofeedback methods; it reduces headache pain in a sufficient proportion of cases to make the method of interest. Biofeedback, like operant conditioning, is a learning method with conditioning aspects. However, emphasis is upon learning techniques of control, and the informative feedback has features beyond ordinary reinforcement.

Another set of practices which reduce pain by psychological means are the techniques of painless childbirth. Two principal methods have been developed: the Read method, known as "natural childbirth" or "childbirth without fear," and psychoprophylaxis ("psychological preparation"), a method based on Russian developments but sponsored in the West by the French obstetrician Lamaze. Because these have some overlap with suggestion, they will be considered further in Chapter 6 in connection with the use of hypnosis in obstetrics.

The Pain Clinic

Because many kinds of pain have frustrated treatment by conventional methods of drugs and surgery, a modern development has been the pain clinic, in which a team of workers familiar with a variety of diagnostic and treatment methods pools its knowledge and skill for the benefit of the patient. The team may have representatives from many different specialties. For example, one of the pioneer clinics, established in 1961 at the University of Washington, had on its staff in 1974 twenty individuals representing thirteen disciplines: anesthesiology, general practice, neurology, neurosurgery, nursing, oral surgery, orthopedics, pharmacology, psychiatry, psychology, radiology, sociology, and surgery. Such clinics are springing up throughout the country as therapists become more aware of the complexity of the pain problem and the futility of hit-and-miss approaches to pain relief. The size of the staff, the amount of time devoted to the clinic by the various specialists, and the range of services available vary from one clinic to another. What the pain clinics have in common are diagnostic and treatment procedures more comprehensive than any one specialist can provide.

The pain clinics deal primarily with debilitating, chronic pains that have incapacitated the patient. Usually there has been a history of many years of inability to work or to function in normal social relationships; many of the patients have spent a major proportion of their time in bed. Often, as many as five surgical operations have been performed in the past, with only temporary relief, if indeed the pain was relieved at all. If the indications of pain exceed what can be attributed to known pathological conditions, or if the evidence of an organic source of pain is uncertain or speculative, the patient may be a candidate for the psychological treatment described above. Contemporary psychologists prefer not to give a disease connotation to such pains by attributing them to hysteria, hypochondriasis, or personality disorders; rather, the pains are regarded as a problem of automatic learning which can be solved by appropriate methods. The pain of such a patient is as real as any other pain; to suggest that the patient is "imagining" it is inaccurate as well as unkind.

Because of the great variety of symptoms involved and degrees of pain reduction achieved, it is difficult to compile statistical evidence of the degree of successes in pain clinics using behavioral modification methods. However, many of the outcomes are dramatic, and the rate of benefit is high. Such positive results are far from easy to achieve. The pain patient remains in the hospital, where his environment is under control, for a month or more; after that, he is treated on an outpatient basis for additional weeks. The program includes an admissions procedure to select patients whose general stability is such that they are likely to benefit from the program. In addition, the home situation must be supportive of improvement; that is, the spouse or other person at home must be able to accept and cooperate in the discipline of the program if the treatment is to be effective. A patient who lives alone or in a troubled home setting is unlikely to profit from the treatment. Once the patient is admitted, his program may include a gradual increase in physical activity and a gradual withdrawal of medication; the regime is designed to remove the reinforcers that have sustained the pain behavior. It is often necessary to initiate a positive program of living a life without pain, for many of these patients have been so long controlled by their pain behavior that they find it hard to live as other people do.

The operant conditioning program in Seattle, under the direction of Fordyce, was initiated in 1967; a report is available on thirty-six patients selected for treatment from those referred between October 1967 and March 1971. At the time of admission, these patients had had their pains for an average of more than 7 years, had been unable to hold full-time employment for more than 3 years, and had undergone an average of 2.7 major operations designed to relieve their pains. All but two had back and neck pains as their primary complaints; one of these two had an elbow problem not relieved by 9 operations, and the other had hip, buttock, and shoulder pain. The results, supported by statistical tests, showed that between admission and discharge there had occurred: (1) a significant decrease in daily medication; (2) a significant increase in walking distance and in other activities involving sitting, standing, and moving about; and (3) increased activity units performed in physical therapy and occupational therapy. Follow-ups averaging two years after treatment indicated that these gains were retained. The program was directed toward the overcoming of handicaps in activity owing to pain—that is, modification of pain-related behavior—rather than toward the reduction of subjectively felt pain. When asked in follow-up to rate felt pain on a 10-point scale, the patients recalled pain at admission as having been at an average level of 8.6; at termination of treatment at 6.0; and at follow-up as at 6.2. Hence it appears that gains in learning to live with pain can be achieved even with moderate reduction of subjective pain.

Related evidence is available from a program guided by Alan Roberts at the University of Minnesota. Many patients who applied for the program were rejected because they showed signs of behavioral disturbance prior to the onset of pain or because an unstable home setting or personal isolation prevented them from receiving the necessary support to maintain the effectiveness of the treatment. In no case, however, was rejection based on the severity of pain or the degree of handicap caused by it. The twenty-four patients who actually entered the inpatient treatment had had an average of 2.25 surgical procedures performed on them previously for the relief of pain and had been largely incapacitated for an average of 4.16 years. Three of the twenty-four dropped out before completing the treatment, and three were still in treatment when this review was made, so the reported outcome is based on the eighteen who completed the course of treatment. Of these, fifteen or 83 percent were able to live normal lives after leaving the six- to eight-week program, with no pain medication, as indicated in follow-ups of up to five years.

It is clear that the psychological contributions to experienced pain are extensive, and that psychological methods frequently achieve pain reduction, as well as the ability to live more normal lives with such residual pain as persists.

Notes

The cultural background of pain, including the observations made by anthropologists, can be found in Melzack (1973) and in Zborowski (1969). The illustration from India comes from Kosambi (1967); that of the Caingang comes from Steward (1946). Current African practices of trephining for the relief of headache, including a motion picture of such an operation, were reported by Melzack (1974).

Drugs and Surgery

Data on patients whose postsurgical pain responds to morphine, to placebo, and to neither are reported by Beecher (1959). The review of double-blind studies showing that pain reduction by placebo corresponds to the effectiveness of the drug for which the placebo substitutes is by Evans (1974), extending an earlier study by Beecher (1959). A thorough study of the placebo effect was completed as a doctoral dissertation by Jospe (1973), who noted the importance of doing placebo studies on patients in preference to laboratory subjects.

Pavlov's study showing that typical responses to morphine could be acquired by dogs as conditioned reflexes is reported in Pavlov (1927).

The action of aspirin and other salicylates is now thought to be primarily peripheral; the analgesic effect is produced by antagonizing amines, kinins, and potassium ions, all of which are pain producers (Barker and Levitan, 1974; Willkens, 1974). That an active agent may be accentuated by its own placebo effect has been discussed by Dinnerstein, Lowenthal, and Blitz (1966).

For discussions of nerve blocks, see the book by Bonica (1959), and later statements such as Bonica (1974b), and Winnie, Ramamurthy, and Durrani (1974). The latter investigators note how frequently the pain diagnosed by nerve blocks originates in the sympathetic nervous system, a source they believe to be too often overlooked.

The quotation on the frustrated neurosurgeon is from White (1968, page 518).

Physical Methods

A short introduction to physical medicine in the control of pain, with references to the scientific literature, is by De Lateur (1974). The reference to "rolfing" came from the San Francisco Sunday Examiner and Chronicle, February 2, 1975 (Pixa, 1975).

The early study of electrical stimulation as a clinical test of the gate control theory is that of Wall and Sweet (1967). The later transcutaneous method has been favorably reported by a number of investigators, including Sweet and Wepsic (1968), Meyer and Fields (1972), and Long and Carolan (1974). Although Taub and Campbell (1974) showed that electrical stimulation did indeed raise the threshold to pain in a laboratory study, they felt that the gate theory was not necessary to explain their findings. In a later report, Sweet and Wepsic (1974) concluded that the effect of suggestion in their method is very great; it might, in fact, be the main component in their successes. A related method—implanting electrical stimulators at selected positions in the dorsal columns—has been reported as successful by Shealy (1974), but he and others (such as Friedman, Nashold, and Somjen, 1974) advise caution in using the method.

Although current reports continue to be optimistic about the effects of external electrical stimulation (e.g., Long and Hagfors, 1975), the history of reported successes and subsequent disenchantments ever since 1858 gives a basis for some skepticism (Kane and Taub, 1975).

James Reston's report on his appendectomy with the aid of acupuncture appeared in the New York *Times* of July 26, 1971; it did much to increase interest in America in the possibilities of acupuncture in relation to pain. The references to auriculotherapy are based on the large book in English by Nogier (1972). The reference to the use of auriculotherapy in Nanking is from Niboyet (1973, p. 155). Melzack's assimilation of some features of acupuncture to pain control through superficial stimulation (and hence to the gate theory) may be found in Melzack (1973, pp. 185–190). His collaborator is apparently less sure, seeing the possibility of a suggestion or hypnotic component in acupuncture (Wall, 1972).

The audioanalgesia study was reported by Melzack, Weisz, and Sprague (1963).

Psychological Methods

Various psychological methods are described by Sternbach (1970).

A general treatment of behavior modification can be found in Bandura (1969). Its use in treating pain is given both theoretical and practical discussion in Fordyce (1973; 1974a; 1974b).

Biofeedback came into prominence after Kamiya (1969) showed that human subjects could gain control over their EEG-alpha brain waves if the waves were amplified so the subjects knew when they were occurring. Brain wave control was found not to reduce pain by Gannon and Sternbach (1971); the results of Melzack and Perry (1975) are indecisive. Applications were soon made to controlling tension headache through relaxing the forehead muscles (Budzynski and others, 1971), and controlling other headaches through warming the hands (Sargent, Walters, and Green, 1973).

The Pain Clinic

The clinic at the University of Washington, its history, organization, and procedures, are described by Bonica (1974c). The data on operant control there are from Fordyce and others (1973). The results at the University of Minnesota are based on a private communication from Roberts (1975), to whom we are grateful for this advance account of his findings. For a report from another pain clinic see Greenhoot and Sternbach (1974).

An interesting question arises in connection with the use of behavioral methods in the pain clinic. Does the patient rid himself of pain, or does he learn to live with it? Some additional comments by Roberts are significant in this connection:

"Part of the regimen of therapy requires inattention to pain, so no formal measures of pain were taken during the therapy. However, after the therapy had been completed, and during the follow-ups, the patients were asked about their pains. For some curious reason, fourteen [of the fifteen successful] reported at the time of leaving that they had learned to live with their pains, but they hurt as much as when they entered the program. Of these same persons, six, when questioned later on, reported that they had had their pain relieved during treatment, and it was now very slight. This discrepancy in the immediate and remembered experience of improvement may tell us something about the subjective nature of the pain experience and the long-term effects of learning to ignore pain signals."

4 Hypnosis in Pain Control

The nineteenth-century revival of interest in hypnosis, still in the form of animal magnetism, rested in part upon its success in relieving pain in major surgery. The first reported case of major surgery was that of Recamier, who performed a major operation with hypnosis in France in 1821. The later work of Elliotson in England and of Esdaile in India has been mentioned in Chapter 1.

It must not be supposed that the introduction of chemical anesthetics alone brought a halt to the use of hypnosis; the practice had met vigorous opposition from the start. In 1842 a physician named Ward amputated a leg while a patient was hypnotized; he reported the successful outcome to the Royal Medical and Chirurgical Society in London. All evidence indicated that the operation was performed painlessly, but the society refused to believe this. Marshall Hall, whose name is familiar in the history of reflex action, moved that the record of the paper's presentation should be struck from the society's minutes because the patient must have been an impostor. Eight years later, on the basis of a rumor, Hall informed the society that the patient had admitted having falsely denied his pain. Witnesses came forward, however, with a signed declaration from the patient himself that the operation had actually been painless.

Fortunately, active antagonism to hypnosis is today no longer prevalent, and its use in pain relief, while not widespread, is increasing. Because it is less familiar than the methods described in the preceding chapter, we are devoting this chapter to its methods and outcomes, chiefly as they are revealed in experimental studies in the laboratory. Specific applications of hypnotic procedures to some representative clinical problems will be discussed in the succeeding chapters.

Procedures Used to Reduce Pain

Those skilled in the use of hypnosis have devised ingenious methods for suggesting the reduction of pain. We shall consider three classes of procedure: first, direct suggestion of pain reduction; second, altering the experience of pain, even though the pain may persist; and third, directing attention away from the pain and its source. These approaches are not mutually exclusive, and they do not include everything that has been done. In the clinical chapters that follow, more details will be given about the use of these and related methods with individual patients, adapting the method to what the patient can do and what he finds congenial.

Most patients are familiar with local anesthetics, often from the experience of having their gums rendered insensitive by a dentist. One direct suggestion is that the painful area—an arm, for example—is getting numb, that it will no longer feel pain or other sensations. For many hypnotizable subjects this is sufficient for them to become insensitive to normally painful stimulation. For other subjects, the suggestion can be made more concrete by asking the person to imagine that a local anesthetic has been injected into his shoulder and is beginning to take effect, the arm feeling like his cheek does after his dentist has injected novocain or xylocain. Imagination may enter into the process in other ways. In one variant the person is told: "Imagine that the nerves to your arm are controlled by switches in your brain. You can turn these switches off. . . . Turn off the switches now, and your arm will be insensitive."

Physicians and psychologists, brought up in the tradition of the physical and biological sciences, feel uneasy about making such unscientific suggestions; some subjects may also object. To counter this uneasiness and yet make use of such reality-distorting suggestions, the practitioner using hypnosis may discuss his rationale very frankly with the subject or patient. The "switches" in the head are of course metaphorical or imaginary, but by exercising imagination in this way, a person can gain control over his pain. The concrete imagery is a support for his effort to gain control. By being entirely open about the procedure, the practitioner steps aside from the role of magician, and the subject is not being tricked or deceived. The highly hypnotizable person finds this exercise of imagination entirely congenial; the less hypnotizable finds in it a way of directing his effort toward control. If the method is too foreign to the subject, another method can be substituted.

It cannot be too strongly emphasized that the scientific use of hypnosis requires that it be treated as a purely naturalistic process; in this respect it differs from pseudo-scientific cults which claim scientific support, and from faith healing, which claims supernatural sanctions. The exercise of imagination certainly belongs within a naturalistic psychology; hypnotic methods, used to stimulate the imagination or to make it serve practical purposes, can be fully explained to the subject so he can accept or reject them just as he accepts or rejects other treatments. Hypnosis is more than a placebo, as we shall see; it does not mask as something it is not. In the same spirit of full disclosure, we object to those who wish to use hypnosis but hesitate to call it by name, for fear of provoking antagonism. Although hypnosis uses imagination, it is not simply the exercise of imagination. We prefer to call a spade a spade, and in that way to gain acceptance for hypnosis in the matter-of-fact manner expected of any scientifically validated procedure.

Another procedure for relieving pain by suggestion directed toward the pain is carried out in two steps. A person already in pain (as distinct from the laboratory subject whose aversive stimulation is about to be produced), may be more easily taught first to reduce sensitivity to pain in some part of the body not now in pain. Consider a person with diffuse head or abdominal pain. If pain sensitivity can first be reduced in a normal hand, he may be convinced that he has some control over his pain sensitivity. Hence the first step may be to suggest that this hand will feel numb and insensitive. The success of this "glove anesthesia" in a nonpained hand can be appropriately tested by stimulating the hand through pinching or pricking with a pointed instrument. When numbness has been achieved and the patient is convinced that he has some control over his bodily sensations, he is ready for the next step—"transferring" the numbness and insensitivity from the anesthetic hand to the place where the pain is felt. This second step is carried out by having the patient rub the painful part with the already anesthetic hand, as a symbol of the transfer.

This is of course an irrational procedure, but it can be explained to the patient so that the hypnotic practitioner is not placed in the role of a magician. A straightforward explanation can be given along the following lines: "You have shown that you can control the feeling in your normal hand. It is easy to locate the sensations in a hand. You can control what you feel in other parts of your body also, but you may not know as well how to direct your attention to them. By rubbing an area to be controlled, you can more easily keep that area in attention and do for it what you did for your hand." There are also experiential reasons which make the act of rubbing plausible: rubbing a pained area has brought some relief before, as in rubbing a forehead to reduce a headache.

Another hypnotic practice can alter pain by displacing it or converting it to something nonpainful. A disturbing pain may not be well localized; such diffuse pain is difficult to manage. Through hypnotic suggestion it is sometimes possible to concentrate the pain into a smaller area, and then to move it from, say, the head or back, to the hands. There the pain, though still felt, may be more tolerable. In some instances, the pain can then be converted as well as displaced. A pain moved to the hand, for example, may be converted to a tingling in the fingers. Skilled modifications can be made in these practices, as we shall note in illustrative cases in the clinical chapters to follow.

Amnesia is a resource available to the highly hypnotizable subject. When pain is intermittent, felt strongly part of the time but absent or greatly reduced during other stretches of time, hypnosis can enable the patient to forget the pain that has been experienced. By eliminating the remembrance of pain, the patient can also eliminate the anticipation of pain to come. In patients who have experienced severe pain, anticipatory dread of future pain increases the discomfort along the way and may aggravate the pain when it comes. The patient can be told that past experiences of pain can be forgotten, and that each recurrent pain will therefore be a completely transient experience. Because the pain is neither remembered nor anticipated, the experience itself will seem to have no appreciable duration and hence be readily tolerated. The pain can even be experienced as a momentary flash of sensation which may go unrecognized as a painful experience.

Directing attention away from pain can be achieved in more than one way. One method is to deny the existence of the painful bodily member. We have utilized this method successfully in the laboratory following reports of its clinical use. Before his arm is stimulated by lowering it into circulating ice water the subject is told, "Think that you have no left arm. Look down and see that there is no left arm there, only an empty sleeve. An arm that does not exist does not feel anything. Your arm is gone only temporarily; you will find it amusing, not alarming, that for a while you have no left arm." The arm is then stimulated by the icy water, and the subject commonly reports that he feels nothing. In a laboratory comparison, the direct suggestion of numbness and the suggestion of an absent arm were found to work about equally well to reduce pain. With each method, some subjects eliminated the pain entirely, others merely reduced it below normal levels.

Other types of fantasy and hallucination can be used to transport the person away from the present in which he is experiencing pain. He may, for example, be returned through hypnotic age regression to an earlier and happier time; while living again in the past he does not feel the pain of the present. Without age regression, he still may find himself in fantasy doing something that he enjoys when he is without pain: climbing a mountain, watching a horse race, fishing in a rowboat, or engaging in science-fiction adventure. Leaving his painful body behind may require little geographical displacement; he may (in imagination) go into the next room to watch television, feeling no pain while absorbed in the (fantasied) program. All these methods make use of the dissociative possibilities within hypnosis, which will be discussed further when we turn to a theoretical interpretation of what happens in hypnotic analgesia (Chapter 9).

Ingenuity in discovering methods for reducing pain may be shown by the hypnotized subject as well as by the hypnotist. Increasingly, investigators are becoming aware that the hypnotic subject is not passive, but actively participates in controlling his own behavior. In one of our experiments, experienced subjects, some of whom had already used their hypnotic abilities to control pain in the accidents of everyday life, showed much play of imagination. They paid little attention to the formal suggestions of the hypnotist that the arm would grow numb when it was stroked, or that it would feel as if it were chemically anesthetized. Instead, as we were told afterwards, each did it his own way. One young woman remembered seeing the Venus de Milo in the Louvre the previous summer; she imagined herself inside the statue, without an arm to hurt. She reported only a slight tingling in her shoulder! One of the young men imagined himself singing a duet with a girlfriend and forgot completely about the experiment. These subjects found it slightly annoying to give a pain report every 5 seconds, but the reports became so automatic that they could simply hear themselves reporting while engrossed in their imaginative involvements at a distance. Other investigators, in asking subjects to think of something else in order to reduce pain, have specifically directed them to listen to a story or to add or count aloud. Such subjects frequently remarked afterward that they would have preferred to use their own methods of distraction.

The methods just described have to do with the reduction of pain *per se*; they are not designed to alleviate fears or anxieties associated with pain. Anxiety reduction may of course be a secondary effect—if pain is mastered, the subject or patient may have less to be anxious about. Hypnosis does indeed have various psychotherapeutic effects, but in the present context we are thinking of the pain experienced as something that hurts, and we are concerned with the manner in which that hurting can be reduced.

Pain Reduction in the Laboratory

In order to study pain experimentally, the first problem is to find a pain severe enough to be relevant to clinical pain, but tolerable for normal laboratory subjects willing to undergo some pain for the sake of contributing to scientific knowledge. The two methods for producing pain that we have used in our laboratory have already been described in Chapter 2. As a reminder, one is the pain produced when the hand and forearm are placed in circulating ice water; it is known as *cold pressor* pain. This pain mounts rapidly, becoming so severe within a minute that we have not found it necessary to expose subjects to the pain any longer than that. The second kind of pain is produced by a tourniquet to the upper arm that cuts off the circulation to the forearm and hand below it. The occluded muscles are then exercised as the subject repeatedly presses a loaded spring device. After the exercise ceases, the pain mounts slowly, but becomes quite severe in a few minutes. Because it is associated with the exercise of blood-deprived muscles, we have called this type of pain *ischemic* pain. The next step is to find some way in which the person suffering pain in the laboratory can report its severity. The simple numerical scale described in Chapter 2 has proved quite satisfactory for measuring both kinds of pain.

When pains produced in the laboratory—either by the cold pressor method or the ischemic method—are measured first when the subject is normally alert and not hypnotized, and then following induction of hypnosis, the pain is not reduced by the mere fact of being hypnotized. The pain is reduced substantially only when suggestions of insensitivity are given in the hypnotic condition. In view of the long clinical history of pain reduction through hypnosis, this general result is to be expected, but the laboratory contributes more precise information.

Pain Reduction as Related to Measured Hypnotic Responsiveness. Not all those who are given suggestions that they will become insensitive to pain can respond positively to these suggestions, and not all people can be hypnotized readily. Are these two related? This is the kind of question that laboratory procedures can be expected to answer. One significant experimental result that is uniformly found is that the amount by which suggestion can reduce pain is positively related to hypnotic responsiveness as measured by the methods described in Chapter 1.

The relationship is not a perfect correspondence: the most hypnotically responsive subjects are most likely to reduce their pains, but not all of them are successful; and the least hypnotically responsive are less likely to reduce their pains by suggestion, although a few of them can. The relationship can be expressed as a correlation of .50 between measured hypnotic responsiveness and reduction of the pain of ice water. What this means more concretely is illustrated in Figure 7, which shows experimental results from an unselected sample of fifty-four college students of limited hypnotic experience. Their hypnotic susceptibility scores were first secured, and then their pain reduction measured. Pain is reduced by one-third or more in 67 percent of the highly hypnotizable, but in only 13 percent of the low group. Even the lows have some success, however; 44 percent of them reduce their pain by 10 percent or more. This means that the relation between pain reduction and hypnotic responsiveness is probabilitistic, with a greater probability of successful pain reduction for those highly responsive to hypnosis. The data do not mean that those unresponsive to hypnosis, as measured by the scales, have no possibility of help through suggestion.

There is no doubt whatever about the reality of pain reduction through hypnosis. Nevertheless, some skeptical writers on hypnosis, through the

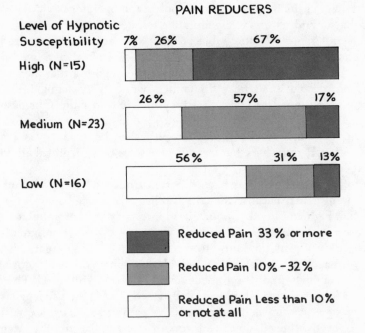

Figure 7. Reduction of pain through hypnotically suggested analgesia as related to susceptibility to hypnosis. The subjects were fifty-four university subjects whose prior experience of hypnosis was limited to a standard test of hypnotic responsiveness following a standardized induction procedure. From Hilgard and Morgan (1975).

emphases within their reviews, have raised doubts about hypnotic pain reduction in the minds of those who read their statements. Hence some of the more convincing kinds of evidence are perhaps worth citing. The main criticism implies that in order to please the hypnotist, the hypnotized person merely tolerates more pain and gives verbal assent to the idea that it has been reduced. According to this interpretation, hypnotic pain reduction is a widespread deception practiced upon the hypnotist by his hypnotized subjects. Because we rely upon the verbal responses of our subjects in describing their pains, this criticism must be answered. One form of answer comes through experiments using simulating subjects, as suggested by Orne (see Chapter 1). Shor was the first experimenter on pain to use instructed simulators, unresponsive to hypnosis, as controls against the truly hypnotizable. The instructed simulators could indeed "playact" as if the shock did not hurt; neither the hypnotist nor the polygraph operator could distinguish their behavior and reports while imitating hypnosis from the corresponding behavior and reports of the subjects who were actually hypnotized. The posthypnotic inquiry, however, in which honest reports were invited from all, gave clear results. The instructed simulators reported that they had felt severe pain despite their false disclaimers while "play-acting." The truly hypnotized continued to insist that they had felt no pain. Our associates performed a small experiment of the same kind in our laboratory a few years later, with the same results; it was not published because it was designed merely to satisfy ourselves that our subjects were being truthful about their pain experiences.

Another experiment has been reported from a different laboratory by Greene and Reyher. Because the criticism has been voiced against the Orne design that high and low hypnotizables represent different populations and hence are not suitable for comparison, Greene and Reyher assigned highly hypnotizable subjects randomly to the hypnotized and simulating groups. They instructed the simulators that they should remain out of hypnosis while trying to fool the hypnotist into believing they were hypnotized. They were to react as they expected hypnotized subjects to react to the pain suggestions. An increasing electric shock served as the painful stimulus; a measure of tolerance level was used along with reports of pain. Despite the attempt to behave like a hypnotized person while not hypnotized, the simulators were less tolerant of the pain under each of the several conditions of the experiment than the hypnotized subjects. For example, under conditions of hypnotic analgesia alone, without the supplementary suggestions given in other conditions, the truly hypnotized increased their tolerance of pain by 45 percent, and the simulators by 16 percent. This means that the shock was more bearable for the truly hypnotized than for equally hypnotizable subjects who were not hypnotized. The differences in objective tolerance were confirmed by the reports given by the subjects after the experiments were completed. These and many other indications deny the interpretation that hypnotized subjects feel pain but report little pain to please the hypnotist.

Because two components of pain have been identified—sensory pain and suffering—it is important to know whether the reduction through hypnosis is general or selective. It might reduce suffering without reducing sensory pain, as is sometimes reported with other procedures. It has been found that, when the subject reports his pain and suffering in the usual way, following the induction of hypnosis and the suggestions that he will be insensitive, *both* pain and suffering are reduced. In highly susceptible subjects, both components yield maximum reports of 0—no pain, no distress.

Hence, in those for whom the hypnotic method is most successful for pain relief, neither pain nor suffering persists.*

Circumstances Affecting Hypnotic Pain Reduction. The susceptibility of the subject to hypnosis is the primary factor affecting the degree of pain reduction to be expected, but several other factors may have some influence.

The first question is whether hypnosis alone, without any suggestions of reduced pain, causes the pain level to decline. This might be the case, because hypnotic induction is a relaxing procedure, and relaxation itself is sometimes said to influence the amount of pain that is felt. Later we shall consider the role of anxiety reduction in the hypnotic relief of pain (page 76), but for the present can report that hypnosis alone, without analgesia suggestions, does not reduce pain any more than it reduces other sensory functions. Through suggestion, the hypnotic subject can be made deaf or blind also, but without special suggestions he hears and sees as well within hypnosis as when not hypnotized. The same thing has repeatedly been found for the experience of pain.

A second question is whether or not suggestions of pain reduction are as successful if they are made in the waking state, without a preceding induction of hypnosis. To answer this question, Evans and Paul conducted a careful investigation using the familiar ice water pain. First they measured the hypnotic responsiveness of their subjects; then they measured the pain reduction for half the subjects without any prior induction of hypnosis, and for the other half following a standard induction. Both groups reduced pain by an equal amount, so Evans and Paul concluded that waking analgesia suggestions were as successful as hypnotic ones. They did find, however, that the amount by which pain was reduced correlated with measured hypnotic responsiveness, just as we had found earlier. The correlations were the same whether or not there had been an induction of hypnosis. These results favor the *trait* interpretation of hypnosis over the *state* interpretation, as discussed in Chapter 1.

It is extremely difficult to conduct a finally decisive experiment on an issue of this kind, because of subtle factors in the selection of subjects, the levels of hypnotic responsiveness represented, and the instructions given to the subjects. We later conducted a related experiment with highly responsive subjects, using taped suggestions to be sure that exactly the same thing was

---

* We shall consider the modification of sensory pain and of suffering at a covert or hidden level in hypnosis in Chapter 9, but the ordinary reports of overt experience are those now under consideration.

said in the same way when the suggestions were given in the waking state and in hypnosis; we found, as Evans and Paul did, that there was a substantial reduction in pain through the waking suggestions. But unlike their results, we found that the amount of pain reduction was increased when the suggestions were given following an induction of hypnosis. One confusing problem in this kind of experiment is that highly hypnotizable subjects —according to their own testimony—readily drift into hypnosis when they follow suggestions such as those for pain reduction. We included in our instructions that they should avoid drifting into hypnosis, and this may have made it more difficult for them to devote themselves fully to pain reduction. The results of the Greene and Reyher experiment (page 70) are consistent with ours. Our subjects preferred the pain reduction within hypnosis because it seemed less strenuous to them. The role of hypnotic induction undoubtedly varies from subject to subject. For many highly hypnotizable subjects, if there is no restriction against spontaneously entering hypnosis, the formal procedures of hypnotic induction may be less important than the suggestions for pain reduction.

A related problem is whether, for those who are susceptible to hypnosis, the depth of hypnosis affects the degree of pain reduction. In an experimental comparison, the same subjects were tested at the usual level, defined by them as a hypnotic scale level of 8 to 10, and on another occasion at a subjective depth of twice this on their scale, that is, at 16 to 20. It was found that subjects unable to reduce the pain of ice water to 0 at the lower depth were also unable to do so at the greater depth. For those already able to reduce pain, nothing appeared to change with depth. At the depths tested, the subject was still in communication with the hypnotist; as noted in Chapter 1, at extreme depths there is little responsiveness to suggestion. Whether or not some spontaneous analgesia might be found at greater depths at which the subject reports a separation of mind and body has not been tested.

The practical question whether a subject can improve in his ability to reduce pain by hypnotic suggestion is related to the general issue of training as a factor in hypnotic responsiveness. It is a separable question, however, because of the possibility that special performances can be improved by training even if there is no general improvement in hypnotizability (Chapter 1, page 9).

Working in our laboratory, Lenox selected subjects who scored very high on the available Stanford scales, including the Profile Scales that tap the most difficult classes of hypnotic behavior. He then proceeded to train them in pain reduction. Subjects were instructed to remove the hand from the ice water at the first indication of pain; hypnotized subjects with analgesia suggestions were gradually able to continue in the ice water indefinitely without pain. They learned also to control the ischemic pain produced by the tourniquet and exercise. Lenox found that subjects reported no pain at all in periods of ischemia up to half again as long as the time to intolerable pain in the waking state. These results confirm that subjects who have considerable hypnotic ability to begin with can profit from special training. That their improvement is somewhat specific to the responses suggested was shown by the finding that these subjects' scores on advanced hypnotic susceptibility tests after the experiment still correlated positively with their scores prior to training.

In a more recent experiment, also in our laboratory, Sachs chose subjects whose scores on the original hypnotic susceptibility test ranged from 3 to 9 on a scale with a maximum of 12. He wished to find to what extent success in training in hypnosis could improve analgesia. The results showed that practice in hypnosis (including experienced but not experimentally tested numbness) improved the amount of tested pain reduction significantly but not dramatically. At the end of the training, none of the subjects reported complete absence of pain in the ice water under suggested analgesia; those more able to reduce the pain in the beginning were the ones who profited most.

On the whole, the best single predictor of success in pain reduction is the amount by which pain is reduced when such hypnotically suggested reduction is first attempted. Measured hypnotic responsiveness is the next best predictor.

Hypnosis is More than a Placebo.   Laboratory psychologists are sometimes accused of elaborating the obvious by exercising great care in demonstrating what practical people have known all along. The charge is quite unfair, even though results do sometimes support what is common knowledge, because many plausible relationships turn out *not* to be found. It is quite obvious, for example, that a placebo must work by suggestion, since it is chemically inert but is thought by the person receiving it to be an active drug. Hypnosis has long been characterized as based upon suggestion. Therefore it would be reasonable to expect placebo responders and hypnotic responders to be the same people. But this turns out not to be the case.

Hypnosis and suggestion are not synonymous. Of course there is a large element of suggestion in hypnotic procedures, but many kinds of suggestion, such as social gullibility, are unrelated to hypnotic susceptibility. Those who believe that a man such as Hitler affects his audience through mass hypnosis are probably wrong, unless they wish to accept a very loose definition of hypnosis. Another kind of suggestion unrelated to hypnosis has sometimes been called impersonal or secondary suggestibility. An example is provided by Binet weights. These are weights arranged in a series, and the subject is to judge each one in relation to the one preceding it. The weights increase regularly in small steps until, at a certain point, they no longer increase and are all alike. Suggestibility is measured by how far into the series of equal weights the subject continues to say "heavier" each time. This kind of suggestibility is unrelated to hypnosis. The mere fact that something involves suggestion does not mean that it will correlate with hypnotizability. Hence it is necessary to conduct investigations that are free to turn out either way.

McGlashan, Evans, and Orne designed an experiment to test for a placebo factor in hypnosis. They used a form of the tourniquet-exercise method in which the subject kept on working as long as he could after the tourniquet cuff was inflated. The exercise was squeezing a bulb to pump water; both time and amount pumped were measured, first to the point at which the subject announced some pain (threshold pain) and then when he could not pump any more (tolerance). The conditions included a normal control without hypnosis, hypnotic analgesia, and a placebo condition. The placebo effect was fairly pronounced for the nonhypnotizable, but not at all for the hypnotizable. Hypnotic analgesia was very effective for the highly hypnotizable, but for the nonhypnotizable it was equivalent only to the placebo. Typical results are shown in Figure 8.

These results do not deny a placebo effect in attempted hypnotic analgesia. For low susceptible subjects—and *only* for them—hypnotic analgesia acts like a placebo; the correlation between the subjective report of pain with placebo and that with hypnotic analgesia was .76 for the insusceptible subjects. The corresponding correlation for the highly susceptible subjects was negligible. Hence we may conclude:

1. For subjects insusceptible to hypnosis, some pain reduction may be achieved through hypnotically suggested analgesia, but it will correspond to a reduction by placebo.

2. For subjects highly susceptible to hypnosis, pain reduction through hypnotically suggested analgesia is far greater than by placebo. For these subjects, the average placebo response is negligible or even negative.

Physiological Concomitants of Hypnotic Analgesia

We have already discussed the difficulties of finding a totally satisfactory physiological indicator of pain (see Chapter 2). Even so, cardiovascular indicators tended to show some correspondence to the subjects who felt pain, because both heart rate and blood pressure increased as the pain mounted. What happens to these and other indicators as pain is reduced by suggested hypnotic analgesia?

For subjects successful in reducing their felt pain, the indicators of pain that are under *voluntary control*, such as crying out, grimacing, and catching

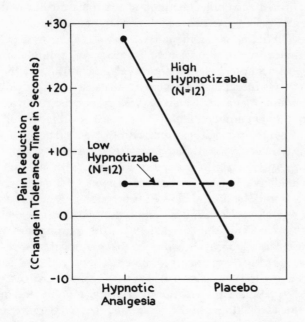

Figure 8. Differential effect of hypnotic analgesia and place-bo on subjects susceptible and not susceptible to hypnosis. Note that high values of tolerance time refer to successful pain reduc-tion. From data of McGlashan, Evans, and Orne (1969), courtesy of Frederick J. Evans.

breath, are consistently found to be reduced more than strictly involuntary responses.

The indicators that are essentially *involuntary* have seldom shown con-sistent reduction under hypnotic analgesia. A subject who is perfectly com-fortable and at ease through suggested hypnotic analgesia may still show a rise in heart rate or blood pressure. The paradoxical finding has been given various interpretations, including denial of the effectiveness of the hypnotic procedures. This is a troublesome logical point involving the definition of pain: if pain is what hurts, then the hypnotic procedures are successful in reducing it; but if one of the persisting physiological indicators is taken as defining pain, then hypnosis is unsuccessful. Sutcliffe, for example, took the position that when subjective pain is reduced but physiological indicators persist, the pain reduction is a "delusion." However, this implies that a physiological reaction to stress defines pain better than a report of what the subject feels. His conclusion may be challenged; the factual summary of the paradox is, however, correct.

We confirmed what others had found—that the cardiovascular changes in hypnotic analgesia were essentially those in normal waking. Whether or not pain was felt did not seem to matter.

Some minor qualifications must be made regarding the absence of physiological concomitants to hypnotic analgesia. With very highly hypnotizable subjects we found the rise in heart rate caused by cold pressor pain to be somewhat less in analgesia than in waking, but the rise was still appreciable. In another experiment, highly hypnotizable subjects were trained by operant conditioning procedures along with hypnotic analgesia suggestions to reduce the pain in ice water. Blood pressure rises were found to be less in hypnotic analgesia than in hypnotic nonanalgesia, although again the rises were not eliminated. Finally, in one experiment in ischemia with highly selected and trained subjects, neither heart rate nor blood pressure rose appreciably as ischemia continued. The latter two findings require further experimentation to determine to what extent the training methods affected the cardiovascular responses. It is known that cardiovascular responses can be influenced directly by operant or biofeedback procedures. These qualifications do not alter the general conclusion that hypnotic analgesia, successful as it is, has very little effect on the underlying, involuntary physiological processes associated with painful stimulation. This is a paradox that we shall have to face in trying to understand hypnotic pain reduction.

These conclusions are compatible with the findings that both pain and suffering are effectively reduced by hypnotic analgesia. The lack of the voluntary components indicates a generally relaxed comfort. The cardiovascular responses are not at all extreme and do not threaten the well-being of the subject. They merely mean that at some level the body is responding to the signals of painful stress upon it.

Relief of Anxiety Not Equivalent to Analgesia

The association of pain, fear, and anxiety has been noted in many contexts. Persistent chronic pain brings with it signs of personality disturbance, in which anxiety and depression may be prominent. One unaccustomed to pain who becomes suddenly exposed to it, as in surgery, is likely to be anxious. Anxiety may not be limited to the fear of pain but may include the possibility of a fatal outcome. It is now rather common to prescribe a tranquilizing drug upon entering the hospital to the patient who is to have surgery. It is possible, therefore, that the calming effect of hypnosis may contribute to its success in reducing pain. However, it would be a grave mistake to assume that the reduction of anxiety, no matter how beneficial to the patient, is the same as the reduction of felt pain.

The many ways of measuring pain contribute to the uncertainty about the relationship of anxiety to pain. Anxiety influences some measures of pain more than others. Anxiety is most likely to influence pain tolerance, and least likely to influence pain sensitivity at threshold. At suprathreshold levels of painful stimulation, anxiety is more likely to influence reports of distress or suffering than reports of sensory pain. These statements can be given greater clarity by comparing the effects on pain reports of tranquilizers, on the one hand, and chemical analgesics, on the other. The tranquilizer acts to reduce anxiety, although it is not an analgesic; the chemical analgesic reduces pain, although it need not reduce anxiety.

Chapman and Feather conducted a series of experiments comparing the effects on pain of a tranquilizer, diazepam (trade name, Valium), both with aspirin, an analgesic, and with a nonactive placebo. Their results can be summarized for our purposes as follows:

1. Tolerance time for a painful tourniquet was increased more by dia- zapam than by aspirin or placebo. If one had only this measure of pain, one might suppose that diazepam was acting like an analgesic.

2. Diazepam reduced the anxiety associated with severe tourniquet pain, even while the pain was mounting (Figure 9). Here we see that the anxiety-reduction and the pain-reduction effects are separable.

3. Diazepam had no effect on perceptual sensitivity near threshold levels of stimulation, as measured with radiant heat pain. The signal detection method was used; no change occurred either in sensitivity or in the measure provided in signal detection of the criterion ac- cording to which the sensory experience was labeled as pain. If one had only these results, the conclusion would be drawn that diazepam has no analgesic value whatever.

At this point the pertinent question is whether hypnotic suggestion acts like a tranquilizer or like an analgesic. Greene and Reyher, using the same measure of state-anxiety that Chapman and Feather used, found no correla- tion between pain reduction through hypnotic analgesia and changes in state-anxiety. Because analgesia was successful, the answer to the question is that hypnosis acts more like an analgesic than like a tranquilizer.

Shor attempted to answer the same question some years earlier in the study already cited, by testing hypnotic analgesia under conditions carefully designed to reduce anxiety. In his pilot studies he found that anxiety had a pronounced effect on physiological responses associated with electric shock. This led him to conduct his main experiment while employing several procedures designed to eliminate anxiety. He found by using the real-simu- lator model that hypnotic analgesia was unrelated to anxiety reduction. That is, the highly hypnotizable subjects were able to eliminate pain entirely through suggested analgesia, while the simulators were unable to do so, even though the physiological signs showed the two groups to be equally relaxed and free of anxiety.

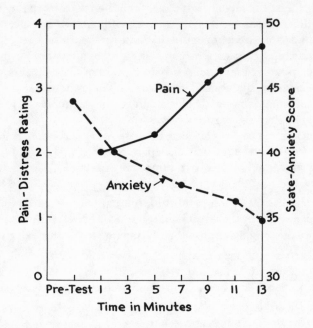

Figure 9.   Separateness of pain and anxiety following a tranquilizer. Tourniquet pain increases over time, while state-anxiety is
decreasing. Modified from Chapman and Feather (1973), combining data from their Figs. 1 and 2.

It is quite possible that pain can be reduced even when anxiety remains
high. Just as pain can mount while anxiety goes down, anxiety can mount
while pain decreases. Maintaining hypnotic analgesia requires some effort by
the subject, even though he knows he is going to be successful in reducing
pain. This effort is accompanied by physiological signs of anticipatory excitement when the subject knows he must soon fight off painful stimulation.
These signs may be interpreted as a form of anxiety, perhaps deriving from a
latent fear that this time control may be lacking. In any case, as shown in
Figure 10, both heart rate and blood pressure increase more when pain is to
be reduced by hypnotic analgesia than when it is to be felt normally at full
value. These measures were taken prior to the exposure to painful stimulation, from subjects who could successfully reduce pain. Hence reduction of
pain and anticipatory anxiety are not incompatible.

The purpose of this discussion has been to present evidence that anxiety
and analgesia are separable components of the total pain experience. Anxiety
is not irrelevant, and hypnosis can control anxiety as well as pain. In some

cases the control of anxiety may be more important than the control of pain. In a brief editorial on anxiety and pain based on his wide experience, Beecher has pointed out that often the basic need is for sedation rather than analgesia, or for sedation plus some analgesia; the common tendency is to overmedicate with narcotics. Recognizing that anxiety is an important clinical symptom in patients with pain, we still must conclude that hypnotic suggestions for pain reduction act primarily as analgesics, whatever other roles hypnosis may play in making the patient more comfortable.

Concluding Remarks on Hypnotic Analgesia

Although laboratory study of hypnotic pain reduction has gained momentum only in the last decade, a few generalizations have been found so consistently that they may be expected to endure. It is clear that laboratory pains of several kinds can be reduced by hypnotically suggested analgesia, but not by hypnosis alone without suggestions that pain will be reduced. Further, the amount by which pain is reduced by suggestions is correlated with measured hypnotic susceptibility; this correlation holds whether the

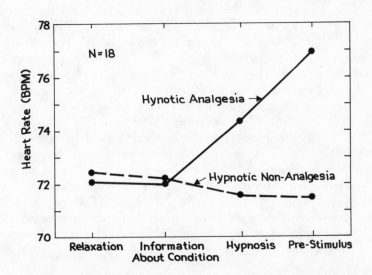

Figure 10. Anticipatory heart rate changes prior to immersion of hand in ice water under hypnosis, with and without analgesia suggestions. The experimental arrangements were those described earlier. Note that the greatest changes occurred in hypnotic analgesia, when subjects anticipate feeling no pain or greatly reduced pain. After Hilgard, Macdonald, Marshall, and Morgan (1974).

suggestions are given in the waking condition or within hypnosis. Highly hypnotizable subjects reduce pain more by hypnotically suggested analgesia than by waking suggestions of analgesia. For insusceptible subjects, hypnotic suggestions are equivalent to the placebo effect, but this is not true for the highly susceptible, who apparently resist the placebo effect.

As with most generalizations, those given above require some special qualifications. Although several experiments have demonstrated that hypnosis does not produce analgesia unless analgesia is suggested, there are some special circumstances within hypnosis in which "spontaneous" analgesia is reported. When hypnosis involves extreme dissociations, such as an arm out of awareness in automatic writing or in a successful "absent arm" suggestion, the member out of awareness may be spontaneously analgesic without any explicit suggestion.

Generalizations about other circumstances affecting analgesia are also emerging. For example, the depth of hypnosis for maximum analgesia appears to be considerably less than that of which the highly hypnotizable subject is capable. The differential effects of various kinds of suggested analgesia have not been studied in sufficient variety, or through a sufficient range of hypnotic potential, to make generalizations that will hold across the board; however, experiments thus far indicate that the highly hypnotizable subject can adapt almost any suggestion to make it operative for him. Experiments with training, both in hypnotic responsiveness generally and in hypnotic analgesia in particular, show that the subject without any talent for hypnosis improves only slightly with training. The subject whose hypnotic abilities are demonstrated from the start can improve substantially, especially in such specific hypnotic skills as pain reduction.

The paradox that hypnotic analgesia reduces subjective pain but does not appreciably reduce the involuntary physiological concomitants of pain sets problems for neuropsychology and neurophysiology. Some things hypnotic analgesia clearly is not—it is not simply a placebo effect, and it is not simply anxiety reduction.

On the whole, the results from the laboratory are by now sufficiently firm to bear upon the clinical applications of hypnosis to be considered in the chapters that follow.

Notes

The early surgical case by Recamier is mentioned by Ellenberger (1970); the episode concerning Ward's painless surgery is in Boring (1950).

Procedures Used to Reduce Pain

The two experimental procedures—direct suggestion of numbness and the "absent arm"—are mentioned as yielding equivalent results by Hilgard, Morgan, and Macdonald (1975). Subjects who preferred to use their own fantasies rather than those suggested by the hypnotist were noted by E. R. Hilgard (1971) and by Barber and Cooper (1972).

Pain Reduction in the Laboratory

That the amount by which pain is reduced correlates with hypnotic susceptibility has been shown by Shor (1959a); Hilgard (1967); and Evans and Paul (1970). A fuller account of the Stanford experiments appears in Hilgard, Ruch, and others (1974).

A review by Barber (1963) of hypnotic control of pain is illustrative of reviews that give the false impression that hypnotic analgesia is largely unsuccessful. See also Barber, Spanos, and Chaves (1974, Chapter 8).

Shor's (1959a) dissertation is only partly reproduced in his best-known account based on it (Shor, 1962b). We have relied on some data from the original dissertation, kindly furnished by Dr. Shor.

That highly hypnotizable subjects can reduce both pain and suffering to zero through analgesia suggestions has been shown by Knox, Morgan, and Hilgard (1974).

Evans and Paul (1970) confirmed in another laboratory the findings of our laboratory that hypnosis does not reduce pain unless combined with suggestions for analgesia (Hilgard, 1969). A finding of no difference in the effectiveness of analgesia suggestions with and without a prior induction was reported also by Spanos, Barber, and Lang (1974). Our finding of a difference with induction for highly hypnotizable subjects is reported in Hilgard (1975c).

The data from the Stanford laboratory on the effectiveness of analgesia suggestions at various subjective depths of hypnosis have not yet been published.

The effectiveness of training in pain reduction, while not precisely measured, may account in part for the results of Lenox (1970) and Sachs (1970), as mentioned in the text of the chapter. The recent work of Sachs (1975) has not yet been published.

That "hypnosis" is not to be identified with "suggestion" is stressed by Hilgard (1973a). The evidence that social gullibility is not involved is from Moore (1964). The distinction between primary suggestibility (the kind prominent in hypnosis) and secondary suggestibility (the kind shown with Binet weights) was made by Eysenck and Furneaux (1945), although Hull (1933) had noted it under different names.

The placebo experiment is that of McGlashan, Evans, and Orne (1969). The data they published were in somewhat derivative form; through the courtesy of Dr. Evans, we obtained the original data and recomputed it for Figure 8; it is presented in this form with his permission.

Physiological Concomitants of Hypnotic Analgesia

That voluntary responses are better controlled than involuntary ones is reported by Sears (1932), Barber and Hahn (1962), and Shor (1962b). The fact that involuntary responses, such as cardiovascular and galvanic skin responses, are not reduced with any consistency has so often been found that a listing of references is almost redundant. Illustrative are Sutcliffe (1961); Barber and Hahn (1962); Shor (1962b); Hilgard (1967; 1969); and Evans and Paul (1970). The minor qualifications come from Lenox (1970); Sachs (1970); and Hilgard, Morgan, and others (1974).

The possibility that hypnotic analgesia might operate as one of the central control mechanisms according to the gate theory has been raised by one of the originators of the theory, Wall (1969). This would require modification of impulses at the level of the spinal cord, which further evidence makes unlikely. See discussion in Chapter 10.

Many psychological problems are associated with pain in patients suffering repeated or persistent pain. Sternbach (1974b), in a book devoted to patients with chronic pain, includes depression as a common symptom. He notes the work of Egbert and others (1964) showing that a preoperative visit by the anesthetist may reduce anxiety enough that the patient may require less medication in the postoperative period.

Anxiety Reduction and Analgesia

Other accounts relating anxiety to pain reduction have referred to such studies as Schalling and Levander (1964), in which young delinquents were found to experience pain associated with anxiety; Sternbach (1965) on the consequence of warning the subject about a possible harmful effect of the shock he was about to experience; and Hill and others (1952) on the increasing effectiveness of morphine if anxiety was high. None of these studies makes for suprathreshold pain the kinds of distinctions that we feel to be important between the sedative effect and the analgesic effect.

The two studies in which tests for anxiety were used along with pain estimates are Chapman and Feather (1973) and Greene and Reyher (1972). Shor's study (1959a; 1962b; 1967) has been cited earlier (page 68). The report on anticipatory rises in heart rate and blood pressure is that of Hilgard, Morgan, and others (1974).

MESMERISM IN INDIA,

AND ITS

PRACTICAL APPLICATION IN SURGERY AND MEDICINE.

BY

JAMES ESDAILE, M.D.,

CIVIL ASSISTANT SURGEON, H. C. S., BENGAL.

" I rather choose to endure the wounds of those darts which envy casteth
at novelty, than to go on safely and sleepily in the easy ways of ancient
mistakings."—RALEIGH.

HARTFORD:

SILAS ANDRUS AND SON.

1851.

Title page from Esdaile's book reporting his use of hypnosis (in the form of mesmerism) on surgical patients in India. Reproduced by Tinterow, 1970.

PART II. *Hypnosis and*
Clinical Pain

Pain is a prominent symptom in cancer, obstetrics, surgery, and dentistry. The source of these pains is related primarily to organic disease, definable stress, or to interventions made in the course of treatment. Pain as a result of disease is represented by cancer; pain as a result of definable stress in an otherwise healthy person is illustrated by obstetrics. In surgery and in dentistry, pains are brought to the physician or dentist because of disease, and some pain is generated by the surgical or dental interventions.

The fields of cancer, obstetrics, surgery, and dentistry have been selected as the most dramatic for our purposes, because the pains have minimal psychological roots; their alleviation by hypnosis produces a convincing demonstration of hypnosis as a psychological method of pain control.

5 Cancer

Despite the many advances in knowledge, cancer remains one of the chief causes of death today; the patient who discovers he has cancer faces a major psychological crisis. Not only is fear of death a source of anxiety, but the reamining months or years of life may be filled with pain, debilitation, and perhaps disfiguration. Hypnotic treatment is not a cure for cancer, but it may improve the psychological and social situation of the patient and make the remaining period of his life more comfortable and agreeable than it would otherwise be. This prospect is one of the most humane promises that hypnosis holds.

In order to give a more concrete picture of what hypnotic treatment is like and what hypnosis can do for a patient, we shall recount the case of one patient treated in our program.

A Patient with Cancer

Mrs. E, aged 42, was referred by her attending physician because of continuous pain in her right arm and hand due to bone metastases from a primary breast cancer. In describing her illness at the laboratory, she reported that she was never free of pain; although codeine took the edge away, the pain never disappeared altogether. Sometimes she was awakened by it at night and could not get back to sleep. She expressed in words what was obvious from her general appearance and from the occasional tears in her eyes—that she felt very depressed. Unable to concentrate on any of her former daytime activities, she tended to be constantly aware of pain and of the implications of her illness.

On this first visit, information routinely obtained included further discussion of the illness, the course of the pain, a brief life history with particular emphasis on the origin of the present problem, special areas of interest, and attitudes toward hypnosis. The patient completed a mood checklist and was administered the Stanford Hypnotic Clinical Scale (SHCS), described in the appendix (page 209).

The pain had begun five months before as a dull ache in the elbow and forearm; it had progressed within a month to a point where it was "terrible." For the past four months, she had a few better days when she needed only a little medication, but more usual were times when she needed codeine every three to four hours.

Married, and the mother of two children, she received genuine psychological support from her family. Many of the interests she described were active athletic ones, now closed to her. She greatly enjoyed nature, particularly scenes and experiences at the ocean. As a child, she had gone often to the beach; this interest had persisted. "I like going into the water, going into the waves, I adore the salt water smell. . . . The waves soothe me. I can sit and watch them forever. It's like eternity. They keep coming and going. I feel buoyant in the water." She loved swimming. "It makes me feel good, like a new person after being tired. It's refreshing, it's relaxing. I love to lie on my back and float." Until the present illness, she had also read widely. She had particularly enjoyed rereading her favorite novels, always with vivid imagery. She had enjoyed close friends.

Asked about her ideas or experiences in hypnosis, she said she knew practically nothing. She had seen it on stage and thought it was exciting. She wanted to be sure that treatment of pain by hypnosis would not make her miss any important shift in her physical condition. She was reassured on this point: not all of her pain would be removed; she would still have signals for correction.

On the hypnotic responsiveness scale designed for clinical use, Mrs. E passed four of the five tests, failing only the test for amnesia. She was asked to keep a log of pain and the times of medication for four days, until the next appointment, at which time hypnotic treatment would begin.

Four days later, after an initial inquiry into the course of the illness, a brief check on her reaction to hypnosis revealed that she thought it a fascinating experience. She was amazed at what she had felt as a child during the regression—"especially the dress with those awful bloomers that my mother made me wear to school."

On a standard of 10 mutually agreed upon as that degree of pain which was barely tolerable, she reported the present level at 8. The hypnotic work was directed toward intervention in this pain. After a brief induction via progressive relaxation and counting, she was regressed to a time at the beach which she had described in the previous interview. She felt she was actually *at* the beach, *in* the buoyant, refreshing waves, and able to smell the salt air.

Hypnosis gradually deepened as the patient felt a greater degree of involvement and success in it. Effort was directed toward inducing glove anesthesia in the unaffected left hand. Gradually she was able to feel that this hand was cold (patient: "I make a snowman in my imagination, or I imagine filling up an ice bucket from the ice maker and sticking my hand in"), and then numb (therapist: "A very cold hand can experience less and less sensation, until it finally feels none"). Often rubbing a numb hand on a painful arm suffices to produce analgesia of the second arm. This did not prove successful for her, however, until anesthesia for the affected right arm itself was suggested in the following way. She was told to imagine that she was putting on a long evening glove, using her numbed left hand; she started slowly at the fingertips to roll on the glove, and moved it over the right hand and up the arm to a point well beyond the right elbow. In this way she achieved complete absence of pain. She was told that, upon awakening from hypnosis, she would retain a discomfort level of 2 on a scale of 10 so that she would always be reminded not to overdo. This would not be enough to bother her or interfere with interesting activities like reading, watching TV, and visiting with family and friends; it was simply a mild reminder to be careful. There were also suggestions that she would recapture the good feelings of buoyancy and freedom she had experienced at the ocean, and that she would carry these feelings with her after the hypnosis was over.

When Mrs. E came for her next visit, she said she had not needed any codeine for the rest of that day. "I could move and stretch my arm, I could put on my wig with two hands"—activities which, for some time, had been closed to her. "My arm and hand were quite comfortable, at the 2 or 3 pain level." On this occasion, the patient learned self-hypnosis along the lines of the hypnosis she had already experienced: first a progressive relaxation by counting; next a production of numbness in the well hand; and finally transferral of this as a glove anesthesia to the painful area. Subsequently she reported success with using the glove whether hypnosis was involved or not. The chart on which she recorded medication showed that her use of codeine had been drastically curtailed.

One problem continued to bother her. If she awakened at night or very early in the morning, she found it impossible to get back to sleep. Since the usual relaxation methods had not solved the problem, and since glove anesthesia had proved so successful in controlling pain, we felt that a method similar to the glove might be useful. After a conference, we settled on a yellow pajama snow suit which in her imagination she would pull up to cover herself. This was a combination of a sleeping-suit which her children had worn as toddlers and a yellow snowsuit that they had worn, which had a hood and was zippered. As she slowly put the suit on, those muscles which were covered would "go to sleep." Finally, after the hood was on, she would turn off the switches in her brain, and everything would grow darker just as it did when she turned off a light switch in the room. By this time she would be asleep. At this point the patient inquired anxiously about being able to wake up when she wanted to. She was reassured that she would always be able to wake up if there was an emergency, when she was called, or when anyone put a hand on her shoulder. Pleasant dreams while sleeping were also suggested. After practicing this procedure successfully several times in the laboratory, she tried it at home. She reported that she had slept so well—"like a baby" —that she hadn't had to repeat it at home after the first night.

The patient was seen a total of seven times during a month. On each occasion, suggestions of relaxation and comfort of mind were stressed: how valuable it was to be able to exert more control over a part of her life, over the pain, and over the insomnia. Judging from the patient's statements, from her cheerfulness, and from a positive shift in the tests of her mood at the laboratory, her mental state had improved markedly. She spent less time thinking of herself, and instead spent more time reading and enjoying the company of family members and friends. The last appointment occurred one month before her death. Unfortunately, contact during this period was lost.

Hypnosis in treatment is not always the same; the approach to the cancer patient may vary from a limited attempt to relieve a specific pain to incorporation of hypnosis into a broader psychological or psychiatric therapy. After digressing briefly to discuss some emotional reactions to cancer, we shall return to more specific problems of pain relief.

At the time of the first contact, Mrs. E was clearly depressed not only by her pain but also by anxiety over the implications of her illness. Anxiety and pain are inextricably woven together in the problems faced by such a patient; at times the anxiety can be more severe than the pain of the disease itself.

Emotional reactions to cancer vary during the course of the disease. Uncertainty, depression, fear of death, despair, dread of protracted pain, changes in body image with increasing weakness, decreasing mental capacity, social isolation either self-imposed or imposed by others who withdraw because of their anxiety—these are some of the contingencies which require a mobilization of ego functions on a scale seldom matched in the life cycle of any individual. There may be other realistic sources of worry, such as the financial security of the individual and of the family. Occasionally there are problems rooted in the past, such as guilt, which complicate the present problems.

Certain types of treatment interventions pose threats too. There are unpleasant side effects, whether from an operation, from radiotherapy, from chemotherapy, or from an increasing dosage of analgesics. Intensive courses of radiotherapy or chemotherapy can produce nausea, vomiting, hair loss, and other side effects; for an individual already partially incapacitated, these constitute difficult and discouraging problems. Tranquilizers and analgesics, prescribed in increasing dosage, may further dull the mind, making ego functions more fragile and social participation less rewarding.

Although the treatment procedures described in Mrs. E's case were initiated for the relief of pain, a review of the case demonstrates that both pain and anxiety were being treated. What were the general treatment approaches?

1. *Support by the therapist encouraged reassertion of ego strength to meet the crisis.* Mrs. E expressed relief at finding someone who would help her with her problems. Psychotherapy, at the level of ego support, assisted the patient in strengthening her existing ego techniques for meeting this critical situation, as well as enabling her to use her talent for imagination and for reliving pleasant former experiences in ways appropriate to the present. She was able to use hypnosis without resistance or conflict after asking a sensible question about the function of pain. As part of our standard procedure we discuss pain with the patient: how it operates as a defense against injury but how, at this point, we need to retain it only as a signal for corrective purposes.

In some patients, anxiety over loss of control must be worked through. Friedman reported an illuminating instance of this nature. A 52-year-old woman with breast cancer had developed extensive metastases to the cervical spine, pelvis, and upper extremity of the right femur. Because the pain was difficult to control with drugs, hypnosis was suggested. Her only objection was that she was unwilling to have anyone dominate her mind and control her thoughts and acts. She was reassured on this point and was invited to submit to an experiment to demonstrate that there would be no loss of consciousness, that she would know at all times what was happening, and that she would not do or say anything contrary to her wishes. Accepting this invitation, the patient was readily placed in a deep trance. Suggestions were then made that she would have amnesia for the name of her husband and for the name of her attending physician. On awakening, she was asked the name of her husband: she gave it promptly. She was, however, unable to give the name of the attending physician. It was pointed out to her that the suggestion of amnesia for the name of her husband, with whom she had lived for thirty years, appeared ridiculous to her; thus she had rejected this suggestion. However, she had no objection to amnesia for the name of the physician. After this demonstration of her degree of control, the patient continued in hypnotherapy with no further resistance. It may be noted that with this patient, glove anesthesia was induced in one hand, then the patient was taught to transfer this anesthesia to any part of the body that was painful by massaging the painful area gently. She was able to induce the glove anesthesia in her hand at will and to control any pain for periods varying from one to several hours.

2. *Relief of anxiety occurred in our patient along with relief of pain.* If the burden of pain can be lifted at least partially by hypnosis, a number of other important steps automatically follow. No longer preoccupied with pain, the individual is free to participate with people and activities; decreased use of narcotics results in less of their depressive effect on mental functioning; with less pain, the patient's prevailing mood is apt to be more cheerful. Anxiety is lessened not only because of relief from pain, but also because of specific posthypnotic instructions (to feel more relaxed, calm, and cheerful) incorporated in the hypnotic work. A more meaningful existence is open to the suffering individual.

3. *Insomnia was overcome.* A troublesome though secondary symptom, the insomnia caused by both pain and anxiety, was relieved. The patient said she could sleep like a baby again and feel refreshed. Such relief of ancillary symptoms occurs frequently. Friedman's patient, for example, had little appetite at the beginning of hypnotherapy, but further suggestions directed toward the problem achieved good results.

4. *Interests were broadened.* The patient can return to interesting activities as he begins to function more normally. The therapist can learn from the patient's personal history about activities he once enjoyed which may again be available. For Mrs. E, such activities included reading, watching TV, and conversing with friends. What the patient can do most satisfactorily depends on his prior interests and enjoyments—such as listening to music, playing a musical instrument, reading, or of participating in games—tempered by what his present physical condition permits. If the patient during his prior life has become immersed in the beauty of natural surroundings, and is capable of short drives through the countryside, this can be a welcome outlet.

Participation in such activities is encouraged both through suggestions in hypnosis and by discussion outside hypnosis. Involvement in daily life activities helps to divert the patient's attention from the illness and the pain. Such involvement can be stimulated by direct suggestion as well as by relief from pain.

5. *Independence from the hypnotist was gained through self-hypnosis.* The stereotype of a patient passively dependent upon the hypnotist is a false picture of the best contemporary treatment practices. Teaching self-hypnosis constituted an essential part of our procedure with Mrs. E, as it does in most cases. The hypnotist showed the patient, through mastery of techniques already used or with changes she preferred, how she could produce the same result through her own efforts. A patient may thus gain a measure of control over situations in which he has previously felt completely helpless. LaBaw described the case of a woman with cancer who was completely immobilized at home by the illness. Through hypnosis—including self-hypnosis—for

control of symptoms, she was able to become mobile again until the day before her death. LaBaw remarked that an important contribution of self-hypnosis was return of maximum control to the patient, permitting the desperately ill person to make constructive use of the days salvaged from pain and the fear of death. He concluded that hypnosis represented a means of helping people die "with their boots on, instead of in a pair of slippers in the hospital."

While self-mastery of the technique is the goal, some patients feel incapable of it or, though capable, resist it. Basic personality factors may promote continued dependence upon outside sources of stimulation and support. Often communication with the hypnotist by telephone maintains sufficient contact. Taped suggestions may be used, or a member of the family may be trained to take over the role of the hypnotist.

Our discussion of Mrs. E's case has shown how much more is happening in hypnotic therapy than pain reduction alone, even though therapy is initially directed toward pain relief. Other aspects of the therapeutic situation must be considered in individual cases, not all of which were important in the case of Mrs. E.

For example, individual attitudes toward cancer based on unusual life experiences may need to be understood before treatment can proceed. Sacerdote reported the case of a 49-year-old woman, a Christian Scientist, with pain from metastatic breast cancer. She was identifying with three women in her life who had been victims of breast cancer; she harbored guilt feelings for not having been firm and outspoken in her faith in order to provide sufficient physical and mental help for them. Sacerdote noted that her continued pain operated as a punishment and expiation for guilt. Others, too, have commented that the guilt-punishment motif sometimes plays a powerful role in the complex etiology of cancer pain. Sacerdote wrote in a later paper that, with experience and understanding, a carefully calculated guess could be made about the guilt which the patient needed to expiate; deep analysis would actually be contraindicated, as it might break down needed defenses. "It is often possible to successfully persuade the patient, in and out of hypnosis, that the amount of suffering which he has undergone may closely balance the amount of guilt he is carrying. At other times, the patient is shown that the emotional causes had taken place such a very long time ago that it would be silly still to be suffering because of them. It is indeed surprising how often these rationalized explanations can be given in very general terms; without even having to know why the patient is blaming himself, an almost immediate abreaction which often constitutes a corrective emotional experience can be elicited."

These accounts should be sufficient to show that successful hypnotic therapy requires a great deal more than skill in the techniques of hypnosis.

The successful therapist, dealing with the life predicament of a cancer patient, must be more than a technician who has mastered a few procedures.

Strategies for Pain Reduction in Cancer

In Chapter 4 we described specific techniques used within hypnosis; these are adapted in many ways to meet the needs of the individual patient. Some methods were described in the case of Mrs. E, such as the use of glove anesthesia transferred to other areas of pain, or of an imagined sleeping garment to relieve insomnia. In what follows, a few widely different examples will be given to show the range of techniques that have actually been used in cancer.

There are numerous approaches even to the familiar glove anesthesia suggestion that so often precedes transfer of the anesthetic effect to some other part of the body. Sometimes a suggestion of warmth or cold is given as a first step in analgesia. With Mrs. E, warmth in the unaffected hand was tried first, unsuccessfully. However, the next suggestion, cold, was successful and could be followed by successful suggestions for anesthesia in this unaffected hand. Rubbing the anesthetic fingertips and hand on the painful hand and arm—a procedure frequently followed—was unsuccessful until the fantasy was added that she was putting on, with the numb hand, a long evening glove to encompass the area and extend beyond the elbow.

Conversion, substitution, and displacement of the pain are frequently used as methods of control. Sacerdote reported the case of a 60-year-old man whose primary lesion was in the throat, with an extension into a large, painful indurated mass involving most of the right side of the neck, jaw, and cheek. After induction, Sacerdote suggested to him that he could experience a pleasant tingling sensation—like a weak, soothing electric current—wherever the tumor extended. The patient was able successfully to substitute the pleasant tingling for the pain.

Erickson treated a cancer patient suffering intolerable, intractable pain with the suggestion of an intolerable, incredibly annoying itch on the sole of her foot. "Her body weakness, occasioned by the carcinomatosis and hence inability to scratch the itch, rendered this psychogenic pruritis all-absorbing of her attention. Then, hypnotically, there were systematically induced feelings of warmth, of coolness, of heaviness and of numbness for various parts of her body where she suffered pain. And the final measure was the suggestion of an endurable but highly unpleasant and annoying minor burning-itching sensation at the site of the mastectomy. This procedure of replacement substitution sufficed for the patient's last six months of life. The itch of the sole of her foot gradually disappeared, but the annoying burning-itching at the site of her mastectomy persisted."

Erickson also reported displacement of pain in a patient dying from prostatic metastatic carcinomatosis and suffering intractable abdominal pain. It was possible to displace this pain to an equal pain in the patient's left hand; in the new location it was endurable, since it did not carry the same threatening significance. The patient became accustomed to the severe pain in the left hand, which he protected carefully. This did not interfere with his full contact with his family during the last months of his life.

Removal from the scene of pain through fantasy may also be used. In the case from Friedman discussed earlier, in which glove anesthesia proved useful, the patient spontaneously experienced a form of floating and soon found that she could float out of her bed. The therapist encouraged this form of dissociation; it soon became possible for the patient to turn around and see herself lying in bed, and not to experience the pain that the patient in bed was having.

This out-of-the-body experience is a frequent manifestation reported by hypnotizable subjects in the laboratory. It can be very useful when suggested for pain control in the clinic.

Erickson also described a patient who, with the onset of agonizing pain, would develop a trance state in response to posthypnotic suggestions. In this trance state she would take herself mentally away from her sick body. She would get into a wheelchair and go into the living room to watch television—free of pain—while her suffering body remained in the bedroom.

It is frequently possible to suggest to the patient that he will return to a time before the present illness began, to an activity in which there was great pleasure and absorption. Patients can relive happy experiences such as camping, backpacking, playing baseball, swimming, or watching favorite television programs. While the patient is in the midst of these experiences, pain goes unnoticed. It is then possible to suggest that, although the experience itself will end, there will be a tendency to ignore any discomfort, and that the feelings of well-being and pleasantness will persist for a long time.

One of our patients was a 14-year-old boy with leukemia, with lesions in the brain, liver, and chest; he suffered from severe chest pain. He could be regressed to a time when he was participating in a Little League baseball game which he thoroughly enjoyed and during which there was no pain. Further suggestions were given that he would continue to be relaxed and feel no pain after he awakened. This technique was usually successful.

Suggestion of pleasant dreams is a way in which the hypnotist can help the patient. Gardner reported the case of an 11-year-old boy with leukemia, first referred because of nausea and vomiting. David gradually developed pain, for which hypnosis also proved helpful. He learned how to induce self-hypnosis, based on relaxation, visual imagery, and arm levitation. He was told that he could have a pleasant dream which he could use as often as he liked. He dreamed that he was an eagle who enjoyed flying powerfully from one safe, peaceful place to another. When anything disturbed him, he could fly off to another place, even safer and happier. At home, when in distress, David successfully continued hand levitation with the eagle dream to achieve quietness and calm enjoyment, sometimes on his own intiative and sometimes on his mother's suggestion, "David, just find your peaceful place." He could shift in this way from a negative to a positive feeling state. There was evidence of the patient's sense of control and mastery gained through hypnosis up to the end of his life.

In our laboratory, we have found that dreams—particularly dreams of flying—help patients to enjoy feelings that range far from drab reality. They can move into an exciting, beautiful, and different world: one patient will hop onto a cloud, while another will find himself piloting his own plane. Feelings such as lightness of spirit and body, as well as a feeling of control, remain with the patient long after the hypnotic session has ended.

Amnesia is yet another technique shown to be useful, particularly with continued episodic experiences of pain. The problem of intermittent, recurrent, severe pain occurs extensively in clinical practice, but has been studied very little in laboratory subjects. Hence, work with amnesia as a method of treatment for pain comes primarily from clinicians.

Erickson describes episodic pain as a construct of past remembered pain, the present pain experience, and future anticipated pain. "Thus, immediate pain is augmented by past pain and is enhanced by the future possibilities of pain. The immediate stimuli are only a central third of the entire experience." Pain also has particular temporal attributes, emotional connotations, and personal interpretations varying from individual to individual.

When pain is of this episodic variety, total or partial amnesia for the pain already experienced can often be induced. As remembrance is dulled or erased, anticipation can also be decreased or eliminated. Patients who have experienced severe pain are prey to anticipatory dread and fear, with apprehension for the future. Such patients can be told that past experiences of pain have been forgotten and that any pain experience will be unexpected and transient.

This technique is useful not only in treating pain in the cancer patient, but also in lessening nausea and vomiting from the intensive chemotherapy regimes now recommended for some neoplasms. Patients may be referred to us because of anticipatory symptoms: in advance of the injection at the hospital, they begin vomiting. Sometimes this happens as the car enters the vicinity of the hospital, sometimes while on the escalator to the treatment floor, and sometimes just as the injection is being given. In addition to these advance symptoms, the expected reaction—nausea and vomiting later in the day—happens far more frequently to these patients. In any given case, amnesia is ordinarily an auxiliary method to others discussed previously. In our work, to help the patients cope with the later excessive vomiting, we may combine amnesia with suggestions for greater interest in outside activities. For example, one 22-year-old patient to whom amnesia was suggested became able to absorb himself again in TV. His vomiting was cut to one-third of the number of times it had been when he first came, and each episode was brief.

In another of our cases, a young woman with Hodgkin's disease had severe nausea and vomiting anticipatory to chemotherapy treatment. It occurred during the hour's trip to the hospital, in the hospital parking lot, and just as the chemical was about to be injected in the treatment room. A rehearsal method within hypnosis prepared her for the sequence of events without nausea or vomiting. She was able to follow the script so successfully as to inhibit all these anticipatory reactions. For example, she reported what happened while being injected. "I looked at the floor when the nurse was actually giving me the treatment to *blank* everything out. . . . I've put what the nurse is doing out of my mind . . . I'm not aware of it . . . I've blanked the person who's *getting* the treatment out of my mind. I'm thinking of my exciting weekend at Yosemite Park."

Amnesia for previous attacks of pain has been successfully combined with hypnotic time distortion by Cooper and Erickson. They taught a patient to experience intractable attacks of stabbing pain—which normally lasted 5 to 10 minutes—as if they were lasting 10 to 20 seconds. The patient was given posthypnotic suggestions that each attack would come as a complete surprise to him; that when the attack occurred he would develop a trance state of 10 to 20 seconds duration; and that after experiencing the pain attack, he would come out of the trance with no awareness that he had been in a trance or that he had experienced pain.

It is evident that the methods available are limited only by the ingenuity of the hypnotist and the imaginative resourcefulness of the patient. This review shows how far we have come from the authoritative commands of a hypnotist who merely tells the subject that he has no pain.

Evaluations of Hypnotic Treatment

As we have noted frequently, if the promise of hypnosis is to be fulfilled, its limitations must also be understood. No therapy is universally successful, but its successes are increased if there has been an appropriate diagnosis and a careful record of successes and failures under specified circumstances. Among the first things we need to know are how responsive a person must be to hypnosis for the treatment to be successful, and how the time of the practitioner can be used most effectively. Evaluation of the outcome of psychotherapy is, on the whole, quite unsatisfactory; hypnosis suffers in this respect along with other treatments. Many reports in the literature cover only a single case, or at most a very few cases, and it is natural that the successes are given more attention than the failures. We shall attempt to assemble such information as is available regarding the outcome of hypnotic treatment when a series of patients have been studied.

Butler, in several reports discussing the problem and giving an account of a series of twelve patients, made a serious effort to classify those who were helped and those not helped by hypnotic treatment. He found that five of the twelve cases were clearly benefited. Some were entirely relieved of pain, others had partial or temporary relief, and some were not helped at all. The situation the therapist had to deal with was frequently more complex than just treating cancer; for example, there were often problems from the past associated with the personality make-up of the individual. Nevertheless, Butler regarded the depth of hypnosis which could be achieved as a deciding factor in the effectiveness of treatment.

"Hypnotic techniques as used in this study did reduce pain, allay anxiety, and aid in organ function; but the results were proportional to the depth, and only five of these selected twelve cases, who were somnambulistic, can be said to be unequivocally benefited by this therapy. The remainder of the patients who could enter a medium trance were helped, but it is doubtful if this improvement is adequate compensation for the time spent to obtain it."

". . . to gain maximum relief for the time spent, one should select patients who enter a deep or somnambulistic trance, for in these patients organic pain and subjective symptoms can be relieved, and, through posthypnotic suggestions, relief may be continued after the period of hypnosis."

Another study bears out the general conclusion reached by Butler. Lea, Ware, and Monroe, reporting on the hypnotic control of intractable pain, listed eleven patients suffering from cancer, only nine of whom could be used in the study. The degree of trance state achieved by each patient was rated as none, light, medium, or deep. The method of hypnotic treatment was to attempt to localize the pain in one pathological area while emphasizing that the rest of the body was normal. In addition, the patient was told that since he had learned to relax, the pain would not bother him so much. Of the nine patients, five showed good to excellent results, and four were failures. Of the two whose results were considered excellent, one was capable of a deep trance, the other of a medium trance. Of the four failures, none achieved more than a light trance. Thus, although no absolute relationship was shown between degree of hypnotic responsiveness and therapeutic results, the trend was clear.

In a large-scale study of hypnosis and cancer, Cangello began with eighty-one patients whom he had treated, seventy-three females and eight males. The study illustrates how difficult it is to do definitive investigation in a clinical setting. In the first place, there is no way of telling just what population the patients represent. These patients ranged in age from 17 to 76 years; we know nothing about the medical, social, or economic factors that found them in the group to be studied. Various circumstances led to elimination of some patients from the group for purposes of quantitative study, so later studies were made on fractions of the total.

An initial session lasting approximately thirty minutes included an assessment of mental ability and of willingness to cooperate as well as a first hypnotic experience. General hypnotizability was measured. Because this is one of the few studies in which such care was taken to assess hypnotizability, the criteria are worth noting: eyelid catelepsy for the light trance; gustatory illusions or glove anesthesia for the medium trance; and complex tactual anesthesia or amnesia for the deep state. We now know that these are criteria of hypnotic responsiveness rather than hypnotic depth. However, in reporting Cangello's work we will use his categories.

Hypnotic sessions lasting about fifteen minutes were carried out during daily ward rounds, commonly at the patient's bed in a multi-bed ward. If hypnotic induction was unsuccessful after these visits (totaling about an hour of attempted induction) the patient was considered unsatisfactory for this treatment. The total time spent with each patient varied from fifteen minutes to two hours, with an average of sixty-six minutes.

Seventy-three of the eighty-one were considered to be successfully hypnotized at some point. Each of these patients received a posthypnotic suggestion as follows: "No reaction, no matter how severe, so far as your illness is concerned, need hurt, upset you, or bother you in any way." Observations by nurses and medical colleagues permitted the results to be evaluated. Thirty of seventy-three had excellent results; twenty were rated good, fourteen fair, and nine poor. The more deeply hypnotizable were more successful in pain reduction, but even the less susceptible were successful in about half the cases. Cangello's group included seven subjects with intractable pain; even for them, four of the five most susceptible to hypnosis found sufficient relief through hypnosis that they did not require surgical procedures.

In order to secure data that might be more objective, Cangello made a special study of twenty-two patients who had been receiving narcotics every four hours for constant pain. This situation permitted narcotic reduction, after hypnotic treatment, to be used as a criterion of success. Slightly more than half of these patients (fourteen of the twenty-two) decreased their use of narcotics to 50 percent or less of what they had been taking. The rest were considered to be failures, so far as the hypnotic treatment was concerned. The hospital routinely used chemical rhizotomy or surgical tractotomy for pain relief when recommended, but none of the patients in whom hypnosis was successfully induced ever required these procedures, even though not all met the foregoing criterion of decreased narcotic use.

Cangello also followed up these patients to find out how long the treatment proved effective. Of the fourteen judged successful by reduced narcotic intake, two had only transient results, lasting two or three days; eight had results lasting at least a week and up to a month; and the remaining four had results lasting from five to twelve weeks. Cangello gives a number of cases in some detail, including six among those successfully treated for pain. He also details miscellaneous cases, including treatment of postoperative anorexias, immobilization of an arm for a skin graft, and other applications of hypnotic practices on the cancer ward not specifically relevant to pain reduction.

No further statistical studies have come to our attention. It appears that, to clinicians, a satisfactory demonstration has been made that cancer pain can be controlled in a substantial number of cases.

The advantage of studies involving larger populations of patients over presentations of individual cases is that failures are much more likely to be reported; an unsuccessful case is unlikely to emerge as a single case report. The results of Butler; of Lee, Ware, and Monroe; and of Cangello show a relationship between hypnotic responsiveness and success in pain reduction. The figure that commonly emerges—about 50 percent of the cases showing substantial improvement—is close to that reported without the statistical basis by other clinicians such as Morphis and Kroger.

Concluding Remarks on Treating the Pain of Cancer

Some committed clinicians distrust large-scale studies and the standardized measurements they call for. Sacerdote, for example, believes that standardized susceptibility scales are too narrow, and that nearly everyone is hypnotizable enough to profit from hypnotic methods. He tends to attribute lack of hypnotic susceptibility to resistance. Chong also feels that depth is unimportant in therapy. However, when the results of larger-scale studies of the clinic are supplemented by results from the laboratory, persistent differences in hypnotizability having little to do with the skill of the hypnotist are found. It is desirable to assess these differences when hypnotic treatment is under consideration.

Writing from another culture, in Singapore, Chong states that good rapport with the patient is as important to the success of treatment as depth of hypnosis. He believes that hypnosis can help at any point in the course of the disease: early, it can help the patient accept the diagnosis and change his attitudes from despair to hopeful toleration; later, it can help to relieve pain and thus lessen the need for narcotics, or it can ease the side effects of radiation therapy. Of the ten cases of cancer treated in Chong's study, three suffered intractable pain from cancer, two suffered from phantom limb pain after amputation of cancerous growth, and one was undergoing deep radiation therapy. Of the three pain patients with intractable pain, two were helped.

Although results to date show that in many cases hypnotic therapy brings relief, the practice of therapy for the pain of cancer could be improved by additional systematic investigations along the following lines:

1. Clinical assessment of hypnotic responsiveness before beginning hypnotic treatment, to determine those patients for whom hypnosis will be an efficient method of therapy.

2. More careful delineation of a range of acceptable, communicable techniques for use by qualified therapists. These should include both techniques of induction and therapeutic practices, including the teaching of self-hypnosis.

3. Establishment of objective indices of improvement to be used in various cancer settings. Useful indices would include reduction in drug use, modification in self-reports of pain on uniform pain scales, and changes in mood or feelings of well-being on regularly administered mood scales.

4. Special studies of the interactive effects of features of the therapeutic program in relation to the course of the disease process, aimed at questions such as the following:

   a. What is the role played by anxiety and other attitudes toward the disease (and toward the prospect of death) in relation to pain? What is the effect of hypnosis?

   b. What is the therapeutic effect of participation in physical or social activities? How can hypnosis encourage these?

   c. Are there side effects of self-hypnosis, involving improved self-image, that contribute therapeutically beyond the hypnotic results themselves? Can family members assist in hypnosis to the benefit of the patient?

   d. Are changes in technique to be recommended as a function of age? (Successes have been reported with a child as young as 4 and with a man as old as 80.)

Despite some limitations in the research on hypnotic pain control in cancer, the evidence is overwhelming that many patients can obtain relief from pain through hypnotic procedures. Sometimes the pain is reduced; sometimes it is completely eliminated. Because use of narcotics can be reduced with hypnotic therapy, the dangers of addiction are lessened, consciousness is less clouded, and the patient is open to experiences that will make life more pleasant, even if the illness is terminal.

Hypnosis should clearly be given an extensive trial, not after everything else has failed, but before heavy doses of narcotics are used and before surgery for pain relief is attempted. The ideal approach would be to start using hypnosis in the early phases of the disease, before pain becomes a disabling entity. In that case, the ability of the patient to hypnotize himself and keep anxiety under control through the course of the disease would aid not only in his general outlook, but probably in the control of pain itself.

Notes

Most clinical literature on the hypnotic treatment of cancer is based on a few successful cases. These demonstrate that the method is successful with some patients and suggest some strategies for the practitioner to try with his patients. However, such cases alone are not helpful in selecting the patients most likely to benefit from hypnosis, or in providing criteria for choosing one technique or procedure over another. We have not attempted to list such individual case reports, except when a special point is at issue.

Because our problem is pain, our discussion of the emotional situation of the cancer patient is rather sketchy, even though we are aware that anxiety and depression may have an influence on felt pain. Asken (1975) addresses the body-image problem caused by a mastectomy performed in the treatment of breast cancer. Facial disfigurements and limb amputations are other illustrations of changes in the body image to which adjustment is difficult. Craig and Abaloff (1974) have shown depression to be a common symptom in a group of thirty cancer patients they studied.

The special problems facing the dying patient have come to the fore in the literature of recent years. Levinson (1975) provides a short history and a thoughtful discussion. His article can serve as an introduction to the field.

The patient whose resistance was overcome when shown that she still retained control was reported by Friedman (1960). The woman who became mobile again after learning self-hypnosis is described by LaBaw (1969). She had had a carcinoma of the breast which had widely metastasized.

Strategies for Pain Reduction in Cancer

The leading figures in clinical control of pain through hypnotic techniques in those whose illnesses are severe or terminal have been Erickson and Sacerdote. Erickson (1959) reported a case in which symptoms could be redirected as new and acceptable perceptions. Later, he assembled his experience into the form of eleven procedures he had used in the alleviation of pain (Erickson, 1967). His cases reported in the text are from the latter source. The time distortion method was developed in collaboration with Cooper and is reported in Cooper and Erickson (1959).

Sacerdote's earlier papers are referred to in Sacerdote (1965). The case reported is from Sacerdote (1970). In two later papers (Sacerdote, 1972; 1974) he deals with the expectations of the patient and their influence on the techniques appropriate in the hypnotherapeutic process. We understand that he is now preparing a chapter on emotional care of the cancer patient, to appear in a book edited by Kutscher.

The case of David, who treated himself through hypnosis and self-induced hypnotic dreaming, was reported by Gardner (1975). Her treatment included more than the dream, but that aspect has been selected here to illustrate a specific technique. For added description of self-hypnosis in children with cancer see LaBaw and others (1975). The amnesia technique is discussed in Erickson (1967).

Evaluations of Hypnotic Treatment

In a series of thoughtful papers published two decades ago, Butler provided a careful discussion of the use of hypnosis in the care of the cancer patient (Butler, 1954a; 1954b; 1955a; 1955b). The quotation is from Butler (1955b, p. 13). He also gave a history of the hypnotic treatment of cancer, with references as far back as 1890 (Butler, 1954a).

The study by Lea, Ware, and Monroe (1960) is a good illustration of what needs to be done on a larger scale, with more careful controls. Their very restricted range of hypnotic techniques may trouble clinicians who prefer to employ a variety of procedures adapted to the individual patient.

Cangello's study, done on one large sample of patients, was separately reported in two papers, Cangello (1961; 1962).

Clinical estimates, such as those of Morphis (1961), must be accepted as only gross approximations. He reported that 50 percent of the patients suffering severe pain in terminal cancer could be helped by hypnosis; he classed the other 50 percent as poor subjects whose pains were better controlled by narcotics. He indicates that about one-fifth of the group that can be helped (10 percent of the total group) can be taken off of narcotics completely, while the others have their requirements reduced. The corresponding figure given by Kroger (1963)—a generalization from his experience without any statement of sample size or patient selection—was that for 60 percent of the patients treated by hypnosis, narcotics could be drastically reduced. Even if these figures were divided in half, they would still mean that a substantial number of patients benefit from the therapy.

Concluding Remarks

Sacerdote's comments are from Sacerdote (1965; 1970); Chong's are from Chong (1968). The very young child is reported by Crasilneck and Hall (1973), the very old man by Hightower (1966).

We are very much impressed by the contribution that the controls used in laboratory studies can make to the clinic, and we are devoting some of the efforts of our laboratory in that direction. A more careful set of diagnostic procedures and a realistic appraisal of the proportion of success to be expected are important not only to the patient but to the physician. A physician attempting to use hypnosis may assume that his technique is faulty if he does not succeed in a high enough proportion of cases, when he may in fact be doing as well as can be expected.

6 Obstetrics

Why a normal process such as childbirth should be so painful is puzzling; many have suggested that the reasons may be in part psychological. Anthropological observations indicate that the behavior expected during confinement varies widely from culture to culture, but the idea that primitive births are painless is probably a myth. In western culture, pain in childbirth has been taken so much for granted that it has been rationalized as in some sense "deisrable;" its reduction, as by chemical anesthetics, has seemed "immoral." This attitude has slowly changed, until the issue we face today is not whether the pains should be reduced, but how. The more favorable attitude toward alleviation of labor pains was given a sanction by England's Queen Victoria in 1853, when Snow anesthetized her for the birth of Prince Leopold. The choice today is between chemical pain reducers and psychological procedures—or, of course, some combination of the two. In this chapter we shall be concerned primarily with the psychological methods, of which hypnosis is one.

There are three principal methods by which the expectant mother may prepare for her confinement in the hope that the delivery will be comfortable without the use of drugs: (1) hypnotic procedures; (2) the method known as *natural childbirth*, introduced by Grantly Dick Read in 1933; and (3) the procedures associated with the *psychoprophylactic* method, introduced in Russia by Velvovski in 1949 and rather widely used in France and elsewhere, often called the "Lamaze method" in America, after the man who helped bring it to France. The three practices overlap in many ways, leading some to believe that they are practically indistinguishable. We recognize the overlap but think it a mistake to gloss over the differences.

From a psychological standpoint, the primary problem once labor begins is pain. In the United States, at least, the solution immediately thought of

103

is chemical pain reducers. However, some cautions must be observed for the protection of both mother and fetus, and anything that reduces the need for chemoanalgesics or chemoanesthetics lessens the risks. Poor-risk mothers —such as those with cardiac or pulmonary disease or with multiple allergies —are particularly good candidates for nondrug methods. When the fetus is threatened, as in a premature birth, reduction of chemicals in the blood may make a difference in survival.

Labor is divided into three stages. First is the period during which the cervix is dilating so the baby may pass through; this is an extended period for most women, and the degree of comfort of the confinement is in part described by the shortness of this period. The next two periods are the passage of the baby through the birth canal—ending with the actual delivery—and, finally, the passage of the placenta or afterbirth. The first stage of labor is variable and may take many hours; the second stage typically takes about half an hour, and the third stage a few minutes. Of course there are more difficult deliveries, such as breech deliveries, which take longer, and caesarean sections in which normal birth is interfered with.

Some surgery is very common in ordinary deliveries to avoid tearing of the vulva as the baby is born. The incision made at this point, known as an episiotomy, is an additional source of pain, especially because it must be repaired after the delivery is completed.

The first six weeks after birth are called the postpartum period; this is the time required to restore the mother to the normal nonpregnant state. Various pains and discomforts are associated with the early postpartum period; in some cases, difficulties with lactation may also arise. Some psychological problems, including major symptoms of depression, may take an extreme form during the postpartum period.

Because most mothers are healthy young women, pregnancy and childbirth can be happy, productive experiences; this is the view that the psychotherapeutic methods seek to emphasize.

Psychophysical Practices in Preparation for Childbirth

The two most widely used practices having clearly defined procedures in preparation for childbirth, without formal hypnosis, are *natural childbirth* and *psychoprophylaxis*. It is quite likely that common use of these methods, particularly Read's method, prepared the obstetrics profession for acceptance of psychological methods and, ultimately, for a more favorable attitude toward hypnosis. Read himself, however, was careful to insist that there was nothing hypnotic about his method. The psychoprophylactic method, at least in its area of origin (Russia), grew out of earlier experiences with hypnosis, so its social history in relation to hypnosis is not the same as in other parts of Europe and in America.

Grantly Dick Read (in later years his name became hyphenated to Dick-Read, and his method became known as the Dick-Read method) believed that something so natural as childbirth should not be painful; he insisted that painless childbirth and natural childbirth were equivalent. He believed that civilization had brought with it the fear of childbirth; fear leads to tension, and tension leads to pain. If fear can be overcome, tension and pain disappear. His later book was entitled *Childbirth without Fear*.

The Read method has three main elements: factual instruction regarding childbirth; physiotherapeutic practices, especially relaxation and breathing exercises; and psychological methods that inspire confidence and carefully incorporate suggestion (but avoid hypnosis). Late in Read's life, in a chapter that appeared posthumously, he was somewhat more tolerant of hypnosis.

Read noted early that some of his patients appeared to be in a trance from the beginning of labor to the end; he attributed this to extreme relaxation rather than to hypnosis, despite the fact that they were both anesthetic and amnesic for the events of the delivery. Others, such as Kroger, readily detected the similarities to hypnosis. A principle of comparison of methods should be stated as a caution, however: *merely because two methods overlap in their psychological consequences does not mean that they are identical*. The methods may be alike in many respects and still differ in important ways. For example, it is quite possible that the Read exercises can be taught satisfactorily to women who, in a strict sense, are not hypnotizable, even if more hypnotizable women achieve a state indistinguishable from hypnosis.

Several large-scale studies have been made of the effectiveness of the Read method. Although too much reliance should not be placed on the exact figures, the reports indicate that about one-fourth to one-third of the prepared mothers required no chemical analgesic or anesthetic for the control of pain; these figures are higher than those for women who were unprepared. Prepared women who required analgesics commonly used less than unprepared women, seldom exceeding 100 milligrams of demerol. The comments of those conducting the studies indicate that they do not regard the elimination of pain as the only purpose of the preparation. They prefer to use as little chemoanesthesia as possible for the benefit of the infant. Thoms, an advocate of the Read method along with "rooming-in," stated that pain reduction was not primary: "Our interest is rather directed toward assuring the woman a psychologically and emotionally satisfying labor experience, and at the same time making it physically safe for both mother and child." Those who have investigated the Read method express personal satisfaction with it as well as the satisfaction of the patients for whom the method was used. Although the data do not completely specify the degree of pain relief obtained, they strongly support the conclusion that relief does occur for some fraction of the women prepared by the method.

The method that has largely supplanted the Read method in the United States is known as the Lamaze method, or psychoprophylaxis. Its history as an outgrowth of hypnosis is worth recounting. Ferdinand Lamaze, a French obstetrician, visited Russia and brought the method back with him to France in the 1950s. By becoming a vigorous spokesman for the method and successfully promoting it in France, England, and the United States, he has given his name to it.

In Russia, an earlier hypnosuggestive method was promoted by the psychiatrist Platonov, director of the School of Psychotherapy in Kharkov. Platonov was interested in the problems of pain, and saw the pains of childbirth as a useful area of study. As a psychotherapist, however, he saw other possible advantages of the hypnotic method, such as a more satisfying mother-baby relationship. He met opposition as he undertook his work in 1923; at first he restricted his efforts to women doctors and medical students who agreed to try his methods. The early procedures, known as hypnosuggestive, caught on strongly after 1936. By that year, Platonov could report 588 cases treated by him and his associates with about 60 percent success. Not all the successful cases were painless, however; other factors were included in evaluation, such as completion of the parturition in generally better condition, with fewer pathological somatic or psychological reactions. The next few years saw a culmination of the use of hypnosis: "hypnotariums" were established in large cities such as Leningrad and Kiev for the delivery of babies by the hypnosuggestive method. There are no precise figures on the numbers thus delivered, but one study indicates that 8000 case reports were published.

The new method, psychoprophylaxis, grew out of the favorable experience with the hypnosuggestive method. It was originated by Velvovski and was officially sanctioned by the Ministry of Health of the Soviet Union in 1951, in a publication called *Temporary Directions on the Practice of the Psychoprophylaxis of the Pains of Childbirth*.

As adopted by Lamaze and his followers, psychoprophylaxis tends to be objective and specific in its teachings, although there is a strong component of suggestion throughout the sessions. Teaching includes what happens in the course of a normal pregnancy; the Pavlovian thesis of relieving pain by eliminating fear; respiratory exercises; neuromuscular control through relaxation; and the appropriate responses during labor and delivery. An important aspect of the process is participation of the expectant mother throughout. The training commonly includes the father, who becomes a participant also.

A careful test of the effectiveness of psychoprophylaxis as practiced in France was conducted by Chertok and his associates. The total study involved more than 200 women, but complete data were obtained throughout pregnancy and confinement for 90 of these prepared by psychoprophylaxis and for 26 unprepared women who constituted a control group. On the basis of a score derived for the "goodness" of the confinement, 49 percent of the prepared women achieved a "good" confinement, as compared with 27 percent of the unprepared group. The prepared women also reported somewhat less pain. Unfortunately, we lack any measure of hypnotic responsiveness within the group; as a result it has not been determined whether those who profit from psychoprophylaxis are the same ones who also can profit from hypnosis.

Although the practitioners of both natural childbirth and psychoprophylaxis admit a component of suggestion in their methods, proponents of each emphasize the differences between the two methods, and even more emphatically their separation and difference from hypnosis. The emphatic distinction from hypnosis may result in part from an antiquated or stereotyped picture of hypnotic practices. Contemporary practitioners of hypnosis do not place much emphasis upon formal induction procedures, and they recognize how much responsibility the subject takes in producing the effects called for. Features in common between the nonhypnotic methods and the hypnotic ones include relaxation, controlled breathing, and reassurances regarding the subject's ability to manage the stresses to be experienced.

One advantage of hypnosis over both the Read and Lamaze methods is its greater flexibility. This may surprise those who think of hypnotists as bound to certain standard induction procedures, but in fact those trained in hypnosis are accustomed to dealing with anxiety, sleeplessness, nausea, and other such problems, besides the problems of childbirth. Because the hypnotic operator has been trained for a wider scope of problem situations, he tends to be more flexible than the individual trained in the routines recommended by Read or Lamaze. The hypnotic operator may incorporate any or all of the techniques used in "natural childbirth" and "psychoprophylaxis" and may develop techniques of his own appropriate to his abilities and to the characteristics of his practice.

Hypnotic Practices

Because they recognized the analgesic effects of hypnosis in surgery, early mesmerists and hypnotists extended its use to childbirth. Through the years, numerous accounts appeared of its use in many parts of the world, but such reports were intermittent until this century. In recent years the literature has increased, in part because the World Wars familiarized so many physicians with hypnosis. This increase has been evident in Germany and Russia as well as in other parts of Europe and in North and South America.

An obstetrician who wishes to use hypnosis in his practice must make a number of choices: when to begin the hypnotic training of his patients; whether to train them individually or in groups; whether to do the hypnosis himself or to have someone else do it for him; and how to divide his attention between early pregnancy, labor and delivery, and the postpartum period. These choices are usually made by personal preference and local customs. Perhaps a useful way to begin is to describe some techniques used by practicing obstetricians.

Group methods are more practical for the obstetrician than for other practitioners because of the greater uniformity in the course of the events with which he deals. Pregnant young women face similar problems in looking forward to their confinement; these common problems and expectations make group methods feasible. The patient whose cancer is suddenly diagnosed and the accident victim have no such affiliation in advance with others whose problems are similar. For the obstetrician, group methods can both conserve his time and utilize the mutual support generated by the patients who share a common experience. Husbands may be included in these sessions, so that they can better understand what their wives are experiencing and can later participate at the time of labor and delivery.

The initial session may consist of a reassuring talk, followed by a group induction of superficial hypnosis. Those women who, for any reason, are uneasy about participating may remain as onlookers; their uneasiness about hypnosis may lessen as they observe the behavior of others and listen to their comments afterward. A later session familiarizes the patients with further induction techniques and permits them to experience a broader range of hypnotic phenomena. It is generally considered undesirable to start these sessions too early; ordinarily, a time in the last two months of pregnancy is judged to be early enough, because anticipation and motivation are then at their greatest. The training sessions emphasize that the purpose of the preparation is not solely to reduce pain, but rather to make the birth a rewarding, participative experience.

When the time comes for the birth process itself, those prepared by experience with hypnosis may themselves initiate procedures they have learned, or they may respond to suggestions given by the obstetrician or by an experienced hypnotist collaborating with him.

The following case, that of Louise, illustrates how much a hypnotically experienced young woman can do for herself. She had found that she could control her pain through hypnosis when she served as a subject in the ischemic pain experiment ongoing in our laboratory. At her request, the investigator in that experiment (Lenox) helped her to learn autohypnosis and self-suggested analgesia in training sessions once a week for two months prior to her confinement. She used counting as a means to find herself in a relaxed hypnotic state; she then concentrated on the idea that any pain would be perceived as a light tingling sensation, "as when your arm has fallen asleep and come to, just a little." This technique had worked for her in the laboratory, and she felt she could use the same method at the termination of her pregnancy.

We had known about this first delivery, in which she used self-hypnosis with an obstetrician who was inexperienced in hypnotic methods. Later, in seeking her permission to describe her experience, we found that she had had a second baby with the aid of hypnosis—this time in another part of the country, again with an obstetrician unfamiliar with hypnosis, and with no hypnotist standing by.

The first pregnancy was very difficult, lasting more than ten months before the delivery of a 11 1/2-pound baby; the labor itself lasted an exhausting thirty-six hours. Self-hypnosis reduced the pain to "light tingling" as expected; she was aware of the contractions, but they were not troublesome. After twelve hours, however, fatigue made concentration on self-hypnosis too difficult. As her attention drifted, she felt occasional pains at first, and then felt pain more regularly. Just before the birth, the obstetrician felt she should be given a caudal analgesic; Louise reported, however, that she had some sensation left even after seven caudal injections. The birth was extremely difficult, and a good deal of surgical repair was subsequently required. During the two hours of this surgery, she had recovered enough to use hypnosis and felt that it improved her comfort. The postpartum period was relaxed and uneventful.

The second pregnancy, two years later, was shorter (nine months), and the labor was shorter also (eight hours); all went quite smoothly despite the 10 1/2-pound baby. Louise had no contact with her earlier hypnotist, but began to practice self-hypnosis again when about six and one-half months pregnant. She practiced irregularly at first, but daily in the last two weeks before confinement. "It also helped me rest and sleep better during those two weeks."

When she arrived at the hospital, her contractions were coming at two-minute intervals; she continued to feel pain while she was inducing hypnosis. As she attained a state sufficiently deep, the sensations turned to the familiar tingling, and as she went deeper all feeling disappeared. "When the doctor asked me questions and I had to come up more, I felt some tingling again. During the last two or three hours of labor I didn't feel even tingling. I *knew* I had contractions because I could feel a little tug or pressure, but nothing hurt."

After the baby's head had already appeared, the doctor gave a saddle block as a precautionary measure because of the history of the first delivery. "It was a bother to me. I didn't need it. I was still under perfect control because I was not tired when the baby was delivered. The saddle block didn't have time to take effect before the baby came. . . ."

As soon as the baby was born Louise felt fine, full of energy. A few hours later she had no discomfort at all with the episiotomy stitches, not even the usual trouble of sitting down on them. "I told myself I would not feel pain in that area; if I were about to sit down on my episiotomy, I went *click* in my mind to cut anything out."

Louise chose to use hypnosis during labor and delivery because of her satisfactory experience with it in the laboratory; she came to the hospital in a similar frame of mind to those who have been prepared by hypnosis specifically for childbirth.

Those familiar with hypnotic control of pain in one context will find that familiar methods recur in other contexts as well. Because there are always some slight differences, we shall risk repeating ourselves by reporting methods used in obstetrics that are similar to those already reported in the treatment of cancer. Obstetric pains are located in specified regions of the body, rather than in the diverse areas found with cancer pain; this makes possible a greater uniformity of practices, although the individuality of the expectant mother must always be recognized. We shall discuss eight characteristics of hypnotic procedures useful in relieving pains connected with childbirth.

1. Training rehearsals for actual labor are extensively employed. This practice, somewhat similar to that used in the Read and Lamaze methods, reduces the anxiety produced by facing an unknown and potentially frightening experience. Because the sequence of events is foreseeable, the obstetrician can give orderly information about what is going to take place. The rehearsals may be given greater reality by being carried out under hypnosis. Cheek and LeCron carry out the hallucination of the actual experience by asking the patient to project forward to the time of the delivery and to signal when she hears the baby cry. This is the happy climax toward which all effort is directed. They also point out that if ambivalence toward the expected baby exists, this pseudo-future orientation may uncover that fact and enable the patient to begin dealing with it.

2. Relaxation is an element in most hypnotic procedures, including induction of hypnosis, deepening of the hypnotic involvement, and combating the tension that may build up during confinement. In an early study of the use of hypnosis in advance of labor, Abramson and Heron hypnotized each of 100 women individually, with emphasis upon relaxation, so that labor could be faced with a calm, detached attitude. They made no serious attempt to induce analgesia; their measure of success was reduction of the time in labor. Their findings suggested that both the first and second phases of labor

were shortened for the 100 prepared women as compared with a control group of 78 women.

The exact influence of various components of training is hard to assess. In a study of 136 first pregnancies and deliveries—30 prepared by hypnosis, 51 prepared by relaxation without hypnosis, and 55 unprepared controls—Furneaux and Chapple found some shortening of labor by the hypnotized women, particularly for the first phase. Based on questionnaire responses, the hypnosis group found the labor less unpleasant than the unprepared control group, whereas the relaxed group found it more unpleasant than the controls. It appears that something about hypnotic relaxation interacted with the effects of relaxation alone to produce a more favorable outcome.

3. Without at first completely ridding the patient of pain, it may be possible to *substitute* a minor symptom for the pain. The secondary symptom is felt in the same location where the pain was originally felt. Louise, for example, successfully substituted a "light tingling" for the pain of her contractions.

4. Another possibility is to *displace* the symptom to another part of the body. For example, the rhythmic contractions felt in the abdomen can be displaced to rhythmic contractions felt elsewhere in the body. August suggests that the patient clasp her hands and tighten them with each contraction. Attention is gradually shifted from the painful abdominal contractions to the painless ones in the hands. A later suggestion that the patient need pay no attention at all to the contractions helps to complete the displacement of all feeling to the hands.

5. *Direct suggestion* of symptom relief may be satisfactory in some instances. Louise told herself she would not experience pain in the area of her episiotomy when she sat down; this direct self-suggestion was successful. Direct suggestion of symptom removal is also used by Cheek and LeCron when they tell the patient she can be "numb from the waist down." Hartland gives the reassuring suggestion that the contractions will not be painful, no matter how heavy or frequent they may be. The only sensations experienced will be a certain amount of discomfort and pressure. Hartland reports that, as a result of such suggestion, many patients remain calm, quiet, and relaxed throughout labor. He also indicates that an episiotomy can be performed painlessly after these direct suggestions.

6. *Indirect suggestions* of pain relief are used in obstetrics as in cancer. Kroger teaches the glove anesthesia method to the patient before the onset of labor. After anesthesia is produced in the hand by stroking and the suggestion of numbness, the patient practices transfer of the numbness from the palm of the hand to other areas—first to the face, and subsequently to the abdomen. When labor begins, the patient has learned the skills necessary to

reduce the discomfort of the contractions. Contractions are felt subjectively as a tenseness of the abdomen; the bearing-down sensations are felt as slight perineal pressure.

7. The practice of *imaginative separation* from the present scene can be used in obstetrics as well as with cancer. August recommends utilization of fantasies that reinstate or elaborate upon pleasant experiences from the past. Because the duration of labor is extended, he recommends fantasies of events taking place over time—such as a trip by car across the country—rather than of a fleeting scene, such as watching a sunset over the ocean. The type of scenario that the patient can create is almost unlimited, provided it is something in which the patient has earlier been involved: a trip to the seashore, hiking, fishing, gardening, singing, and playing the piano are just a few possibilities.

8. *Posthypnotic suggestions* can be given at any stage. They are intended to reduce postoperative pain and discomfort, to make the whole experience satisfying, and to provide a positive and confident attitude carrying into the postpartum period.

Notwithstanding the many possibilities for extensive preparation just described, hypnotic procedures can be used in delivery with patients who have received no previous instruction in hypnosis. Good results have been reported, with a minimum of professional time required. Schibly and Aaronson, for example, reported the use of hypnotic methods on a routine basis in the deliveries of seventy-eight out of ninety-three residents in a home for unwed mothers. The patients had no preparation prior to the onset of labor. The investigators felt that the results were quite good and that the method could be recommended to others. To satisfy themselves that the analgesia was complete, in seven cases they performed and repaired the episiotomy with no chemical analgesia whatever. This number did not reflect the maximum that might have been done in this way, for they routinely used an anesthetic for the episiotomy except in the few cases done to satisfy their curiosity about the hypnoanalgesia.

Most practitioners who use hypnosis in the course of delivery find it congenial to inject a local anesthetic for the episiotomy. Such an anesthetic cannot cause any damage to the child, and it relieves the obstetrician of the need to determine just how anesthetic the patient is.

Even after repair under a local anesthetic, an episiotomy may be painful, as any repaired tissue in a sensitive area is likely to be. Women prepared for it by hypnosis tend to find this pain or discomfort lessened, as in the case of Louise.

Lactation is another problem of the early postpartum period for mothers who wish to nurse their babies. There is anecdotal evidence that hypnotically prepared patients may be influenced by suggestion to lactate more promptly. It is known that tension may inhibit lactation via the pituitary gland. The relaxation afforded the prepared patient may thus result in the prompter flow of milk. Another beneficial result of hypnosis said to occur in the postpartum period is a good relationship among father, mother, and newborn, resulting from a happy participative relationship in the birth experience.

Benefit to the baby was shown in a study by Moya and James comparing newborn infants delivered under hypnosis to newborn infants from mothers given varying amounts of analgesics or local anesthetics. Careful study of the acid-base balance during the first hour of life showed that the hypnosis group of babies had a significantly greater ability to recover from the asphyxia of birth than the nonhypnosis infants.

Successes with Hypnotic Analgesia

Evidence that hypnosis is successful in reducing pain and in otherwise making childbirth a more satisfying experience for the mother comes both from individual cases and from a few statistical studies which indicate the range of usefulness of the method. After another illustrative case, we shall turn to the statistical studies that yield kinds of information individual cases cannot.

It may be noted that successful caesarean sections performed with the aid of hypnosis but without chemoanalgesia are among the more convincing as to the effectiveness of hypnosis. Some illustrations will be given in the chapter on surgery, because, so far as the problems of pain are concerned, the caesarean section is essentially a surgical procedure.

Although as scientific evidence individual reports may not be as important as controlled studies, they do furnish insight into the quality of the experience for the person whose experience it is. Here is another illustration of a patient who was highly motivated because it was her own choice to try hypnosis. The case is reported by Crasilneck and Hall:

> A 32-year-old physician who had had two previous pregnancies asked if we would use hypnosis during her third pregnancy. Her obstetrician was in agreement, as her first two pregnancies were marked by prolonged labor of about eighteen hours accompanied by much distress and pain. She responded well to hypnosis and was seen once a week during her pregnancy. Her labor started at 9:00 A.M. and hypnosis was induced immediately. Three hours later she delivered a normal 7 1/2-pound male child. Some of her recorded comments were "I feel relaxed—no tensions, no fears, no anxieties . . . I know the pain perception should be pretty rough at this point . . . but I am comfortable . . . very comfortable . . . just a dull pain . . . like having a period and

yet I normally have a low pain tolerance . . . I should be perceiving pain but I'm not . . . I almost feel like a 3+ drunk, relaxed, lethargic, but my brain is functioning so clearly, only a tight band about my abdomen occasionally . . . I just don't give a damn!"

She did not require nor was she given any anesthetic other than hypnosis during labor and the repair of the episiotomy. Her final comment was "No one could ask for an experience in which the pain was so intense during my first two deliveries and yet completely blocked this time."

Although the statistical studies of the obstetric use of hypnosis suffice to establish its effectiveness for a number of women, they are all unsatisfactory on two counts. First, most such studies lack any precise information regarding the hypnotizability of successful and unsuccessful patients; as a result, it is not known whether any preliminary screening would improve efficiency in the use of the method. Second, the studies commonly lack any satisfactory index of the pain felt. Because of an unwarranted hesitation to use subjective estimates of pain, investigators have sought such "objective" measures as reduction in the amount of chemoanalgesia or chemoanesthesia required. On the presumption that those suffering the most pain would demand the most relief, a correlation can be expected between the amount of medication required and the pain felt. This correlation is of course imperfect, not only because the response to analgesics is not uniform, but also because the response to the patient's requests depends upon the physician and the nurses. In this clinical setting, the usual "double-blind" procedures are inappropriate; as a result, it is difficult to know how much the dosage depends on the patient and how much on those in control.

Of course, some self-selection of patients is bound to occur when an obstetrician is known to use hypnosis in his practice. Hence a general percentage of success must not be taken as a population figure, but only as an indication that for a substantial number of women such successful deliveries are possible. August, some of whose methods have been mentioned, reported on 1000 consecutive deliveries for which he was responsible. Of these, 850 were done with hypnotic analgesia and 150 without. Major anesthetics and analgesics were available to patients who requested them. Of the 850 cases in the hypnotic analgesia group, 58 percent required no medication whatever, 38 percent used only analgesics such as demerol, and only 4 percent (36 of the 850) requested either a local or a general anesthetic.

Because of the unreliability of such "objective" methods of measuring success as the duration of labor or the amount of analgesics or anesthetics required, other researchers have turned to the patient's own estimate of the amount of pain felt. A study from Russia when the hypnosuggestive method was fully acceptable, reported by Katchan and Belozerski in 1940, gives rather good evidence on 501 cases. The two clinicians were more interested in discovering which method was suitable for which woman than in making a case for the effectiveness of the hypnotic method in general. According to their own statement, their prediction of favorable or unfavorable outcome of their treatment was wrong in 61 percent of the cases. Their general conclusion was that complete analgesia was obtained in 29 percent of the cases, partial analgesia in 38 percent, doubtful results in 12 percent, and failure in 21 percent. The complete and partial analgesia successes represented positive results with 67 percent of the group studied.

In a 1962 study of 210 pregnant women, Davidson included a careful estimate of their felt pain. The women were divided into three groups of 70 each on the basis of preparation: first, a control group receiving no training; second, a group taught autohypnosis in preparation for labor; and third, a group taught relaxation by exercises and controlled breathing—the Read method. By assigning numerical values to the four levels of pain reported by Davidson—0 for "no pain," 1 for "slight pain," 2 for "moderate pain," 3 for "severe pain"—we have been able to compute a mean for each of her groups. In the first stage of labor, the mean for the control group was 1.95, moderate pain. Those prepared by physiotherapy reported their pain as 1.58—below that of the control group—but the autohypnosis group was lowest of all at .83. In the second stage, when all pains were reported as more severe, the control and physiotherapy groups were practically alike (at 2.56 and 2.67), close to the upper limit of the scale; the autohypnosis group, with a mean of 1.43, was still near the scale value for slight pain. Davidson concluded that the time spent antenatally in hypnotic preparation (averaging about 1 1/2 hours per patient) was certainly worthwhile for the benefit produced. The hypnotic preparation appeared more successful in the relief of pain than the Read method, which showed no advantage over the control group at the time pain was most severe.

Another study, by Rock, Shipley, and Campbell, was done with a non-volunteer group of twenty-two subjects who had no training in preparation for labor and were in active labor when hypnosis was first attempted. The hypnosis was commonly carried out in the patient's own bed in a noisy environment; the only privacy was that afforded by cloth partitions that could be used to separate the bed from its neighbors. The conditions, so far from ideal, show that hypnosis can still be effective even in adverse circumstances. The time the practitioner spent in inducing hypnosis was only twenty minutes; the total time added by the hypnotic procedures was estimated at only forty-five minutes beyond that devoted to control patients not receiving any hypnosis. Those patients who were hypnotized rated the labor and delivery as less painful than the nonhypnotized controls by a significant amount. In a study of this kind, one would like to have additional controls—such as someone spending the same amount of time in nonhypnotic reassurance with the patient. Such a control is provided in part by the nonhypnotizable patients, for whom the hypnotic procedures serve essentially as if nonhypnotic. The fact that sixteen of twenty-two, or 73 percent of the total group, gave good reports of their labor and delivery indicates that some of those low in hypnotic responsiveness must have found the treatment helpful. To give proof of the role of hypnosis, added controls would be necessary; as they stand, the results of the study suggest a practical effectiveness.

The ideal study of hypnosis in childbirth would combine the features of studies we have discussed, along with one measure that is lacking in nearly all those in the literature: a measure of hypnotic responsiveness. For some purposes the practicing clinician does not need such a measure. Hypnotizability may not be essential because those who are not hypnotizable can profit from the relaxation, just as many profit from physiotherapeutic or psychoprophylactic preparation. It would be well to have the question answered, however, for some patients fail to profit from the nonhypnotic preparation methods also, and they may be the ones who are the least responsive to hypnotic procedures. In the study by Rock, Shipley, and Campbell just discussed, an effort was indeed made to measure the hypnotic responsiveness of each subject. A few simple tests were made, so their results could be related to the satisfaction expressed by the patient with her labor and delivery. The four tests were eye closure, heavy hand, hand levitation, and glove anesthesia; each was scored as $-$, $\pm$, or $+$. By assigning values of 0, 0.5, and 1 to each of these and then adding them, the hypnotic responsiveness of each of the twenty-two subjects can be assigned a numerical value between 0 and 4.0. We have computed such values for the hypnotized patients. Of the twelve who scored above 2.5 on the responsiveness scale, the labor and delivery were rated as "good" by ten, or 83 percent; of the ten whose responsiveness was below 2.5, six, or 60 percent, rated their experience as "good." In such a small sample this difference is not statistically important, but it is in the expected direction. It is worth noting that all five patients whose scores were above 3.5 rated the labor and delivery as "good."

Conclusions Regarding Hypnosis in Childbirth

The evidence is clear that for many women hypnotic preparation can provide for a comfortable, participative labor and delivery. The mother is aware of what is going on and can assist in the birth process with a minimum of pain. The outcome appears to be good for the mother and the newborn infant, not to mention for the father, if he has shared in it all. The exact proportion of women who can benefit cannot be specified, but of those who wish to have their babies with the help of hypnosis, a substantial fraction are likely to be successful.

The large percentage of patients who, with hypnotic preparation, require little or no medication indicates that the approach holds benefits even for those who are little hypnotizable by ordinary standards. This may perhaps be explained in the same way as the successes also achieved by supposedly nonhypnotic methods such as natural childbirth and psychoprophylaxis. When hypnosis is used, the less hypnotizable probably reap the benefits that all can achieve from relaxation and fear reduction, while the more hypnotizable receive the further benefits of hypnotic analgesia. These conclusions are partly conjectural, however, because the least well established relationship is that between successful prepared childbirth and measured hypnotic susceptibility.

Notes

The matter of childbirth pain in primitive cultures has been discussed by Freedman and Ferguson (1950). An excellent history of the use of hypnosis in obstetrics can be found in the book by Chertok (1959); this source also gives the background of the nonhypnotic methods for reducing pain in childbirth and relates them to hypnosis. The bibliography of 587 titles includes many citations to the Russian literature not available in English. Another useful review, citing 116 references (with little duplication of those in Chertok) is by Hoffman and Kopenhaver (1961).

The reference to Queen Victoria's anesthesia for childbirth is from Hingson and Hellman (1956), as cited by Chong (1963).

Psychophysical Practices in Preparation for Childbirth

The Read method of "natural childbirth" or "childbirth without fear" is described in his books, Read (1933; 1944—second edition, 1953). There was a background for natural childbirth in progressive relaxation (Jacobson, 1929), but Jacobson (1954; 1965) was critical of the techniques that Read recommended. A later indication that Read adopted a more tolerant attitude toward hypnosis was in a posthumous publication (Read, 1962). Some studies of the Read method are: Roberts and others (1953), based on 1043 prepared deliveries compared with 3000 unprepared ones; Thoms and Karlovsky (1954), reporting on 2000 cases, but more specifically on 968 whose use of analgesics and anesthetics during delivery was carefully recorded; and de Soldenhof (1956), based on 1000 prepared cases. Thoms' comment is from Thoms (1950).

Others have assigned a greater place to suggestion in Read's method than he cared to give: for example, Kroger (1953); Mandy and others (1952).

The history of the Lamaze method as an outgrowth of the Russian developments is well given in Chertok (1959; 1973). The Russian source available in English is Velvovski and others (1960). The figure of 8000 case reports is found there. Lamaze and Vellay (1957) have a book in English on their methods. In America a popularization of the method by Bing (1969) has had a following.

A third method, besides those of Read and Lamaze, is that of autogenic training. This derivative from the German experience with hypnosis in the 1920s was practiced over many years, and for many purposes, by Schultz; since his death, it is being carried on by Luthe (as an example, see Schultz and Luthe, 1969). In his wide travels, reviewing the work of thirty clinics using psychophysiological preparation for childbirth in Europe and the United States, Buxton (1962) included visits to Germany where autogenic training was being used in obstetrics (see, for example, Prill, 1956). Buxton's book is a useful summary of the practices of 1960. Although he credited hypnosis with lending techniques to the nonhypnotic methods, he was evidently unfamiliar with modern hypnosis, for he believed that the hypnotized woman was not aware of what was going on in her labor and delivery.

The shift from hypnosuggestive methods to psychoprophylaxis took place gradually in Russia; hypnosis continued to be used for the more difficult cases. The official sanction of psychoprophylaxis began with a report issued by the Ministry of Health (1951). Later, at a congress in Kiev in 1956, the word "pain" was dropped from the name of the method; the expectation of painlessness had apparently led to too much frustration on the part of the prepared women.

The large-scale study of psychoprophylaxis carried out in a Paris hospital by Chertok and his associates is reported in Chertok (1973). An opportunity arose to relate the success of psychoprophylaxis to suggestibility by at least one measure that was taken (the body-sway test); unfortunately, the money ran out and that part of the analysis was never completed.

Hypnotic Practices

For fuller accounts of hypnotic practices as developed by the various authors cited, see the books by August (1961); Cheek and LeCron (1968); Hartland (1971); and Kroger (1962; 1963).

The comparison of length of labor following preparation by hypnosis to its length without such preparation was reported by Abramson and Heron (1950). The other study mentioned in this connection is that of Furneaux and Chapple (1964).

The study of routine deliveries with the aid of hypnosis in a home for unwed mothers was reported by Schibly and Aaronson (1966).

August, among others, believes that lactation may be facilitated by the suggestions of the hypnotist near the termination of delivery.

The study indicating more rapid recovery from birth asphyxia for babies delivered by hypnosis was done by Moya and James (1960). James (1960) points out that the more powerful drugs not only depress the baby but prolong labor. The seriousness of the effects of local and regional anesthesia during labor upon the newborn infant is brought out in a recent study of sixty firstborn infants three days after birth by Standley and others (1974). Their paper also provides a review of the pertinent literature.

We have not undertaken to deal critically with the many ancillary problems associated with difficult pregnancies and labors, although there is a considerable literature which makes claims for the helpfulness of hypnosis. For example, there are reports of the hypnotic control of premature labor and the resulting threat of abortion, by Hartmann and Rawlins (1960); Logan (1963); and Schwartz (1963). The opposite effect, inducing labor when the time is appropriate, has also been reported (Rice, 1961). Some hypnotic practitioners believe the benefit of hypnosis to be greatest for "high risk" women who, for medical or psychological reasons, are most likely to have trouble. Ordinary healthy and well-adjusted young women, for whom hypnosis is somewhat inconvenient, might as well be handled by ordinary hospital routine; they believe it is the "high risk" patients who particularly need the benefits hypnosis can provide (Cheek and LeCron, 1968).

Successes With Hypnotic Analgesia

The patient whose satisfaction with hypnosis is described was reported by Crasilneck and Hall (1973). The study of 1000 consecutive deliveries was reported by August (1961). We have felt no obligation to assemble all the studies that have been made; most show rather similar results, but are not necessarily representative of the population of all pregnant women. One quite substantial study by Gross and Posner (1973) compared the results of 200 cases delivered by the same obstetrician before he became interested in hypnosis with 200 subsequent cases in which he routinely used hypnosis. The later cases were essentially unselected—except that they may have been partially self-selected in coming to an obstetrician known to use hypnosis. He rejected only 5 percent of the later 200 consecutive cases, because of a history of emotional instability or because of personal or religious objections to hypnosis. The hypnotic group used analgesics less frequently both in the first stage of labor and in the postpartum period; a comparison for the delivery period would be inappropriate because anesthetics had been used routinely in the control group. However, 62 percent of the hypnotic group received no chemoanesthesia during delivery. The authors report great "morale" benefits in the hypnotic group.

The Russian study is that of Katchan and Belozerki (1940), reported in the Russian language, and available to us only through the account given by Chertok (1959, pp. 42–45).

Davidson's (1962) dissertation is well designed and well presented. Although it showed psychophysiological preparation by the Read method to be partially successful in the first stage of labor, the hypnotic methods were successful in both stages. Too much point should not be made of these relative advantages, especially because the obstetrician conducted the hypnosis training sessions, whereas other therapists and midwives in the hospital conducted the nonhypnotic ones. We wish we knew something about the hypnotic potentialities of those successful by either method! The Rock, Shipley, and Campbell (1969) study appeals to us because measures of both hypnotic responsiveness and pain were included, but the study does not contain sufficient cases to make results statistically significant, however plausible they may be.

7   Surgery

For most people, an operation is in the realm of the unknown and is associated with anxiety and tension. Numerous fears are connected with anesthesia and surgery: fears of suffocation, of not awakening, of mutilation, and of what organ damage or disease may be found during surgery. In addition there is the stress of separation from the familiar home and family members, and substitution of a strange environment with many new procedures. It goes without saying that many patients are suffering from some degree of pain prior to surgery, and that they anticipate pain after the operation is over.

The modern hospital staff is aware of the patient's psychological reactions as well as his physical needs. It is good hospital practice for the anesthesiologist to visit the patient the night before the operation to foster greater rapport and reassurance. Surgeons, too, attempt to explain more to their patients than was formerly the case. There is, of course, much reliance upon sedative and analgesic drugs to relieve anxiety and tension prior to the major anesthetic to be used in the surgery.

How might hypnosis be useful in the surgical setting? The answer is that it presents a broad spectrum of possibilities for relief in surgical patients. It has been utilized before, during, and after surgery.

1. Preoperatively, hypnosis may help to overcome apprehension and anxiety about the anticipated anesthesia and surgery. In addition to minimizing these negative attitudes, it can frequently help to induce a calm, quiet state of mind. Sometimes hypnotic analgesia can aid in control of the pain at this stage.

2. Operatively, hypnosis may produce analgesia and anesthesia, thus reducing or replacing chemical anesthetic agents.

3. Postoperatively, hypnosis may afford a more comfortable transition from the operative phase to convalescence. Posthypnotic suggestions can help raise the pain threshold so there may be less need for postoperative narcotics. Such suggestions may help reduce nausea and vomiting or stimulate more adequate breathing and coughing. In addition, hypnosis can aid in producing better morale.

A further beneficial aspect of hypnosis is that its contribution to the relief of pain is combined with the relief of anxiety. When hypnosis is used primarily as an anesthetic during the operative period, the patient usually receives reassurances in regard to his state of mind, in addition to the major effect of analgesia.

We have already noted (in Chapter 1) that for a brief time a century ago, hypnosis demonstrated its effectiveness as an anesthetic in surgery. At that time, the medical profession as a whole looked askance; when chemical inhalants were introduced, the use of hypnosis in surgery died out. This does not mean that it was not employed again in the intervening years, for many case records of successful hypnoanesthesia are scattered through the literature. Our own interest, however, is in current practices, so we shall emphasize the reports of the last twenty years. They give an encouraging picture of the place hypnosis has earned for itself in surgical services.

Hypnotic Procedures and Practices with the Surgical Patient

Hypnosis can be used in the preoperative period, within the operation itself, and as an aid to postoperative recovery. These three phases form a whole, so good morale during the preoperative period may make the operation itself go more smoothly and may persist in the postoperative period. Hence, even as we discuss what the hypnotist does in each phase individually, we shall respect the fact that each phase influences that to follow.

A more relaxed state of mind in the preoperative phase affects both the operative and postoperative phases; during surgery and recovery the patient is apt to remain more settled in mind and better able to cooperate. Prior to the administration of anesthesia, many therapists use specific posthypnotic suggestions to the effect that comfort and well-being will occur after awakening.

Once hypnosis has been used to control preoperative anxiety, it is likely to be invoked to control further anxiety in the operating room and during the postoperative period. This is, of course, a natural development. For some patients, such repetition is necessary to counteract the constant buildup of anxiety. Further, once a method is successful, it is wiser to chance overuse than to underestimate the need for reiteration.

When hypnosis is begun during the preoperative phase, the familiar practices of hypnotic induction may be used. Anesthetists and surgeons who use hypnosis agree that they prefer such advance preparation when circumstances permit. If the patient comes to the hospital several days in advance, as in some cases of heart surgery, brief hypnotic sessions can be given daily. When hypnosis is to be used during the operation, a unique feature of the patient's preparation is the *rehearsal technique*, in which the operation is carried out in pantomime, and everything is explained to the patient. In the following specimen conversation given by Kroger, the patient is hypnotized and positioned in a bed as if on the operating table.

"Now your skin is being sterilized." (At this time the abdomen is swabbed with an alcohol sponge.) "I am now stretching the skin and making the incision in the skin." (The line of incision is lightly stroked with a pencil.) "Now the tissues are being cut. Just relax. You feel nothing, absolutely nothing. Your breathing is getting slower, deeper, and more regular. Each side of the incision is being separated by an instrument." (The skin and muscles are pulled laterally from the midline.) "Now a blood vessel is being clamped." (A hemostat is clicked shut.). . . .

Some hypnotists carry the rehearsal so far as to have the patient hallucinate a date of recovery and readiness to return home.

It should be noted that when hypnosis is used as the major anesthetic for surgery, the patient is not unconscious; hence the same description of what is happening that was used in the rehearsal is given to the patient again during the operation itself. Cheek recommends that this information be given the patient during the operation even when general chemical anesthesia is employed; for, as we shall see, there is some uncertainty about how much conversation is processed in some manner by the anesthetized person.

Children are more hypnotizable than adults, so they are particularly good candidates for preoperative hypnosis, whether or not chemical anesthetics are also to be used. Marmer found a workable method for preparing children for ether anesthesia in tonsillectomy. Prior to induction, he ascertained the child's interests, likes, and dislikes. Most children liked to watch television; some preferred to watch movies or sports. At the time he was writing about his cases, one program many enjoyed was "Lassie," an episodic drama featuring a heroic collie dog. A child would be asked to close his eyes and then to imagine he was viewing a television screen, watching the program. The program might be suggested: "Lassie is walking up the hill with Jeff. It is a quiet, peaceful day and Lassie is feeling very good, but she is getting a little tired and sleepy. Now Lassie is lying down in a very comfortable position, and she has closed her eyes. She likes the calm, peaceful feeling it gives her. Notice how tired Lassie is, how very drowsy she is. She is beginning to feel sleepy. She is so drowsy that she is falling asleep. Lassie is going to take a nice long nap and she is going to remain asleep until she is awakened. Lassie is breathing deeper and deeper and falling fast asleep." The child would respond to the indirect suggestion by becoming relaxed and hypnotically responsive. At this point a posthypnotic suggestion could be given about well-being and comfort, as well as about being able to swallow readily when the operation was over.

This preparatory stage merges gradually into the inhalation of ether. When the ether is started, the anesthetist continues: "Lassie is fast asleep and is breathing very deeply. Now a wind is blowing across her face, and she is breathing in and out more deeply. This is a strong wind and carries with it a funny but pleasant odor, the odor of a strong wind. Deeper and deeper breathing. In deeply and out deeply. Fast asleep, fast, fast, asleep." At the termination of the operation, posthypnotic suggestions of well-being and comfort are again repeated. Marmer adds an amusing and instructive incident about a 7-year-old girl, the first on whom he used hypnosis. When she was still asleep two hours after the operation, he recalled that he had said Lassie would not awaken until told to. He said, "Lassie just woke up; she opened her eyes, took a deep breath, and ran away." At that point the patient woke up.

Reactions to anesthesia produced in this manner are said to be quieter and more peaceful. The child is more responsive and cooperative during the procedure, and recalls the experience afterward as a satisfying one.

Practices vary widely. Some have found that, with children, hypnosis can eliminate preanesthetic medication, or at least reduce its dosage enough to prevent any untoward effect on respiration. Different methods may be used with children of different ages. Betcher in describing his methods, recommends that with all children there should be a get-acquainted period so that the child's preconceptions and fears can be understood. As an induction technique for children from 3 to 8 years, he recommends "pretending," on the grounds that the child at this age enters the world of make-believe so easily. "See that rabbit over there? He's so tired. Show him how to close your eyes and go to sleep." For children, 9 to 14, the technique involves television viewing, similar to that described by Marmer. For a child of 14, the induction can be essentially that used with adults. Although he used hypnotic procedures in conjunction with general chemical anesthetics, Betcher indicated that needs for both preoperative and postoperative sedatives had been reduced.

Children are especially likely to feel helpless and frightened when in the hospital. They are separated from their familiar surroundings for perhaps the first time, and do not know what to expect. Such children, even as young as 3 or 4 years, can be aided by hypnosis. Children who have sustained accidental injuries may be in a state of excitement in addition to their apprehension over the coming surgery; they, too, may be helped by hypnosis.

The following accounts of individual patients indicate some special preoperative problems that can be met with the help of hypnosis.

A 42-year-old woman admitted for a thyroidectomy because of an exophthalmic goiter was extremely apprehensive and greatly upset from fear that she would die during the operation. Marmer had several brief hypnotic sessions with her in the hospital that day; she was able to reach a deep level of hypnosis. Posthypnotic suggestions resulted in a very marked reduction in anxiety and in restful sleep that night without medication. The next morning the patient was still calm. She was again hypnotized before being taken to the operating room. With a combination of hypnosis and chemical anesthesia, the one and one-half hour operation was completed smoothly. Posthypnotic suggestions were given that the patient would have no distress; that she would feel comfortable; that she would swallow easily; and that food and drink would be retained. Upon request, the patient herself removed the endotracheal tube through which she had been breathing artificially; she awakened immediately. Her postoperative course was uneventful.

Another of Marmer's patients, about to have her gall bladder removed (cholecystectomy), was convinced that her heart would stop, that she would not be able to get her breath, and that she was going to die. The more excited she became, the more she felt that this was already beginning to occur. Marmer listened, gained her confidence, and explained more about the hospital, the surgery, and the anesthesia. All of this helped somewhat, but she did not really calm down until he listened to her breathing with his stethoscope and began suggesting that she would breathe more deeply, easily, and gently, and that she would relax completely and feel more confident, secure, and drowsy. Soon her pulse rate decreased from 140 to 80 per minute.

On the morning of surgery, suggestions were again used to control symptoms of impending panic. The cholecystectomy was performed successfully and, with further posthypnotic suggestions given after surgery was completed, the patient had an uneventful postoperative course.

One of Betcher's patients, a 56-year-old man who had entered the hospital for repair of a hernia, was agitated and extremely apprehensive. On the night before the operation he expressed fears that he would be unable to withstand the procedure and would die. Physical examination showed no organic abnormality other than the hernia. Through hypnosis, it was possible to induce such a calm, relaxed state in this patient that he required no sedation that night nor preoperatively the next morning. At the time of the operation, hypnosis was induced and a spinal anesthesia administered. During the procedure the patient, conscious but not in pain, closed his eyes and remained completely relaxed. The patient was given posthypnotic suggestions for comfort, and no analgesic agents were necessary postoperatively.

For hypnotic analgesia to work effectively during the surgical procedure itself, it is not enough to have the patient hypnotized when the operation begins. Maintenance of the hypnotic response while surgery is in process must be optimal, especially if hypnoanesthesia is the major anesthetic. The principal recommendation is that relaxing instructions, reassurances, and informative statements about what is happening should continue throughout the operation. There is little reason to be apprehensive about a hypnotizable patient suddenly becoming aroused; if a temporary lapse occurs, the hypnotist can assist or the patient can restore hypnosis for himself. The patient is free to request some chemoanalgesic supplement. In any case, he is not likely to turn from no pain to excruciating pain because of a spontaneous loss of hypnotic control. Some hypnotists prefer to keep in communication by having the patient give finger signals when circumstances prevent him from talking. He can easily raise one finger to reply "yes" to an inquiry, and another finger to reply "no." The question of how much the patient hears at the deep planes of chemical anesthesia is unsettled, but it is a wise caution to say in the patient's presence only things that would be helpful for him to hear. Posthypnotic suggestions favoring a restoration of normal functioning and feelings of well-being may be given while the surgery is still in progress.

Most of the cases already discussed have indicated that hypnosis used preoperatively or within the surgery itself had aided the postoperative course as well. Patients tend to be more relaxed, to feel less pain, to be generally more cooperative toward procedures necessary for the healing process and for their own feelings of well-being.

Several studies of the recovery phase have reported on many patients, in contrast to the emphasis on fewer specific cases in studies of surgery itself. The reasons for this are not hard to find. In the first place, the postoperative situation is more uniform than the circumstances prior to or during the operation. Surgical patients enter the hospital with or without pain, electively or in emergency, facing operations which differ greatly in seriousness and risk. Quantitative study of the pain and its hypnotic reduction under these circumstances would be unusually difficult because of the many dissimilarities from case to case. This situation changes somewhat following the operation. All patients are likely to be uncomfortable after anesthesia and surgery, whether the surgery is minor or major. The patient's morale and willingness to undertake normal activities can influence his recovery rate. These are the kinds of problems toward which the hypnotist has commonly addressed himself, and on which he can obtain some evidence.

One puzzling problem is distinguishing between the use of suggestion following induction of hypnosis and suggestion without any formal hypnotic procedure. In many situations the issue is not important; as we have seen from laboratory studies, waking suggestion produces results comparable to hypnosis in hypnotically responsive individuals. Although hypnosis adds something to suggestion—especially for the more hypnotizable—many of the benefits of hypnosis can be obtained through suggestion alone when the context is favorable, as it appears to be in the postoperative setting.

Several studies offer immediate reduction of requests for narcotic pain relievers on the first postoperative day as evidence of the benefit of hypnotic suggestions. Although our reservations about the reliability of narcotic intake reduction as scientific evidence hold here as well as in obstetrics (see below), frequent reports of 25 to 45 percent reduction in postoperative chemoanalgesia are not to be ignored.

Much that can be done with the aid of hypnosis can be done without it, provided that the same attitudes are communicated to the patient. A good illustration is furnished by a study by Egbert and his associates, in which ninety-seven patients were divided into two groups, neither of which was treated hypnotically. One group, however, was given special education by the anesthetist about what to expect postoperatively, based on the nature of the surgery. This group was also given encouragement about recovery. The other group lacked this instruction and support. The researchers found that postoperative narcotic requirements were reduced for those who had received the special attention. Such a study indicates that hypnotic suggestions are in the right direction, whether or not they are unique; the study does not, of course, imply that hypnosis does nothing more than can be accomplished by simply reassuring the patient.

Wolfe and Millet made a very large study of the consequences of giving therapeutic suggestions to the patient while still under general chemical anesthesia. The suggestions were given near the time of completion of the operative procedures, usually as subcutaneous tissues were sutured. Interviews with 1500 consecutive unselected patients who underwent anesthesia and were given the suggestions showed that 50 percent were without postoperative discomfort; and another 10 percent developed discomfort only at a site removed from the area of the operation. According to the authors, such a distant or displaced pain does not distress the patient to the same extent as the pain expected from the operation. Since the study lacked a control, however, one must take the authors' word that the degree of discomfort was far less than usually found. The fact that reassurance can be given effectively under deep levels of anesthesia is of interest, however; it is demonstrated also in the next study, by Pearson.

Pearson relied particularly on an earlier discharge from the hospital as evidence of the postoperative role of suggestion. Suggestions were given only when the patient was in a surgical plane of anesthesia—that is, under deep, chemically produced general anesthesia. To the extent that the results of this study are valid, they support the contention that the deeply anesthetized person is more accessible to words spoken in his presence than is ordinarily believed. The investigation was in the form of a double-blind placebo experiment in which the surgeons, anesthetists, and others involved in patient care did not know which tape had been played to the patient through earphones. Each patient in the "suggestion" group received suggestions via the tape on how to handle specific items in the postoperative period. The tape also contained statements, repeated and strongly emphasized, that if the patient would relax and follow the suggestions, faster recovery from the illness would follow. The placebo tapes contained music or were blank. Of eighty-one patients for final evaluation, forty-three received suggestions and thirty-eight received no suggestions.

The results indicated that during the postoperative period, surgeons could not differentiate between patients who had received suggestions and those who had not. There was no difference in the use of narcotics between the two groups, but the patients who had received the suggestions were discharged an average of 2.42 days sooner than the control group. The mean postoperative stay for the suggestion group was 8.6 days; for the no–suggestion group, it was 11 days. The author concluded that there is evidence that patients in a surgical plane of anesthesia can hear and respond to suggestions.

The personal concern of the hypnotic practitioner for the patient has often been cited as one influential factor in overcoming fear of surgery and making convalescence easier. It has been said that the introduction of general anesthetics may in effect have lessened the interest of the surgeon in each patient as a person with problems of his own. By the very nature of his procedures, the practitioner of hypnosis comes to recognize the individuality of the patient. One surgeon, Kolouch, has emphasized in his writings the problems of the frightened surgical patient, the subjective factors in postoperative recovery, and the mistakes that may occur when personality problems of the patient are ignored. His observations, although not translated to statistical comparisons, are based on a large number of patients who have accepted hypnosis as an adjuvant to chemoanalgesia in surgery. In one study, he based his account on 254 patients (116 male and 138 female), who had accepted hypnotic treatment while undergoing 269 surgical procedures. Comparison with patients not receiving hypnosis convinced him that hypnotic treatment was of benefit both subjectively and objectively. The patients receiving hypnosis seemed to need less pain-relieving drugs postoperatively, and their stay in the hospital tended to be shorter.

Kolouch begins his treatment prior to the operation to neutralize any irrational fear of the surgery. One of his patients, a 46-year-old man, had a recurrent inguinal hernia. Returning for treatment four years after an earlier repair, he was very nervous, lacking confidence in surgery and surgeons. He feared the prospect of another anesthetic. The patient was willing to try hypnosis; he proved to be a good subject and entered hypnosis very rapidly. His fear of anesthesia was explored within hypnosis. Regressed to age eight he relived a frightening experience in which, without any prior explanation, an anesthetist and surgeon held him down, put him to sleep with ether, and removed his tonsils. After giving expression to these fears, the patient awakened reassured. While still hypnotized he was given optimistic preoperative suggestions, and developed a realistic image of the forthcoming anesthesia and surgery. A rehearsal of the actual operation was given, so the patient would be fully prepared. He was given suggestions that postoperative discomfort would not bother him; that he would be hungry; that his bowels and bladder would function normally; and that as soon as he felt capable of looking after himself he would leave the hospital. Aroused from hypnosis, the patient felt relaxed, refreshed, and very confident. As soon as the effect of the spinal anesthetic disappeared, he was able to move about and enjoyed a full diet. The patient was very enthusiastic over his experience.

When Hypnosis is the Preferred Method

Hypnosis is not widely used in major surgery today; the convenience of both general and local anesthetics is such that hypnosis is seldom to be recommended as the sole anesthetic. There are times, however, when the use of chemical agents is unwise or is dangerous to the patient. In such instances, hypnosis may be the preferred agent for controlling pain.

One patient who was in very poor condition to use chemoanesthesia was a pregnant woman, two weeks overdue for delivery, described by Winkelstein and Levinson. She presented a case of medical emergency diagnosed as a fulminating preeclampsia—a rapidly accelerating toxic disorder that may lead to convulsions and coma in connection with pregnancy and childbirth. The patient was obese, weighing 287 pounds, with a markedly swollen face, hands, and ankles. She complained of a severe headache, nausea, and vomiting. Her blood pressure, already high at 190/130, had risen rapidly to 230/160 in spite of medication intended to lower it. It was decided that her baby should be delivered by caesarean section. The anesthetist and surgeon agreed, however, that either general or spinal anesthesia would be dangerous. General anesthesia was rejected as presenting too great a threat to the baby. In view of the extreme elevation of the blood pressure, especially with the diastolic pressure at 160, spinal anesthesia was contraindicated because of the possibility of vascular collapse and resulting shock. Since tremor of the hands and legs was already present, local infiltration anesthesia was also considered potentially dangerous, lest the extra stimulation of local injection should precipitate a convulsive seizure. Under these circumstances, hypnoanesthesia seemed to present an opportunity for a safer procedure.

The patient was easily hypnotized. No more than four minutes were spent in induction, and about two minutes more in the development of complete anesthesia. During the operation, suggestions were continued. After the baby was delivered, the patient's blood pressure dropped to 180/120. Hypnoanesthesia continued after delivery, and both uterine and abdominal wounds were repaired with only the inhalation of exceedingly small amounts of nitrous oxide.

Chemical analgesics may be considered dangerous because of pre-existing cardiovascular pulmonary disease. Anderson reported that a 71-year-old patient needed an abdominal exploration because of possible cancer. The presence of advanced emphysema and intractable asthma made an inhalation anesthetic unwise. Hypnosis was an acceptable alternative. For two weeks, the patient was seen daily; he was able to develop deep hypnotic trances, and was given periodic rehearsals of the operative procedures under hypnosis. In the operation he maintained hypnosis during the incision of the skin, fascia, and muscles down to the opening of the peritoneum. With further hypnotic suggestions, the peritoneum was relaxed and the abdominal cavity entered. Exploration revealed a common duct stone, but the antici-pated cancer was not found. During the abdominal exploration, "due to vagal and sympathetic reflexes," the patient partially broke the hypnotic trance; 5 cc of 2 percent thiopental (pentothal) was administered. The patient was given suggestions that he would have no postoperative pain but would instead feel quite comfortable. He complained of no pain after the operation.

Four patients described by Werbel illustrate the use of hypnotic an-algesia for patients considered poor risks for chemical anesthetics. One of these was a 49-year-old woman who needed skin grafting for treatment of a leg ulcer, but who had severe coronary artery disease marked by frequent episodes of cardiac arrest. During the first operation, in which a thick crust covering the wound was excised, hypnosis, demerol, and atropine were used analgesically. Within the second operation, however, hypnosis was the sole anesthetic agent in a procedure lasting one hour. A split thickness graft was removed from the patient's left thigh with a dermatome and sutured over the prepared ulcer bed. The patient, after awakening, had no recollection of the operation. This may be attributed to posthypnotic amnesia rather than to total unconsciousness during the operation. There was no postoperative pain.

Unsuccessful cases utilizing hypnosis as an anesthetic are less likely to be reported. Werbel mentions a situation of this type, however, in which abdominal surgery was attempted under hypnotic anesthesia. Prior to the surgery, the patient had attained hypnotic depth and analgesia which permitted a 1½-inch needle to be plunged into the calf of one leg without any demonstrable evidence of pain. As soon as the skin incision was made for surgery, however, the patient complained of pain and a general anesthetic had to be substituted. Werbel adds, "It is perhaps only fitting that an unsuccessful case be described in this paper so that all may know that, in abdominal surgery, hypnosis used as an anesthetic agent is unsuccessful more frequently than it is successful."

Finer and Nylén reported that hypnosis was the sole preoperative, operative, and postoperative analgesia in a burn case in which there was danger of cardiac arrest. Skin grafts were taken from both lower legs with the electrodermatome and applied to severely burned areas on the hands, arms, and both thighs. The patient, who had received only 30 minutes of advance training in hypnosis, reported no anxiety or pain during or after the operative procedure. Four months later, decubital ulcers were excised and grafting completed on four occasions with hypnosis as the only analgesic agent.

Many patients cannot achieve satisfactory anesthesia through hypnotic suggestion. What is the consequence when such patients are considered poor risks for chemoanesthesia? The answer is that in these cases the amount of the chemical needed may be reduced by hypnosis, so the danger to the patient is less.

Sometimes hypnotic analgesia may be used to avoid repetitive medication with chemoanalgesics. Patients who have been severely burned often require multiple debridements (as preparation for further grafting, removal of tissue that has not properly healed), changing of dressings, and repeated skin grafts. The side benefits of hypnosis may prove advantageous in such situations.

The case of a 30-year-old man with thermal burns covering 45 percent of his body surface was cited by Crasilneck and Jenkins as illustrating the appropriateness of hypnotic treatment. The patient had become increasingly fearful of the frequent anesthetics needed for dressing changes, the painful manipulation of his extremities, and debridements. Because of his fears and complaints, it was decided to substitute hypnoanesthesia. With the aid of hypnosis, bandages could be changed and the areas extensively debrided without any perception of pain prior to, during, or following the procedures. With further surgery under hypnosis, a donor split-thickness skin graft was removed from the patient's leg and placed on the burned areas, which had again undergone extensive debridement in preparation for these grafts. There were no problems during this extensive procedure under hypnosis.

A 10-year-old girl with severe third degree burns of neck, anterior chest, and both upper arms presented several problems, as described by Betcher. Dressings were changed under hypnosis. An operation was necessary to release severe contracture scars of the neck, which had forced the chin onto the sternum with complete inability to extend the neck; hence, insertion of an endotracheal tube was impossible because of the acute angle of head flexion. Consequently, general anesthesia via the endotracheal route was ruled out and hypnosis was substituted. The patient was found to be susceptible and, after a rehearsal, the operation was successfully carried on with the aid of hypnosis until the head had been released sufficiently for some chemical anesthesia to be administered.

Sometimes patients appear for emergency surgery who should not be given chemoanesthesia. A person who has just eaten a substantial meal presents a special problem if general anesthesia is necessary following an accident. One such accident happened to an 11-year-old girl while skating, just after she had eaten a large steak dinner. As reported by Bernstein, she fractured her hand badly, displacing the right radius and fracturing its lower end (known as a Colles fracture). It was unwise to wait the six hours normally required for emptying of the stomach. Furthermore, after an accident food may remain in the stomach longer than normal because of pain or anxiety. The physician induced hypnosis, using relaxation suggestions and an hallucinated TV program; the patient experienced no pain while the repair took place. Recovery was excellent.

A patient who presented an obstetrical emergency illustrates the advantage of having available someone familiar with hypnotic procedures. A woman expecting a baby had been poorly handled on the ward of the hospital. She had been there for hours with an impacted breech before Cucinotta, as the ward consultant, became aware of her. At that time she had a high fever, a systolic blood pressure of over 200, and a heart rate of more than 150 beats per minute. She evidently needed a caesarean operation, but the anesthetist refused to give any general chemoanesthesia, and the operation under local anesthesia was not judged feasible. Hence Cucinotta, who was to do the surgery, determined to use hypnosis. Although he had not seen her before and she was completely naive to hypnosis, he hypnotized her during the ten to fifteen minutes in which he was scrubbing and preparing her abdomen. The record obtained by the anesthetist during the course of the operation showed that the vital signs steadily returned to normal despite the progress of the surgery. A normal infant was delivered, and the mother's recovery was uneventful. The record was later reviewed by a senior obstetrician who described it as remarkable.

Occasionally a patient requests hypnosis on the basis of a prior successful experience. Bowen, for example, had used hypnosis in his practice of psychiatry and had successfully hypnotized himself. When he required a transurethral resection, he insisted on having the operation done under hypnosis alone. He subsequently published a report based on his own experience. In the previous year he had used hypnosis to relieve the pain of a fractured right ankle, and he had no doubt about his ability to use it successfully again. The night before the cystoscopy he put himself into a hypnotic state three times, planting the thought that with the introduction of the cystoscope there would be a warm, gentle sensation rather than any pain. He slept well; the next morning on the operating table he induced the hypnosis and felt only the warm, gentle sensation. Following this success, he had the transurethral resection two days later with self-hypnosis as the only anesthetic. All he felt was the same warm, gentle sensation, with no pain.

A satisfactory experience of childbirth with the help of hypnosis (discussed in Chapter 6) may lead a woman to wish hypnotic analgesia when other surgery is required. Taugher described two cases of women who, after having their babies with the aid of hypnosis, later requested that surgical procedures be done under hypnosis. A 25-year-old woman had a tonsillectomy in which the only drug was atropine sulfate, 0.4 mg; under hypnosis the patient's tonsils were dissected, but all she reported feeling was pressure and pulling. In the second instance, the 26-year-old patient requested hypnosis for a curettage because of her excellent experience during delivery. She received only atropine sulfate, also 0.4 mg. Like the first patient, she reported no pain either during the procedure or afterwards.

This tendency to use self-hypnosis once it has been learned was demonstrated in a group of highly hypnotizable subjects in our laboratory. After a training course which enabled them to participate in experiments, they were questioned later as to any use they had made of the training. It was found that several had adapted it to the relief of headaches, dental pain, and pain in fractures and minor operations.

The variety of cases that come to the attention of the surgeon (and the anesthesiologist) is almost infinite, and in selecting a few examples of special conditions favoring hypnoanalgesia we mean only to suggest the range of possibilities.

Sometimes heightened sensitivity to drugs or allergies to them lead to a recommendation of hypnoanalgesia. Ruiz and Fernandez report a case of a cataract extraction performed under hypnosis. The operation had previously been abandoned because of the patient's sensitivity to all local drugs and to general anesthesia. In the three sessions in advance of the operation, this patient was able to attain anesthesia at superficial and deep levels of hypnosis. The operation involved the corneal incision, iridectomy, and eight sutures. During this time the patient was completely relaxed, showed total loss of sensibility but preserved the oculomotor reflexes. There were no signs of pain, and the patient recalled no pain. The total time involved was 25 minutes.

There are some circumstances in which the surgeon wishes to explore neurological responses without the interfering effects of a chemical anesthetic. Crasilneck and his associates noted a case in which it was desirable to monitor the EEG during a lobectomy in order to determine that the site of epilepsy had been incised. A temporal lobectomy was performed on the 14-year-old epileptic patient under hypnosis and the EEG was monitored without the disturbing effects that would have been produced either by inhalation or intravenous injection. In this case, chemicals were not avoided altogether; procaine was used for the incision in the scalp, and 100 mg of thiopental was injected during the surgery.

Such cases as those just presented, in which hypnosis is preferred when it can be used, provide a sound basis for the judgment that hypnotic analgesia is a technique that should be available, either in an adjunctive capacity or, if necessary, alone.

Hypnotic Suggestion as the Sole Anesthetic

As we have seen, hypnotic procedures are commonly given a place along with chemical agents by those who favor hypnoanalgesia or hypnoanesthesia; hypnosis is not expected to displace chemical anesthetics. At the same time, the demonstration that major surgery, with the patient entirely comfortable, is *possible* under hypnosis overcomes some of the skepticism associated with its ancillary uses. By studying the circumstances in which a highly hypnotizable patient in surgery becomes free of pain through hypnotic suggestion alone, we have a basis for comparison with the laboratory investigations previously reported.

Once a surgeon has used hypnosis repeatedly in his practice he does not report a case in the literature unless it presents unusually interesting features. For that reason published cases cannot be used as a basis for estimating the frequency with which hypnotic analgesia is used. We have, however, listed some of the surgical conditions in which hypnotic suggestion has served in the capacity of sole analgesic or anesthetic, as reported in the past two decades. These are tabulated in Table 2.

Although four of the patients received some nonanalgesic chemical agent (a tranquilizer, a sedative, or a relaxant), no case is included in which there is any doubt that hypnosis or suggestion was alone responsible for the reduction of operative pain. To satisfy any who may think of those drugs as contaminating, those cases in which non-analgesics have been used are noted with an asterisk in the table; the other cases proceeded without reported medication of any kind as part of the preoperative or surgical procedures.

In some instances, the demonstration was made in order to show that it was possible. The caesarean section of Kroger and DeLee falls in this category, as does the breast tumor excision later reported by Kroger. In that case the patient, with whom he had no prior contact, was selected for him; he had the opportunity for a single training session with her before the opera-

Table 2. Some Operations in which Hypnotic Analgesia or Anesthesia or Anesthesia was used with no Chemical Analgesics or Anesthetics, 1955–1974.

Type of Operation	Reference	Type of Operation	Reference
Abdominal Surgery		*Genitourinary continued*	
Appendectomy	Tinterow (1960)		
Caesarean section	Kroger and DeLee (1957)	Vaginal hysterectomy	Tinterow (1960)*
	Taugher (1958)	Circumcision where phimosis present	Chong (1964)
	Tinterow (1960)*		
Gastrostomy	Bonilla, Quigley, and Bowers (1961)	Prostate resection	Schwarcz (1965)
		Transurethral resection	Bowen (1973)
Breast Surgery		Oophorectomy	Bartlett (1971)
Mammaplasty	Mason (1955)		
Breast tumor excision	Kroger (1963)	*Hemorrhoidectomy*	Tinterow (1960)*
Breast tissue excision	Van Dyke (1970)	*Nerve Restoration*	
Burns		Facial nerve repair	Crasilneck and Jenkins (1958)
Skin grafting, debridement, etc.	Crasilneck, McCranie, and Jenkins (1956)	*Thyroidectomy*	Kroger (1959)
	Tinterow (1960)		Chong (1964)
	Finer and Nylen (1961)		Patton (1969)
Cardiac Surgery	Marmer (1959a)	*Venous Surgery*	
	Tinterow (1960)	Ligation and stripping	Tinterow (1960)
Cataract Excision	Ruiz and Fernandez (1960)	*Miscellaneous*	
		Removal of tack from child's nose	Bernstein (1965b)
Fractures and Dislocations	Goldie (1956)	Repair of lacerated chin in child	Bernstein (1965b)
	Bernstein (1965)		
Genitourinary		Removal of fat mass from arm	Scott (1973)
Cervical radium implantation	Crasilneck and Jenkins (1958)		
Curettage for endometritis	Taugher (1958)		

*Some nonanalgesic medication used during preoperative or surgical procedures.

tion was telecast at the annual meeting of the New York State Society of Anesthesiologists in 1956.

Hypnosis and Chemical Anesthesia

Because chemical analgesia and anesthesia and their hypnotic counterpart serve some of the same purposes, confusing issues arise over their relative advantages and disadvantages.

Current practice with regard to chemical agents dictates that the anesthesiologist visit the patient prior to final decision with respect to the drugs and anesthetics to be used. The chemical agents used will vary with the patient's previous condition, current use of pharmacological agents, and his preferences. Ordinarily some premedication is given, so the patient comes to the operating room awake but drowsy, with little anxiety, and prepared to cooperate. Quite apart from specifically hypnotic procedures, sole reliance need not be placed on medication to produce the desired effect. An investigation of premedication with and without a preoperative visit by the anesthetist by Egbert and his associates showed that the drug (pentobarbitol) alone, although it increased drowsiness, did not reduce "nervousness" or anxiety as much as the visit alone. In fact, apart from drowsiness, the visit alone was about as satisfactory as the visit plus the drug, according to the anesthetists' judgment of adequate sedation at the time the patient entered the operating room.

For readers who are unfamiliar with the terminology used in anesthesia and analgesia, a short digression may be in order. *General anesthesia* denotes a loss of consciousness in addition to loss of sensation; a *local anesthetic* produces a regional loss of sensation without loss of consciousness. *Analgesia* refers to a loss of pain, without reference to the loss of other sensations. General anesthesia can be induced by the *inhalation* of anesthetic vapors such as nitrous oxide, ether, cyclopropane, or halothane, or by the intravenous *injection* of thiopental (trade name Pentothal), with appropriate supplementation. Thiopental, like other barbiturates, is not an analgesic, and therefore must be supplemented by inhalation or by spinal anesthesia. A *spinal anesthetic* involves the injection of a normally local anesthetic into the spine.

Local chemical anesthetics are in wide use; they are familiar to most people through their use in the dentist's office. They are usually given by injection. The most familiar is probably procaine (under the trade name of Novocain), which is administered subcutaneously. The main characteristic of a local anesthetic, of which there are many others, is that it makes a particular region of the body anesthetic without causing loss of consciousness or loss of sensitivity in other regions.

Anesthesiologists administer drugs within surgery for purposes other than pain reduction. Some promote muscle relaxation; some reduce secretory activity in the respiratory and alimentary tracts. Hence, although hypnosis may be the only anesthetic used in a surgical procedure, some nonanalgesic drug may occasionally be used, as noted in Table 2.

When the hypnotist speaks of using hypnosis as a substitute for a general anesthetic, he does not intend to imply that the patient would be unconscious. One difference between a general chemical anesthetic and hypnosis is that no matter how "asleep" the patient is under hypnosis, he is not unconscious; he is always able to respond to the hypnotist. The only sense in which the anesthesia is "general" is that the whole body may be without sensitivity. In some respects the "general" anesthesia of hypnosis is more like a widespread local anesthetic: sensitivity can be preserved where desired, as in proprioceptive sensations that are available to the patient when he responds with finger signals to the hypnotist's questions. The use of the metaphor of sleep by hypnotists has led to some misunderstanding about the degree to which the hypnotized person—who may not suffer at all from surgical pain—retains responsiveness in other respects.

Although by definition the patient has not reached a surgical plane under a general anesthetic unless he is unconscious, the question as to when he is fully unconscious under chemical anesthesia is not readily answered. The anesthesiologist has tests for various planes of anesthesia, but these are in terms of reflex responses, such as eyelid, eyeball, or pupillary responses; the decrease of respiratory movement; or the disappearance of muscle tone. Naturally, a person whose breathing is no longer under his control is in no condition to reply verbally to a question, even if he can hear it. However, a patient paralyzed by anesthetics, though unresponsive, may not be unconscious at all. For instance, it is well known that nitrous oxide, when used as a general anesthetic with relaxants, may permit the patient to recall the conversations of the surgical team. Hearing what is said may be amusing or frightening to the patient—depending, no doubt, on the content of the conversation.

As pointed out earlier (page 127), there are some indications that even in a deep plane of surgical anesthesia, the patient may respond to suggestions affecting his postoperative recovery. Hypnosis has proved to be a useful method in facilitating the recall of things said by the surgeon or anesthetist under deep anesthesia.

In one of the more carefully controlled studies, Levinson arranged an experiment that could be carried out in the operating room. Anesthesia was induced by a combination of chemical agents, including pentothal, flaxidil, ether, nitrous oxide, and oxygen. The patient's EEG was monitored to indicate that the anesthesia was profound. At a signal, the anesthetist stopped everything, saying audibly that the patient's lips were too blue, and that he was going to give more oxygen. He then pumped the rebreathing bag and said that everything was now all right and that the operation should proceed.

Each of ten patients, known to be hypnotizable, had an operation in which the above scene was enacted. When interviewed a month later, the patient remembered nothing of the operation in the normal waking state. He was then hypnotized and told to relive the operation. The kind of report obtained may be illustrated by a verbatim report from one of the patients. During the hypnotic recall session, the hypnotized subject was told to raise one finger when the operation was starting, and to signal later if anyone was talking. When talking was first indicated, the following conversation occurred:

"Who is it, who's talking?"

"Dr. Viljoen. He's saying my color is gray."

"Yes?"

"He's going to give me some oxygen."

"What are his words?"

"He said I will be all right now."

"Yes?"

"They're going to start again now. I can feel him bending close to me."

The experiment was not uniformly successful, but four of the ten subjects were able to repeat words spoken by the anesthetist. Four others became anxious about reliving of the operation and woke from hypnosis. Two reported that they had heard nothing.

Whether or not the recall could have been produced by methods other than hypnosis is not the issue; it is the fact of recall of a conversation within deep anesthesia itself that is significant. Cheek, who has repeatedly called attention to the possibility of such recall, tells of a patient anesthetized with sodium pentothal followed by fluothane and nitrous oxide. The operation was a vaginal hysterectomy, and Cheek had assured the patient that there would not be excessive bleeding. In hypnotic recall of the operation afterward, she reported her agitation at hearing a second doctor remark, "the blood is ready." Cheek's main point is that surgeons should be very careful about what is said in the presence of an anesthetized patient.

The relation of this matter to hypnotic anesthesia is twofold. First, from a theoretical standpoint, the difference between general chemical anesthesia and hypnotic anesthesia may not be so great as at first supposed. Second, from a practical point of view, the hypnotist's habit of continuing to make comforting and reassuring remarks within the surgery itself receives further justification.

Just as drugs are often used in combination, so hypnosis may be combined with drugs, as several of the previous cases have shown. Although hypnosis alone might in many cases be substituted for chemical agents, it is usually reassuring to the patient to know that chemicals are available and that the surgeon or anesthetist has no objection to their use if he requests them.

The severity of the surgical operation to be performed naturally affects the amount of pain reduction required; this will be reflected also in the degree of success when hypnotic analgesia is used. An informative study was made some years ago in a casualty hospital in London. All the cases in one month were treated without hypnosis. In the following month, the same routines were followed and the same anesthetics and analgesics were available, but hypnotic suggestions were routinely added in all cases. The procedures which took place included incisions, removal of foreign bodies, suturing, nail avulsions, and orthopedic reduction of fractures and dislocations. In all instances the proportion of patients completing the procedure without anesthetics was higher in the hypnosis group; the results were not of critical significance, however, except for the orthopedic patients. Only five of twenty-seven in the group without hypnosis had their fractures or dislocations reduced without anesthetics, whereas twenty-six of thirty-eight in the group with hypnosis had theirs reduced without any chemical agents. Many of the patients in the orthopedic group were children, one as young as 3 1/2. The high hypnotic susceptibility of children may account for the large proportion of success with hypnosis in this procedure. The very young child referred to had a dislocated shoulder. She entered hypnosis readily to dream of playing her favorite game with a friend. Within 5 minutes she was in a deep, relaxed hypnotic sleep. She groaned once as the bones were realigned, but awakened smiling after the plaster had been applied. She told her parents she had had a nice dream, and had no memory of the procedures.

There are various estimates as to the proportion of patients who could tolerate major surgery under hypnosis without any chemical assistance. Kroger's figure of 10 percent seems to be about the maximum that has been claimed. Wallace and Coppolino suggested that "our percentage of success in the complete substitution for chemoanesthesia has been less than the previously quoted 10 percent. . . . 10 percent is an oft-repeated but unsubstantiated quantity, and the true percentage of successful cases is much below that figure." Marmer, who had said earlier that only about 10 percent can reach a level deep enough for performance of a surgical procedure without chemical agents, added in 1963, "Few of us would guarantee to produce surgical hypnoanesthesia in one in a hundred unselected cases." He remarked that surgery under hypnoanesthesia is difficult for two reasons: first, it is hard to produce and maintain hypnoanesthesia; second, it is difficult to attain sufficient muscular relaxation. "The muscular relaxation of hypnosis cannot be compared with the profound deep muscular relaxation produced by chemical muscle relaxants in order to meet the demands of the surgeon during a prolonged intraabdominal procedure." Marmer noted that most operations performed under total hypnoanesthesia have been those which do not require extensive or deep muscular relaxation, such as operations on the breast, thyroid, and heart. Even in caesarean section, nature had provided a nine-month period for total stretching of the abdomen. He felt that it would be almost impossible under hypnosis to attempt removal of a spleen, repair of a perforated viscus, or an abdominal perineal resection. "It would require an extremely rare patient and an unusual hypnotist to accomplish this."

Hypnosis is known as a valuable resource for relaxation, so its rejection on the basis of insufficient relaxation may seem surprising. Marmer's conviction that the relaxation produced by hypnosis is not enough for most abdominal surgery could very well be overlooked. If he is correct, however, the necessity for an extraordinary degree of continuous deep muscular relaxation, difficult to achieve through hypnosis, represents a limitation on the use of hypnosis in surgery. This consideration should not limit use of hypnotic procedures in cases in which pain reduction is more important than the achievement of deep muscle relaxation.

One of Marmer's cases illustrates the adjunctive use of hypnosis with only a minimal amount of chemoanesthesia. A 39-year-old woman, hospitalized for a mitral commissurotomy,* had experienced several episodes of cerebral emboli during the previous year, with recovery. She was an excellent hypnotic subject; after two sessions in advance of surgery, she was able to produce anesthesia of the chest wall. On the morning of surgery she was taken to the operating room, in the hypnotic state in response to a posthypnotic suggestion. Hypnosis was deepened by way of a prearranged signal, and 100 mg of thiamylal sodium—a rapid, short-acting barbiturate similar to thiopental—was injected intravenously. The vocal cords were sprayed with 5 percent hexylcaine topical solution (a surface anesthesia to prevent possible laryngeal spasm) so an endotracheal tube could be put into place for the administration of oxygen. Throughout the procedure 100 percent oxygen was given. To insure that the patient would remain quiet during the first valve fracture, she was given intravenously 30 mg of succinylcholine, a muscle relaxant given to make the operative field quieter. The patient was able to open her eyes on command after each of the three attempts at valvular fracture. At the end of the two-hour operation, she was given posthypnotic suggestions with regard to comfort, relaxation, and the ability to breathe deeply and cough adequately. When asked to awaken, she responded immediately. She made an uneventful recovery, requiring no narcotic drugs postoperatively.

---

* This is a sectioning of the fibrous ring surrounding the mitral oriface in the heart for the relief of mitral valve stricture.

In an abdominal exploration with the patient under hypnosis, Anderson reported that after successful incision of the skin, fascia, muscles, and peritoneum under hypnosis, the patient's trance was partially broken, so thiopental had to be given intramuscularly. Thus the problem was presumably not insufficient analgesia for cutting of skin and peritoneum, but maintenance of the hypnotic state over time.

There is no great mystery why mild doses of analgesic drugs make hypnotic analgesia available to more people. Because mildly hypnotizable people far outnumber the very hypnotizable, and because pain reduction through hypnosis is correlated with hypnotizability, chemical assistance helps the less hypnotizable to gain the full advantages of hypnosis. Such chemical analgesia need be given only at the more critical times. For a person who is relaxed and confident throughout an operation, the occasions of severe pain are not very frequent; if he can be helped over these stumbling blocks, the rest of the course is easier. Pain can be expected when the skin is incised; when the peritoneum is incised; and when there is pulling and torsion of the abdominal organs. Suturing of the peritoneum and of the skin are further occasions for pain. But much of an operation is essentially painless, even if the patient is only slightly responsive to hypnoanesthesia. Some of the chemical aids which may be administered have effects unrelated to pain, such as producing a relaxed area where deep relaxation is needed. These statements are not meant to minimize the importance of hypnotic pain reduction for those who can achieve it. No one doubts the pain of dermabrasion of the face, of burns, or of setting compound fractures, all of which can be completely controlled by hypnosis for some patients.

Concluding Remarks on Hypnosis in Surgery

Anesthesiologists and surgeons have demonstrated that for some highly hypnotizable people, hypnosis can be the sole anesthetic for major operations. Under certain conditions, and for some patients, it is the method of choice. The extra benefits beyond pain reduction—composure, confidence, and cooperativeness—extend the usefulness of hypnosis to many patients of moderate hypnotic responsiveness who lack the ability to reduce pain completely.

Further investigations along the lines suggested below should help to answer some of the puzzling questions that remain.

1. The relationship of individual differences in susceptibility and the motivations of the patient facing surgery to the success of hypnotic analgesia has never been satisfactorily determined. We need answers to two questions: For whom should major surgery be attempted with hypnosis alone, as an elective procedure? For whom, when hypno-

anesthesia is the method of choice, is its use alone likely to prove dependable? In the many cases in which hypnosis can readily be supplemented by chemicals as necessary, this issue is not a crucial one for the practitioner.

2. Can more efficient techniques be developed to save the time of busy professional people? Although hypnotic training through tapes and the teaching of self-hypnosis have saved time in other contexts, these methods are probably less applicable to surgery, where the problems often arise without much advance warning. In any case, there is so much advantage in personal contact between the patient and the surgeon or anesthesiologist that the necessary time is probably well spent.

3. The whole surgical team—including the member interested in hypnosis—should perhaps devote more attention to the postoperative phase, rather than relying solely on posthypnotic suggestions given in the preoperative or operative phases. During the preoperative phase the patient has immediate worries and concerns—his present pains, and anxiety over the forthcoming operation. As a result he may not be ready to listen to suggestions for postoperative comfort. Similarly, during the operation his concern is with the present. After the operation, fresh hypnotic reassurance can be added to whatever has been given in the way of posthypnotic suggestions. By directing the patient's attention to optimistically undertaking the activities of normal life, the hypnotist can improve morale, aid in planning, and make a difference in the rate of recovery.

Whether used frequently or only occasionally, hypnosis has much to contribute to the surgical team. Both surgeon and anesthesiologist would do well to be familiar with it; they need not be experienced in hypnosis themselves to obtain the assistance of someone qualified to help.

Notes

Chapters on the use of hypnosis in surgery appear in the major books on the clinical uses of hypnosis, such as those of Cheek and LeCron (1968); Kroger (1963); and Schneck (1963). There are closely related books on hypnosis in anesthesiology, such as Coppolino (1965); Lassner (1964); and Marmer (1959c).

Kroger's rehearsal technique in preparation for surgery utilizing hypnosis, used successfully by others as well, is described on p. 187 in his book. The quotation is taken from that source. Hallucinating the date of recovery is recommended by Cheek and LeCron, p. 164. The danger of careless conversation while the patient is thought to be unconscious was noted by Cheek (1964).

Marmer's work is repeatedly cited in the pages of this chapter. The sources used are Marmer (1959a; 1959b; 1959c; 1961; 1963; 1969). As an anesthesiologist he has responsibility for deciding, in collaboration with the surgeon, when hypnosis is to be recommended.

Betcher's work with children is reported in Betcher (1958). The usefulness of hypnosis in correcting the fears of children as they approach surgery has been noted by, among others, Daniels (1962) and Hoffman (1959), who discusses the 3- or 4-year old children.

The studies of the effects of suggestions on the recovery phase are those of Wolfe and Millet (1960), Pearson (1961), and Kolouch (1962; 1964; 1968).

Reduced postoperative use of pain relievers has frequently been reported following hypnotic preparation. Specimen studies are those of Laux (1953), who reported a 34 percent reduction in narcotics on the first postoperative day for forty urologic patients; Papermaster and others (1940), who arrived at a figure of 43 percent reduction in narcotics for thirty-three patients recovering from various operations; and Bonilla, Quigley, and Bowers (1960), whose nine patients undergoing knee surgery in a military hospital required 25 percent less demerol than the forty previous patients who had undergone the same operation without the help of hypnosis.

The study conducted by the Harvard group of anesthesiologists headed by Egbert, showing the importance for postoperative recovery of direct reassurances without hypnosis, is Egbert and others (1964).

When Hypnosis is the Preferred Method

The pregnant woman in poor condition for her caesarean was reported by Winkelstein and Levinson (1959). The abdominal exploration done with hypnosis because of cardiovascular problems was described by Anderson (1957). Additional poor risks were described by Werbel (1967). The burn patient presenting danger of cardiac arrest was reported by Finer and Nylén (1961). Additional, similar experiences were reported by Finer (1967). Further burn cases mentioned in the chapter are those described by Bernstein (1965a); Crasilneck and Jenkins (1958); and Betcher (1960).

Schafer (1975) has reported on 20 cases in a burn unit. The success in pain reduction was clearly related to degree of hypnotizability. Of the 11 of 20 who achieved a clinical rating of 4 or 5 (high) on the Orne and O'Connell (1967) diagnostic rating scale, all but one showed substantial pain reduction through hypnosis; of the four who rated 1 or 2 (low) none was helped. The others fell between.

The girl who came for emergency treatment on a full stomach after a skating accident is described by Bernstein (1965b). The emergency obstetrics case of Salvatore Cucinotta is unpublished; it is here recounted with his permission. The obstetrician who reviewed the patient's records was George Hoffman, who kindly called the case to our attention.

The self-report on a transurethral resection is by Bowen (1973).

The women who requested their surgical procedures—one a tonsillectomy, the other a curettage—without chemoanalgesia because of their success with hypnosis in childbirth, were presented by Taugher (1958).

The cataract extraction under hypnosis because of unfavorable sensitivities to chemical agents was reported by Ruiz and Fernandez (1960).

The exploration for the site of epilepsy was reported by Crasilneck, McCranie, and Jenkins (1956), and Crasilneck and Hall (1973).

Hypnotic Suggestion as the Sole Anesthetic

The references to the studies summarized in Table 2 are all given in the table; the descriptions of individual patients are from the same sources.

Hypnosis and Chemical Anesthesia

The recommendation that the anesthesiologist visit the patient before the final decision with respect to the anesthetics is standard in modern textbooks, such as Dripps, Eckenhoff, and Vandam (1967). The study of the importance of a preoperative visit by the anesthetist is by Egbert and others (1963).

The matter of an awareness on the part of the deeply anesthetized patient that may, in some instances, be recovered later has been reported by Levinson (1967), and in a series of papers by Cheek (1959; 1964; 1966).

The study in the casualty hospital was done by Goldie (1956). Caution is required in interpreting a study of this kind because the general reassurances of the physician-hypnotist, coupled with a strong invitation to use less pain-killer, could account for many of the differences found. The difference with the orthopedic children was statistically significant. In the language of statistics, the difference was significant at the .001 level.

The uncertain estimates of those who could have major surgery done under hypnosis begin with the 10 percent given by Kroger (1957) and cited approvingly by Marmer (1961), but later rejected as too high by both Wallace and Coppolino (1960) and Marmer (1963), whose quote is from that source, p. 118.

Maintaining hypnosis over time was noted as a problem by Anderson (1957). The successful use of hypnosis in dermabrasion is illustrated by Ecker (1959).

8 Dentistry

Many dentists became familiar with hypnosis during World War II, and after the war a number of them joined together to further their interest in hypnotic practices. War casualties frequently appeared with damage to the oral cavity that had to be repaired near the front, where chemical anesthetics might not be available. Hypnosis was sometimes the answer.

In a prisoner-of-war camp near Singapore in 1945, conditions were primitive and very little anesthesia was available. Surgical procedures were attempted with the aid of hypnosis in twenty-nine cases, of whom twenty proved to be capable of deep hypnosis, and four of superficial hypnosis. Three were insusceptible, and the other two were treated by suggestion alone without any attempt at producing a hypnotic condition. Dental extractions were performed on twenty-three of these patients, including many multiple extractions. On being aroused from hypnosis, the patient commonly expressed surprise at finding himself in the operating theater. He refused to believe that a tooth had been extracted until he located a gap in his teeth with his tongue. Postoperative pain was reported by only two of the patients.

The effort by dentists to use less painful methods in treating patients has a long and continuous history, not only in hypnosis but in chemical anesthesia as well. The first reported case of a tooth extracted under hypnotic anesthesia was given by Oudet in 1837. In 1842, ether was used for the extraction of a tooth. Dentists were among the first to use nitrous oxide ("laughing gas") in their practice, beginning in 1844.

The modern dentist thinks of his task as including more than the standard procedures associated with dentistry, such as filling cavities, straightening teeth, extracting, and constructing dentures. He prefers to think of his task as emphasizing the treatment of *people* who have dental problems; when he uses hypnosis, it is often in this larger context.

Hypnotic Relief of Pain and Anxiety

Fear, tension, apprehensiveness, hostility—these are some common attitudes of patients toward dentistry. Anxiety may be free-floating and general—with or without avoidance of specific objects and experiences—or it may be channeled into symptom formation, as in dental phobias or pronounced gagging that interferes with the course of treatment.

Are sedatives the answer? Sedation can be accomplished chemically, but chemicals cannot re-educate the patient to enable him to respond more positively to dental treatment. Unlike major surgery of other kinds, dental treatment can be expected to recur again and again; thus negative reactions may be cumulative if not counteracted. An increasing number of cases have been recorded to show that this process of re-education can be facilitated by hypnosis, so that dental anxiety is markedly lessened.

Dentists have used two major methods to reduce patient anxiety through hypnosis. The first method treats anxiety directly and symptomatically, relying largely on relaxation and reassurance during hypnosis; results with this method are often quite satisfactory. In the second method, the dentist is aware of the psychological nature of the problem, which may be rooted in the past. He may be tempted to use psychiatric methods for uncovering anxieties, but it is not considered appropriate for him to step outside the dental role for which he has been trained.

Severe dental anxieties and phobias commonly arise from one of two sources. One cause may be previous unpleasant experiences with dentists, often dating from childhood, that have produced a kind of conditioned aversion. The second common source is a vicarious experience transmitted empathically from a significant person who, at some earlier time, excitedly and fearfully related an unpleasant experience with a dentist—again, usually during the patient's childhood years. Such a patient's anxieties and fears may actually enhance his pain once dental procedures begin. Hypnosis functions to prepare the patient for his dental treatment, in part by separating the present from the past.

Two cases may be used to illustrate these methods of dealing with anxiety prior to dental procedures. The first case used reassurance; the second involved some uncovering through age regression.

In the first case, reported by Golan, a 29-year-old woman came to the dentist trembling and sweating profusely. She had not seen a dentist for nine years and was "frightened to death." She had an acute alveolar abscess in one of her few remaining teeth, and obviously required treatment. The dentist obtained a brief case history which assured him that chemical anesthetics would not be contraindicated. He then carried out a brief hypnotic session. Many of the overt signs of her anxiety disappeared promptly with hypnotic relaxation, and this was called to her attention. Next it was explained that whatever happened in the past to frighten her had occurred many years ago, and that she need no longer have any of these reflex actions based on what belonged to another time. By explaining psychosomatic processes, the dentist enlisted the patient as part of the healing process; he pointed out that she was able to do something for herself in this situation. The trance was terminated with a posthypnotic suggestion that whatever was done would be accompanied by a minimum of discomfort. X-rays were taken without emotional incident. Hypnosis was again induced and the patient was given a novocaine block; reassurances were continued, with suggestions that the procedure would be efficient, that healing would go well, and that she could practice relaxation at home. The initial treatment went uneventfully, and the patient returned for the additional sessions required, each time with simple hypnotic induction procedures that took little time. Although the possible roots of anxiety in the past were mentioned, no effort was made to explore the past under hypnosis; the treatment consisted essentially of relaxation and reassurance.

In the second case, the dentist went somewhat further in his probing than usual. A girl of 18, treated by Stolzenberg, needed a statement that her teeth were in satisfactory condition as part of a college entrance requirement. Her teeth were in obviously poor condition, yet she would not permit even a routine examination of her mouth with mirror and explorer. She eventually agreed to hypnosis, entered a satisfactory hypnotic condition, and was age-regressed to determine the origin of her dental phobia. As a young child the patient had been sitting at the dinner table when her sister had returned from the dentist, crying hysterically and relating how the dentist had cut her mouth with a drill. The patient was instructed to recall the incident out of hypnosis, in order that the dentist could discuss it with her. He pointed out that the sister's trouble was very temporary; she had, in fact, returned a number of times to the same dentist without complaint. In this way he prepared the patient to face the present situation. Acceptance of the explanation reduced the patient's fears so she found no difficulty in going on with her treatment.

In the first case described, hypnotic reassurance was continued within the dental procedure, even though a local anesthetic was given to reduce the pain. Hypnosis continued to calm the anxious patient and raise her pain threshold. There is no clear demarcation between the preprocedure phase and the procedure phase of hypnotic treatment. Because it is during the dental procedure itself that sensory pain must be controlled, a special discussion of hypnosis specific to pain control will follow later. Here we wish to emphasize the role of anxiety generated by earlier expectations of what is going to happen. We find that when dental procedures begin, hypnosis continues to be a valuable ally even though the pain itself may have been dulled by chemicals.

A 5-year-old girl, reported upon by Kroll, had a double intraventricular septal defect of the heart and severe pulmonary hypertension. Although she was referred for dental work under general anesthesia, she was not a good candidate for it. She came to the dentist violently resistant to medical or dental treatment—an ill and frightened child. In her first session, various hypnotic techniques were used to gain her cooperation while a series of X-rays were taken. All this was, of course, painless, and her attitude was greatly improved by the time she came for her next appointment. During the second visit a light trance was induced and she "watched" her favorite television program while the examination took place. The restorative treatment itself began on the third visit. The patient was premedicated with meperidine as the more seriously involved teeth were treated, and occasionally received chemical anesthesia by infiltration and block. By combining hypnotic and chemical treatment over a six-month period, some teeth were saved that would have been sacrificed had everything been done at once under a general anesthetic. The patient's response to hypnosis was variable, and use of alternative approaches was sometimes necessary. However, she invariably returned in good spirits after the first visit.

Another case involving the conjoint use of hypnosis and chemical anesthetics was reported by Bernick. A 13-year-old boy had an uncontrollable dread of needles and of being put to sleep. His parents reported that he had undergone a series of rabies injections at the age of six which left him thoroughly frightened of a doctor's needles. Previous dental work had been done under general anesthesia; the inference is that something connected with that experience led to his fear of being put to sleep. For this patient, the details of hypnotic treatment through successive sessions have been reported, so one can visualize the steps involved. After the X-rays during the first session he was hypnotized by the traditional eye fixation technique. One hand was then made anesthetic by suggestion, and he was told that he would be able to transfer this insensitivity to his mouth in the next session. At the beginning of the next session he was hypnotized, and the analgesia established in the hand was transferred to the area of the mouth to be worked on. Suggestions were continued that he would feel no discomfort, only pressures. When aroused from hypnosis, he was pleased that all had gone well and that no needles had been necessary. In a subsequent session, after the patient was hypnotized and analgesia established as before, the dentist explained that he needed more profound insensitivity to treat a particular tooth. This was done in order to prepare the patient for the more protracted oral surgery to follow, in which an injected anesthetic was to be used. This time the boy said he did not object to receiving a local anesthetic by injection. In a final session, the patient was sent by the first dentist to an oral surgeon for removal of an impacted bicuspid under local chemoanalgesia. The original dentist had implanted a posthypnotic suggestion that the patient would enter a relaxed hypnotic state in the oral surgeon's chair and would awaken from the state when the surgeon had completed his work. The surgeon later remarked that this was one of the most relaxed patients he had ever had.

What is the role of hypnosis once the dental procedure has been completed? If hypnosis has been used to produce analgesia, there is the question of how long the analgesia should endure. One method is to give a suggestion for terminating the analgesia at a later time. In one such case reported by Owens, a periodontal curettage was completed under hypnosis and hypnotic analgesia. The technique used was to visualize switches in a control room, which would turn off pain in any of the four quadrants of the mouth; no anesthetic supplement was used. Because the dentist did not want sensitivity to return promptly, he gave the suggestion that the analgesia would last for 24 hours before sensitivity was restored to normal.

Although the usual hypnotic practice is to unify the treatment experience as much as possible, beginning before the dental procedures proper and continuing into the recovery period, the following case shows that hypnosis can occasionally be used specifically during the recovery period, even for the first time. A female patient had all her upper teeth posterior to the right and left cuspids extracted under local anesthetic by another dentist before she came to the attention of Thompson, who was familiar with hypnosis. The patient's problems were compounded by a sinus perforation near the first molar on the left and by development of two "dry sockets." These proved to be very painful; five days after the extractions the patient still had no relief from pain and could not rest or eat properly. When hypnosis was proposed, both the original dentist and the patient readily agreed, because they were willing to "try anything." The patient was hypnotized deeply within two minutes, and the whole treatment time was twenty minutes. Under hypnosis she listened carefully to a rationale for what she had to do: first, pain was no longer needed as a warning signal, so she was free to relinquish it; second, the healing process required that she get rest and nourishment; and third, as she became more relaxed her circulation would improve, and this in itself would help the healing process. After the dentist-hypnotist repeated these points in varied ways, the patient was aroused from hypnosis with suggestions of well-being and self-confidence. Her pain was completely relieved; she was able to eat and sleep normally. She indicated that what she had been told under hypnosis seemed reasonable and therefore easy to accept and respond to.

The judgments of the patient and the dental practitioner as to the success of procedures used are not always the same. One patient of Thompson's with a history of frequent "dry sockets" (technically known as *alveoalgia*) was referred for emergency extraction. The purpose of the adjuvant hypnosis in this case was to increase circulation as well as to reduce pain. A local anesthetic was also employed. Definite suggestions to control bleeding were given—the blood was to enter the sockets and thicken and clot there to promote healing. Suggestions of rest and nourishment for proper healing were added. The dentist was pleased that no "dry sockets" developed, but the patient complained of pain; as further treatment sessions followed, the patient remained unhappy about what the dentist considered a normal healing rate. The dentist thought that the complaints were related to the meaning to the patient of losing her teeth, but felt it improper to delve further into the psychological aspects of the case. She did not communicate her tentative interpretations to the patient.

The foregoing cases illustrate the use of hypnosis in dentistry, without any insistence that hypnosis should be used alone, and in full recognition that its role in relaxation and anxiety reduction may be as important as its role in pain reduction, because local anesthetics are convenient and effective.

Hypnosis and Chemoanalgesia

A large fraction of dental patients can be managed readily by premedication, local anesthetics, and optimal operative procedures. Hypnosis can be most useful with "problem patients" who cannot be so managed—especially the nervous, frightened patient. As Moss puts it: "The primary use of hypnosis in dentistry is to 'normalize' the patient so that we can manage him as we do our other patients." Because of the ready availability of local anesthetics, most dentists who use hypnosis employ chemoanalgesics along with it, unless there are special contraindications.

It is a matter of scientific interest to know to what extent dental pains can be controlled by hypnosis alone, without the use of any chemoanesthetics whatever. To illustrate this less common practice, a few of the cases reported over the last decades are listed in Table 3. Some of these cases have already been referred to in other connections; some others will be given in more detail in what follows.

Occasionally a patient asks for hypnosis because of an aversion to drugs based on his lifestyle; this of course provides a favorable motivational background. A case of Weyandt's, a man of age 65, was a member of a health organization which advocated vegetarianism, organically fertilized soils, and avoidance of medication. He had been wearing a partial upper denture, but now his seven remaining maxillary teeth were to be removed and a full upper denture provided. The first session was devoted to an explanation of all procedures, illustrated by a skull model displaying the anatomy of the oral cavity. This was followed by practice in hypnosis, induced through eye closure followed by arm catalepsy. At the next session, impressions for the patient's full upper dentures were obtained, and hypnosis was induced again.

Table 3. Some Case Reports of Dental Procedures with Hypnosis as the Sole Anesthetic.

Source (in chronological order)	Patients	Nature of Procedure
Traiger (1952)	(a) 4-year-old (b) 9-year-old	(a) Pulpectomy and pulpotomy (b) Four pulpotomies during 3 hrs.
Crasilneck, McCranie, and Jenkins (1956)	Woman patient	Complex procedures on 5 occasions, each lasting 2 hrs.
Lucas, Finkelman, and Tocantins (1962)	Hemophiliacs (4 cases)	Extractions
McCay (1963)	Male physician under self-hypnosis	Extraction
Secter (1964)	Patient in spontaneous trance	Extraction of two mandibular premolars
Petrov, Traikov, and Kalendgiev (1964)	(a) Woman, age 35 (b) Woman, age 20 (c) Woman, age 25	Extractions, including one difficult case lasting $1\frac{1}{2}$ hours
Owens (1970)	(a) Woman, age 35, with multiple sclerosis (b) Woman, age 41 (c) Male, age 49	(a) Extraction of 2 abscessed teeth (b) Extraction of 2 abscessed teeth (c) Periodontal curettage
Radin (1972)	Adult male; chemoanesthesia contraindicated	Extensive extractions on repeated occasions, including suturing
Weyandt (1972)	Male, age 65	Seven teeth extracted

This time anesthesia was produced. The patient's right thumb was made numb by suggestion, and this numbness was transferred to his palate and ridges. The dentist tested the effectiveness of the anesthesia suggestion, complimented the patient on his cooperation and skill, and then terminated the hypnosis. At the next session the waxed-up denture was tried and necessary corrections made. After this, a simulation was carried out under hypnosis of everything that was to be done to prepare the mouth for the full upper denture. The patient was hypnotized by a prearranged signal, his upper jaw anesthetized as before, and everything was rehearsed, including posthypnotic suggestions regarding swelling, pain, and healing. Aroused from hypnosis, he was again praised, and arrangements were made for the next session. In the crucial session everything proceeded as planned; the procedure was completely painless without any chemoanalgesia. The teeth were extracted, some areas sutured, and the denture inserted, to be kept in overnight until postoperative treatment the next morning. The patient slept comfortably and complained of nothing; there were no signs of swelling or bleeding. Apart from minor adjustments of the occlusion on the denture teeth, all went well; the sutures were removed five days later. A month afterward, when the patient returned for some work on his lower teeth, he reported that the denture felt fine and that he was able to eat whatever he wished.

Sometimes a patient's preference for hypnosis is based on an unfavorable reaction to local anesthetics, as reported by Crasilneck and his associates. A 36-year-old woman had previously reacted to procaine with edema of the face and body, urticaria (hives), nausea, and vomiting. As a result, even minor dental procedures had been carried out under general anesthesia. Because of her unfortunate experiences, she had refused to return to her dentist; by now most of her teeth had developed cavities. She needed a series of sessions with her dentist, and it was judged impractical to place her under a general anesthetic each time. A psychologist familiar with hypnosis was consulted to determine whether she would be an appropriate candidate for hypnosis. A personality evaluation indicated that she was relatively free of emotional symptoms other than her extreme fear of dental procedures. After a discussion, hypnosis was induced; she proved to be an excellent subject and was soon capable of reaching a profound hypnotic state. Thereafter, on five separate occasions, dental procedures lasting approximately two hours each were successfully performed. On all five occasions the patient achieved analgesia through hypnotic suggestion. She was free of all pain and apprehensiveness. Eventually her fears of dental procedures were greatly diminished, so she could accept minor procedures without hypnosis.

If the physical condition of the patient precludes use of chemical anesthetics, hypnosis alone may very well be the preferred method. Radin reported on a 49-year-old male patient who came with rheumatic heart disease, increasing dyspnea, palpitation, swelling of the ankles, and a fever of 100.0°F. He required extensive extractions. Before the dental work could be undertaken, he needed additional medication for his heart condition; although still a poor risk, he improved sufficiently so that the course of extractions was begun. Fortunately, he proved to be a good hypnotic subject; the procedures were carried out under hypnosis, with no general or local anesthetic and no chemical treatment, although penicillin was used to prevent further infection. Extractions were performed on May 9, 23, and 30, followed by a treatment session on May 31 because of a hemorrhage of tooth sockets. Additional extractions were done on June 27 and July 4—four teeth were extracted and sutured in the latter session. The sutures were removed under hypnotic treatment on July 11. On July 18 the final three extractions were made and sutured. The work was completed on July 25 with the removal of the sutures. This extensive series of extractions, covering nearly three months, was carried out comfortably under hypnosis in this high-risk patient.

These three cases all involve unusual conditions, but they show that hypnosis used alone can be effective, even in difficult dental procedures. Many routine procedures in which hypnosis can be used effectively alone, including minor surgery and the control of bleeding, do not find their way into the literature.

Individual case reports do not give any assurance that generalizations based on them will be widely applicable to other cases. They show what is possible, but they do not in themselves indicate the range of applicability of the procedures.

There are few satisfactory studies in which groups of unselected dental patients have been studied to show how hypnosis compares with chemoanalgesia. If the aim of the hypnosis is merely to relax the patient in preparation for dental procedures carried out with local anesthetics, Moss has claimed that some degree of success will result for over 80 percent of the cases. Of course, such a figure is not very informative. A dentist committed to hypnosis finds it useful in a whole range of dental procedures; Jacoby, for example, tabulated the kinds of dental problems treated in 308 patients during 1214 sessions. However, he reported nothing about the degree of hypnotizability of the patients in relation to the success of hypnosis, nor anything about the use of chemoanalgesia.

A study by Pollack used a large sample of patients to show that fairly simple suggestions reinforcing a topical anesthetic helped to calm the dental patient. The investigator divided 500 patients into four groups. Some patients received the topical anesthetic, with and without supplementary suggestions; others received the placebo (a nonanesthetic antiseptic) with and without the suggestions. The study showed that a calming effect occurred for the patients who received the anesthetic combined with the suggestions. This enhancement or supplementation of a chemical agent is doubtless one of the roles that hypnotic suggestion can serve.

A recent study by Gottfredson bears upon some previously unanswered questions. It relates dental procedures done with hypnosis as the sole anesthetic to the measured hypnotic susceptibility of the patient, and it compares the effectiveness of hypnotic anesthesia with that produced by a local anesthetic. Ratings by the patients themselves in the midst of treatment were used to assess the amount of pain felt. In this study, a dentist and a psychologist addressed problems of clinical practice in the same way that the problems of pain are studied in the laboratory.

The quantitative aspects of the investigation will be considered first, followed by some typical case studies from it. A dentist, although not himself familiar with the use of hypnosis in dentistry, offered to make consenting patients available to a psychologist. The latter performed the hypnosis and conducted the study. Of twenty-nine patients contacted, twenty-five volunteered to participate, even though it meant having at least one of their regular dental sessions with hypnosis as the only anesthetic. For comparison, another session utilized a local chemical anesthetic. These two sessions were randomized, twelve patients having hypnosis before the local, thirteen in the inverse order. The order did not significantly affect the findings. The subjects were first tested on the Stanford Hypnotic Susceptibility Scales; twelve were classified as highly susceptible (scores of 8 to 12), six as medium (scores of 5 to 7), and seven as low in susceptibility (scores of 0 to 4).

As a measure of the pain involved in the procedures, subjects reported their felt pain while the work progressed by raising as many fingers as necessary to describe the pain on a scale from 0 (no pain) to 10 (intolerable). This made verbal reports unnecessary.

Actually the chemical anesthetic was available to the subject if requested, even when the procedure was being attempted with hypnosis as the anesthetic. One of the first findings was that nine of twelve, or 75 percent, of the highly hypnotizable completed the treatment under hypnosis without any chemical supplement. Only five of the thirteen medium and lows, or 38 percent, managed without any supplement.

The amount of pain reported during the procedures carried out with hypnosis correlated −.39 with measured hypnotizability. This means that the more hypnotizable the subject was, the less pain he felt. Here, then, a clinical study documents the same relationships that have been shown in the laboratory with artificially induced pains. For both the high and medium-to-low groups, more pain was felt under hypnosis than with the local anesthetic, a result that is not surprising under these circumstances (Figure 11). Only the highly susceptible group came close to the chemical anesthesia in their level of pain reduction through hypnosis. Anxiety was also measured, but the results were both complex and confusing, so no attempt will be made to summarize them here.

Although the quantitative results are informative, much of the richness of the study is added by the case studies that follow.

Most of the treatments in the dentist's office required only drilling and restoration of teeth, but two subjects required extractions. Both were highly

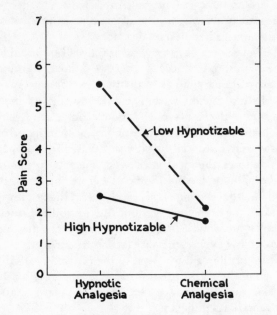

Figure 11. Pain felt within dental procedures under hypnotic and chemical analgesia, with subjects grouped according to measured hypnotic susceptibility. (From Gottfredson, 1973)

hypnotizable according to the results of the susceptibility test. The first of these was successful, the second was unsuccessful; their contrast gives an indication of differences that are encountered.

The successful extraction was with a 29-year-old male who had a fully developed lower molar to be removed. Other work was to be done as well. After he was hypnotized, there were first thirteen minutes of drilling on another tooth; then an impression for a crown was taken. Next, with hypnosis deepened, the extraction was undertaken. It was a difficult extraction because the roots were curved, making it necessary to remove some of the overlying bone structure in order to remove the tooth. The patient remained calm throughout; his average pain was 2, and the maximum pain report was 5. He reported that other wisdom teeth had been extracted with local anesthetics, but that this experience under hypnosis was the easiest one for him. He stated his preference for hypnosis over chemical anesthesia.

The unsuccessful attempt was with a college girl of 18. She was scheduled to have her wisdom teeth extracted, but she came to the appointment and announced that she was going to postpone removal of the teeth because of the expense. The dentist offered to defer his bill because he felt that delaying treatment might harm her teeth; after some hesitation, the decision was made to go ahead. Although she had earlier scored 10 of 12 on the susceptibility scale, she had not felt herself deeply hypnotized at that time, and now responded little to hypnosis. The procedure was attempted under hypnosis, even though she reported her hypnotic state to be very light; she soon reached a pain report of 10 and required chemical anesthesia. The extractions under the local anesthetic were uneventful and unemotional, although the patient reached a pain state of 6 and required an additional injection. The success of the highly hypnotizable, as measured by the susceptibility scales, is only probabilistic; that is, the chance that a subject who measures high on the scale will produce a satisfactory hypnotic anesthesia is greater than the chance of one low on the scale, but the success is not a certainty. In practice, measurement of susceptibility on the scales would be supplemented by clinical judgment of the effectiveness of hypnosis in reducing the patient's pain.

A more profound hypnosis is required to relieve pain without chemical supplements than for hypnotic procedures to control anxiety. One case was that of a 14-year-old girl who had unpleasant prior experiences with dentists. She refused to go back to the dentists who had treated her, but was persuaded to try a different dentist. Even during the initial examination, with no drilling or other painful stimuli, she was so agitated that the dental assistant had to hold her down physically. The patient proved susceptible to hypnosis and was calmed by hypnotic suggestions; however, she experienced enough pain during treatment to request a chemical anesthetic because hypnosis alone did not suffice. Under a combination of hypnosis and chemical anesthetic she remained calm and the treatment was routine. Interestingly, when chemical anesthesia was used alone she again became agitated and required hypnosis to quiet her; neither hypnosis alone nor the anesthetic alone was effective. In subsequent sessions the dentist continued to use hypnosis along with the chemical anesthetic, even though the experiment was over.

When a procedure is performed under light hypnosis without chemical anesthesia, the question of "heroism" arises: has the subject resolved to endure the pain without calling for the chemical supplement? Another possibility is that a subject who is not hypnotizable may, by strong voluntary effort, turn his attention away from the pain and actually feel it less. This latter possibility was illustrated by one subject who was essentially unresponsive to hypnotic suggestions. Induction of hypnosis for the dental procedures was attempted, but the patient reported no feeling whatever of being hypnotized. Still, during the drilling of several teeth, he reported a pain no higher than 2 for eight minutes. When, however, the dentist began work on a tooth with a missing filling the patient found it very sensitive. He raised all fingers in a pain report of 10 and asked for an injection of the chemical anesthetic. Following both treatment sessions—hypnotic and chemical—he said he was satisfied with hypnosis as an anesthetic. If he made sufficient effort to concentrate on the hypnotist's suggestions, he was able to direct his attention away from the drilling and block the sensation of pain. However, this effort was difficult to sustain, and when his attention faltered he could feel the drilling. When the nerve in his sensitive tooth was hit, he panicked. This finding is similar to that reported by our laboratory subjects when they compared pain reduction by an effort of attention without hypnosis, to their experiences when hypnotized. For the highly hypnotizable subject within hypnosis, pain reduction is essentially effortless; the nonhypnotizable subject (or the hypnotizable subject in the waking state) requires considerable effort to achieve comparable results.

The effortless nature of the response was clearly illustrated by one highly hypnotizable subject in Gottfredson's study. He had the chemical treatment first and experienced mild discomfort, but did not require a second injection of anesthetic. During the hypnotic treatment he reported feeling "dead to the world;" yet he responded readily to requests to turn his head, open his mouth wider, and so forth. His average pain report during eighteen minutes of drilling was 1.1, compared with 1.3 during chemical treatment. His final estimate was: "From today's experience, I would say hypnosis would be more appropriate than a chemical anesthetic in every case." The dentist judged that the hypnotic and chemical treatments were about equally effective for this patient.

Dental Problems other than Pain

The dentist familiar with hypnosis finds it useful in treating problems other than pain. We have already noted the intimate relationship between anxiety and pain. Many problems take specific forms such as gagging, excessive salivation, blood flow, bruxism (teeth grinding), and tongue thrust against the teeth. We do not propose to discuss these problems in any detail, but they deserve some mention in order to keep the dental use of hypnosis in proper perspective.

One of the more troublesome problems that the patient may bring to the dentist is that of gagging as soon as anything is inserted into the mouth. Normally, reflex regurgitation occurs only when something is accidentally introduced into the trachea; it thus protects the person against choking. The "trigger" lies so deep that the reflex does not typically affect the dentist's work in the oral cavity. For some patients this "trigger" point has moved forward through conditioning to the lips, the tongue, or other areas touched in dental examinations; unless controlled, the gagging makes dental procedures impossible.

Fortunately, patients capable of only light hypnosis can learn to eliminate the gagging response so the dental work can proceed. Control can be achieved in many cases by direct suggestion, but sometimes more complex methods, including "uncovering" techniques, must be used.

Weyandt reported a man of 40, a heavy smoker with a smoker's cough, who was unable to tolerate any dental treatments without an anesthetic because of his extreme gagging. He was enthusiastic about trying hypnosis, and after some prior explanation, he achieved a light hypnotic state with eye fixation, eye catalepsy, and hand levitation. He was then given direct suggestions that anything done in his mouth would be tolerated without annoyance or discomfort. The first test was the taking of X-rays; because of violent retching, this had previously been impossible without injection of a local anesthetic. Now, however, the X-rays were accomplished without any difficulty. Roused from hypnosis, the patient said, "It's the first time I ever enjoyed a dental visit." During subsequent years the patient underwent a number of complex dental procedures with the aid of hypnosis, always with ease and comfort.

Sometimes control of gagging can be achieved promptly through direct suggestion; sometimes the suggestions must be given in more complex ways over a period of time; and sometimes the roots of the problem must be uncovered, as in the following case reported by Erickson, Hershman, and Sector. The subject was a young man who volunteered for a demonstration of the treatment of gagging before a workshop dealing with hypnotic techniques. He proved sufficiently responsive to hypnosis, but could not control his gagging in response to direct suggestion. An "uncovering" technique, used on the spot in this first contact with the patient, revealed that his problem began in childhood with an excessive dose of castor oil. After eliciting this information, the hypnotist was able to assure the subject that the castor oil problem belonged to the past, and that he no longer need be troubled by it, now that he knew the history of his problem. This succeeded, and the subject no longer gagged.

One of the patients in the experimental study previously cited produced so much saliva that the dentist had difficulty completing his work. The hypnotist said to the hypnotized patient, "You are salivating too much, and I want you to stop it." He was inexperienced in such suggestions and was amazed that the saliva flow stopped immediately. The method was not tried on other patients, so the general effectiveness of such a direct suggestion could not be assessed. However, clinicians commonly indicate successes in relation to this symptom.

Bleeding may present either of two problems: too much, as in hemorrhaging, or too little, as in dry sockets. Some of the cases discussed previously have indicated the successful control of dry sockets.

Newman has reported a woman of 43 years who was a chronic bleeder in the dentist's office. Following one extraction, she bled for eight hours. Subsequently, she presented herself with a broken upper left lateral incisor that required extraction; the dentist was confronted with a problem. Somewhat reluctantly the patient accepted the idea of hypnosis; through a relaxation procedure, she achieved satisfactory anesthesia of the right arm and hand. The dentist planted the suggestion that she was not naturally a bleeder by showing her that when she pricked her hand with a needle, she felt no pain and did not bleed. When extraction was performed on the following day, it was only necessary to give indirect suggestions that the bleeding would stop. The bleeding stopped within a minute after the extraction was completed. Roused from hypnosis, the patient said she felt so good that she wished to return to work. Two days later she reported that there had been no bleeding on the day of the surgery, and that she felt normal and wonderful.

Any surgical treatment of hemophiliacs presents a severe problem; dental extractions are commonly preceded by the transfusion of blood or plasma—or both—or of plasma fractions. For many patients, however, hypnotic procedures such as those described by Lucas and his associates may greatly reduce or eliminate the need for transfusions. The hypnosis is not used alone, but is combined with protective splints and critical packing of sockets. A 41-year-old male hemophiliac came with severe dental caries and gingival recession; X-rays showed moderate to severe bone loss and some apical infection. He had been admitted to the hospital many times since childhood for bleeding episodes. A fracture of the nose when he was seven had produced severe bleeding for forty-two days. Previous tooth extraction had led to long periods of hospitalization with many transfusions of blood and plasma. By use of methods in which hypnosis played a significant role, two teeth were removed on each of two separate occasions; healing was satisfactory, and no transfusions were necessary. A report on 114 extractions done in 24 hemophiliacs indicated no abnormal bleeding in any case.

How the control of bleeding is achieved as a consequence of suggestion is by no means clear. It may be a secondary consequence of the general relaxation achieved under hypnosis; or it may be related to the specific control of vasomotor responses that can be developed through hypnosis and biofeedback, as in the selective control of hand temperature. One experimental attempt to control the temperature of the gums directly through hypnosis found the subjects convinced that they had achieved such control, but the objective evidence was against any vasomotor change. More experimental work needs to be directed to this problem in order to clarify the clinical successes.

A habit that may come to the attention of a dentist is thrusting of the tongue against or between the teeth, perhaps in contact with the lower lip or the inside of the cheek. This is a consequence of an abnormal swallowing pattern; tongue thrusters are unable to be quiet while eating and attempting to swallow, and many are nagged as children because their mouths tend to hang open. The effect upon appearance is objectionable in the older tongue-thrust patient. The persistent habit results in repeated pressure against the teeth which in turn leads to malocclusion; this brings the child to the dentist. One investigation by Barrett and von Dedenroth reported twenty-five such cases in which hypnotic treatment was successful when more conventional methods failed. The conventional method of treatment, practiced by some speech therapists, involves learning normal swallowing by deliberate, conscious control of the process. The investigators state that this is ineffective in many cases because 90 percent of the swallowing is done when the subject is unaware of it. This instructional phase is important, however, even if it fails to break the habit.

The second, or hypnotic, phase is important in difficult cases. Once the patient is hypnotized, essentially the same instructions are repeated that were used in the effort at conscious correction; now, however, the suggestions emphasize that the control will occur even when the swallowing is not being attended to. The study reported success in all twenty-five patients, in one to four hypnotic sessions. The overall time devoted to the symptom ranged from fifteen minutes to one and one-half hours.

Teeth grinding, known technically as *bruxism*, can create serious problems. Graham reported the case of a 26-year-old woman who complained of jaw pain in the morning resulting from extensive teeth grinding at night. A dental hospital had made a special denture to prop open her mouth to prevent grinding, but she had ground the denture into her gums, which were sore and lacerated. She was tense and anxious because, in addition to the presenting symptom of bruxism, she suffered two or three attacks of migraine each week. Five years previously, she had been involved in a bus crash; her grinding had started about a year after the accident, and her migraine a little later.

The patient proved to be a responsive hypnotic subject. The first session was devoted to teaching relaxation; it ended with specific instructions for relaxing before going to bed. Although no reference was made to the headaches, they disappeared after the second visit, and she began sleeping better. The teeth grinding, however, continued. The patient was regressed to the time of the bus accident, and apparently obtained some relief from the emotional expression that occurred. She reported that, at the time, her breath had been knocked out; she had wanted to scream, but could not. The dentist told her to have a scream in the office; she did so, and afterward felt better. The grinding stopped and her morning pain was gone. The results were enduring.

In fulfilling his professional duties, the dentist occasionally reports that, following hypnotic treatment for his purposes, other pains not usually classified as dental pains may disappear. One illustration is the disappearance of migraine headaches in the young woman being treated for bruxism.

Another illustration of such a beneficial by-product of hypnotic treatment is a case of tic douloureux (facial or trigeminal neuralgia), reported by Golan. Because the trigeminal nerve innervates the teeth, the extraction of teeth is sometimes resorted to when other methods fail, in the hope that the patient's pain may be relieved. A 77-year-old male had undergone numerous treatments, some successful for a time, but always followed by recurrence. He had recently been referred to a dental service by the neurology service, and had four teeth removed. He experienced an attack of his typical paroxysmal pain when the sutures were removed. An infraorbital local anesthetic relieved the attack, but within a week the symptoms were as severe as ever. Suggestive therapy was subsequently undertaken during weekly visits; the therapist's goal was to convert the pain sensations to a heavy feeling, which the patient spontaneously altered to a "feeling of pickiness." Medication was discontinued, and emphasis was placed on viewing daily life as a pleasant experience. His pains disappeared partially at first, but soon were entirely gone, and new dentures were fitted without incident. His symptoms recurred once when he struck his nose with his fist during sleep; this brought on his old attack. Treatment by hypnosis controlled his attacks, first during the hypnotic state and then outside it. The interpretation is that at least some cases of tic douloureux must have an emotional component that hypnosis may correct.

The literature on dental hypnosis contains discussions about the extent to which the dentist should deal with problems that might belong to the psychiatrist. The dentist is trained to deal with problems of the oral cavity, but if he meets anxiety over dentistry, gagging, or bruxism with psychosomatic roots, what is the next step? Clearly, he must treat his patients; if their symptoms are related to dental problems which interfere with dental procedures, he attempts to resolve them in his office. If he detects that the patient has deeper problems that might be helped by psychotherapy, he refers the patient to an appropriate psychotherapist. The issues are matters both of expertness and of professional ethics; there are obviously many borderline cases, as the preceding case studies indicate.

Concluding Remarks on Hypnosis in the Relief of Dental Pain

Although we are concerned particularly with the relief of pain, other problems met by the dentist are so intimately related that the pain problem cannot be completely separated. In fact, it is very common for dentists who use hypnosis to inject local anesthetics to control pain and to include chemical vasoconstrictors along with the injection in order to control bleeding. These methods are so convenient that there is little reason to displace them. Hypnosis serves to reduce fear and anxiety, and incidentally to raise the pain threshold; it may have ancillary effects in controlling bleeding and aiding postoperative recovery. Because the more severe stresses of the pain are controlled chemically, the advantages of hypnosis are available to practically all dental patients, despite individual differences in susceptibility.

At the same time, some cases arise in which chemical anesthetics are not advised; it is fortunate that hypnosis alone is often very successful in reducing dental pain. The evidence is quite clear that for highly hypnotizable subjects who are sufficiently motivated, hypnosis can serve as the only anesthetic for dental procedures which are normally quite painful, including difficult dental surgery.

Notes

The role of dentists in furthering the use of hypnosis after their experiences in World War II is recounted in the chapter by Moss (1963b) which appears in the book by Kroger (1963). The dental report from the prisoner-of-war camp near Singapore is that of Sampimon and Woodruff (1946).

Hypnotic Relief of Pain and Anxiety

Of the two methods for treating dental anxiety or dental phobia—the direct method and the uncovering techniques—the latter is more controversial, because most dentists lack training in psychodynamics. The case from Golan (1971) is one of three cases he reported. He used some psychological interpretations of present symptoms without delving into the patient's past. The next case, from Stolzenberg (1961), is one of two cases in which he utilized age regression. It may be noted that, in the case reported, he hit upon something definitely related to the patient's present attitude toward the dentist; he used age regression merely to ascertain some facts in her history. The facts were interpreted in a straightforward way in the waking state. There can be no objection to using regressive techniques in this way, but too much searching into the past, as though the dentist were doing a psychotherapeutic exploration, is not to be recommended. If the dentist finds a case in which the psychological background relates in a complex way to the fear of dentistry, he might well seek the advice of someone better trained than he in psychodynamics. Most cases can be handled by methods strictly within the dentist's sphere of competency, as in the next two cases of Kroll (1962) and Bernick (1972).

Owens (1970) indicated that suggestions could prolong analgesia for 24 hours.

Thompson's cases were both reported in her paper, which states very well the rationale for suggestion in dentistry (Thompson, 1963).

Hypnosis and Chemoanalgesia

The thought that hypnosis serves to "normalize" the patient who is not ready for dental procedures is from Moss (1963a); the quotation is from that source (p. 111).

The cases listed in Table 3 were all treated without chemical analgesia or anesthesia. They are not presented to propose more general use of hypnosis in this manner, but merely to add to the large body of testimony of the reality of hypnotic pain reduction.

The patient who, because of his other commitments, prefers dental treatment without medication, is psychologically well prepared to accept some nonmedication method of pain reduction. The case discussed in the text was reported by Weyandt (1972).

The woman who required hypnosis because of prior unfavorable reactions to procaine was reported in Crasilneck, McCranie, and Jenkins (1956).

The patient with a history of rheumatic heart disease, for whom hypnosis was the preferred method, was reported by Radin (1972).

The imprecise figure of 80 percent of patients for whom hypnosis can be helpful was asserted by Moss (1963b). The range of procedures involving hypnosis was reported by Jacoby (1960).

The large sample study of Pollack (1960) was not strictly a hypnotic study at all, but it showed that simple suggestions could have some calming effect beyond that of a topical anesthetic alone, even if the suggestions were not strong enough to enhance a placebo effect.

The unpublished dissertation by Gottfredson (1973) represents a model design for a clinical study controlled as an experiment. The subjects were assigned randomly to chemoanalgesia and hypnotic analgesia, so no personal preference was involved in the choice of treatment; assignment was also independent of the kind of dental procedure to be faced. Hypnotic responsiveness was tested on scales not specific to the dental experiences. Ratings of pain felt were obtained in the midst of the treatment rather than recalled afterwards. The limitations of the study are those that are inevitable in clinical practice: not all patients underwent equally painful procedures, and the total numbers, although adequate for the purpose, permit only tentative generalizations. The correlation of $-.39$ between hypnotic susceptibility and felt pain is marginally significant with twenty-five cases; it does not differ significantly from the correlations between pain and hypnotizability found in laboratory studies. The cases reported are from the same study.

Dental Problems other than Pain

The smoker with a smoker's cough who was relieved of gagging is reported by Weyandt (1972). The control of gagging is commonly demonstrated in workshops illustrating hypnosis in dentistry; success is commonly achieved in a single session before an audience. The case reported is detailed in a book by Erickson, Hershman, and Sector (1961), covering a wide range of hypnotic applications in medicine and dentistry.

Excessive salivation, a problem that is met rather frequently, is illustrated by one of the cases from Gottfredson (1973).

The chronic bleeder was reported by Newman (1971). The study of hemophiliacs is by Lucas, Finkelman, and Tocantins (1962), supplemented by Lucas and Tocantins (1964). The possibility of vasomotor control through hypnosis is illustrated by the hand temperature studies of Maslach, Marshall, and Zimbardo (1972), Roberts, Kewman, and Macdonald (1973), and Roberts and others (1975). The change in subjective temperature of the gums without vasomotor changes was found by Clark and Forgione (1974).

Tongue thrust was investigated by Barrett and von Dedenroth (1967), bruxism by Graham (1974). The tic douloureux case was reported by Golan (1971).

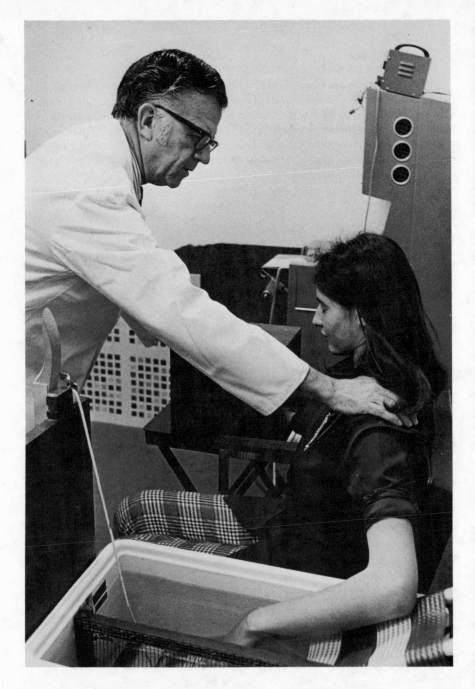

Overt and Covert Pain in Hypnotic Analgesia. The hand in ice water may feel no overt pain following suggestions of hypnotic analgesia. With his hand on the subject's shoulder, however, the experimenter can tap a hidden part of the person that reports covert pain being felt at some level. From the Stanford Laboratory.

PART III. *A Perspective on the Hypnotic Control of Pain*

It was recently discovered that a hypnotized person who *overtly* felt no pain or distress from either cold pressor pain or ischemic pain could be shown to have felt considerable *covert* pain, especially sensory pain. Distress was frequently absent both overtly and covertly. The discovery of this discrepancy between overt and covert pain solved some paradoxes in understanding hypnotic analgesia, but raised some new questions as well.

As a conclusion to this survey of experimental findings and their interpretation, along with the review of clinical pain reduction in cancer, obstetrics, surgery, and dentistry, the final chapter consists of a summary and an appraisal of the future of hypnosis in relation to pain and other therapies. Although many aspects of pain have been omitted in this survey, the firmness of the results in the areas studied gives promise for a wider use of hypnosis in the future.

9   Hidden Pain and its Interpretation

We have referred earlier to a paradox found when pain is reduced by hypnosis: felt pain may be reduced while the involuntary physiological indicators of pain may persist at nearly normal levels. Does this mean that pain is registered at some level but ignored? Is the person who is successful at reducing pain through hypnosis merely deploying his attention away from the pain? Is the pain felt but immediately forgotten through some sort of amnesic process? Is the subject in an unusual state in which some subconscious part feels the pain, but the rest of him is unaware of it? These puzzling questions are intimately involved with the organization of mind and consciousness; the answers are of more than academic interest. The realities underlying the answers bear upon the practical treatment of pain, the nature of postoperative shock, and the recovery from painful episodes.

The Discovery of the "Hidden Observer"

A new complication within hypnosis came to our attention through an observation made almost by chance, and not perceived immediately as related to pain at all. The instructor (E. R. H.) was conducting a classroom demonstration of hypnotic deafness. The subject of the demonstration was a blind student, experienced in hypnosis, who had volunteered to serve; his blindness was not related to the demonstration, except that any visual cues were eliminated. After induction of hypnosis, he was given the suggestion that, at the count of three, he would become completely deaf to all sounds. His hearing would be restored to normal when the instructor's hand was placed on his right shoulder. To be both blind and deaf would have been a frightening experience for the subject, had he not known that his deafness was quite temporary. Loud sounds were then made close to the subject's head by banging together some large wooden blocks. There was no sign of reaction whatsoever; none was expected, because the subject had, in a previous demonstration, shown lack of responsiveness to the shots of a starter's pistol. He was completely indifferent to any questions asked of him while hypnotically deaf.

One student in the class questioned whether "some part" of the subject might be aware of what was going on. After all, there was nothing wrong with his ears. The instructor agreed to test this by a method related to interrogation practices used by clinical hypnotists. He addressed the hypnotically deaf subject in a quiet voice:

"As you know, there are parts of our nervous system that carry on activities that occur out of awareness, of which control of the circulation of the blood, or the digestive processes, are the most familiar. However, there may be intellectual processes also of which we are unaware, such as those that find expression in night dreams. Although you are hypnotically deaf, perhaps there is some part of you that is hearing my voice and processing the information. If there is, I should like the index finger of your right hand to rise as a sign that this is the case."

To the surprise of the instructor, as well as the class, the finger rose! The subject immediately said, "Please restore my hearing so you can tell me what you did. I felt my finger rise in a way that was not a spontaneous twitch, so you must have done something to make it rise, and I want to know what you did."

The instructor placed his hand on the subject's right shoulder, and the following conversation took place.

"Can you hear my voice now?"

"Yes, I hear you. Now please tell me what you did."

"What do you remember?"

"I remember your telling me that I would be deaf at the count of three, and could have my hearing restored when you placed your hand on my shoulder. Then everything was quiet for a while. It was a little boring just sitting here, so I busied myself with a statistical problem I have been working on. I was still doing that when I suddenly felt my finger lift; that is what I want you to explain to me." The whole procedure was recounted; what had happened was puzzling to all concerned. The subject was brought out of hypnosis.

At this point an important innovation was introduced. In the laboratory we had been doing some experiments on automatic writing; we had found that material not in the subject's awareness could be recovered through the writing of a hand placed "out of awareness" of the subject by suggestions under hypnosis. It seemed worth testing with this highly hypnotizable subject whether, by analogy, "automatic talking" might yield similar results.

Hence, with the subject hypnotized again but able to hear, the instructor spoke as follows:

"When I place my hand on your arm like this [he demonstrated] I can be in touch with that part of you that listened to me before and made your finger rise—that part that knew what was going on when you were hypnotically deaf. When I question that part, it will be able to answer me and tell me what it knows about what happened. But this hypnotized part of you, to whom I am now talking, will not know what you are saying—or even that you are talking—until, out of hypnosis, I shall say, 'Now you can remember everything.' All right, now I am placing my hand on your arm."

The following conversation ensued: "Do you remember what happened when you were hypnotized and what the hypnotized part of you reported?"

"Yes." (This very literal response is characteristic of this subject when hypnotized. If a question can be answered "yes" or "no," it gets no more extensive answer without further probing.)

On further questioning he repeated much of the earlier conversation, including his surprise at his finger's lifting.

"Does the part to whom I am now talking know more about what went on?"

"Yes."

"Tell me what went on."

"After you counted to make me deaf you made noises with some blocks behind my head. Members of the class asked me questions to which I did not respond. Then one of them asked if I might not really be hearing, and you told me to raise my finger if I did. This part of me responded by raising my finger, so it's all clear now."

The instructor then lifted his hand from the arm. "Do you remember what has happened in the last few minutes?"

"You said something about placing your hand on my arm, and some part of me would talk to you. Did I talk?"

The subject was aroused from hypnosis and told that he would remember everything. He then recalled all that had happened and had been said.

This unplanned demonstration clearly indicated that a hypnotized subject who is out of contact with a source of stimulation (in this case auditory) may nevertheless register information regarding what is occurring. Further, he may be understanding it so that, under appropriate circumstances, what was unknown to the hypnotized part of him can be uncovered and talked about. As a convenience of reference, we speak of the concealed information as being available to a "hidden observer."

It should be noted that the "hidden observer" is a metaphor for something occurring at an intellectual level but not available to the consciousness of the hypnotized person. It does not mean that there is some sort of secondary personality with a life of its own—a kind of homunculus lurking in the shadows of the conscious person. The "hidden observer" is merely a convenient label for the information source tapped through experiments with automatic writing, and here through the equivalent, automatic talking. Just how the split in consciousness may be explained will be discussed later in this chapter; first we shall address ourselves to empirical findings.

Covert Pain in Hypnotic Analgesia

We soon saw the applicability of the foregoing observations to our pain experiments. We turned promptly to studying the covert experiences in cold pressor pain and in ischemic pain, the laboratory pains we had used extensively in studies of hypnotic analgesia.

Covert Pain and Suffering in the Cold Pressor Test. As noted above, experiments on automatic writing were already being conducted in the laboratory. A numerical task was performed by a hand out of awareness, while the subject was consciously naming colors from a chart in front of him.

The adaptation of this experiment to pain was to have an automatic writing report on the covert pain intensity, while the subject, with his other hand in ice water, was verbally reporting essentially no pain at the overt level. The first subject on whom we tried this was a young woman experienced in hypnosis; she had no difficulty reducing the pain completely in one arm, while keeping the other arm out of awareness for the purposes of automatic writing. She was familiar with our usual pain scale from earlier experiments —0 for no pain, up to 10 for a pain so severe that she would wish to remove her hand from the water; she would count beyond 10 if asked to continue in the water after that level was reached.

The subject was hypnotized and instructed to feel nothing in the water; she verbally reported "0" on all successive requests for reports at 5-second intervals. She had been instructed under hypnosis to use the same numerical reporting scale with her hand out of awareness, but she would not be aware of what the hand was writing. While she was overtly reporting "0," the hand out of awareness was writing scale values for increasing covert pain—"2", "5", "7", "8", "9". The "hidden observer" was reporting essentially normal pain while the hypnotized part of her was feeling no pain at all!

Automatic writing is a cumbersome technique for questioning a hypnotized subject; so, beginning with this same subject, we applied the automatic talking method, using a refinement of the instructions given in the deafness demonstration. With this method, the pilot pain subject told us that, while her hypnotized self had felt no pain, the hidden part had felt pain of about the same sensory intensity as that produced by the cold water without hypnosis. However, the covert pain bothered her much less—at this hidden level within analgesia—than overt pain bothered her in the normal waking state.

After another pilot subject was tested, with similar results, we designed a more careful experiment with moderately high hypnotizable subjects. We wished to determine, first, how general these findings regarding pain would be, and second, how generally applicable "automatic talking" would be. It was not feasible at this stage to use subjects who were incapable of hypnotic amnesia and automatic writing, so the experiments were limited to subjects in approximately the upper 10 percent of hypnotic responsiveness. The methods used were outgrowths of those already described, with some minor changes. We wished to get an accurate picture of the development of pain perception at the covert level, simultaneously with that at the overt level in hypnotic analgesia; for this, we needed something easier to record in an orderly way against time than automatic writing with a pencil. Hence we substituted for the pencil a device rather like a small computing machine, in which the numerical report could be given by means of two keys—one key would be pressed for tens, the other for digits. This device yielded an objective record of the covert pain, simultaneous with the verbal report of overt pain.

In the hypnotic analgesia condition, the covert report through automatic talking was obtained retrospectively. The arm was first removed from the ice water, dried, and returned to normal, then the subject was asked, through the hidden observer method, what the maximum pain was that had been felt. This invariably agreed with the covert pain reported on the keys, and was frequently higher than the overt pain reported verbally in hypnosis. In the waking analgesia condition, the pain reported by key-pressing was not covert, because no hypnosis was involved. In that case, a truly covert report could be obtained only retrospectively. After the waking suggestion part of the experiment was over, the subject was hypnotized and, through the automatic talking technique, was questioned about any covert pain that might have been experienced. In practically every case, this covert pain equalled the overt pain in this condition (Figure 12).

The results for the twenty subjects in the experiment can be summarized as follows. Under waking suggestion of analgesia, the maximum overt pain reported fell from a mean of 14.2 to 8.5 on the scale—a reduction of 40 percent. In this condition the covert pain and the overt pain were the same. Under hypnotic suggestion of analgesia, the maximum overt pain fell to 4.2, a reduction of 70 percent from the normal waking pain, or nearly twice the reduction under waking suggestion. The covert pain revealed by automatic talking averaged 7.3, however—significantly higher than the overt pain. The

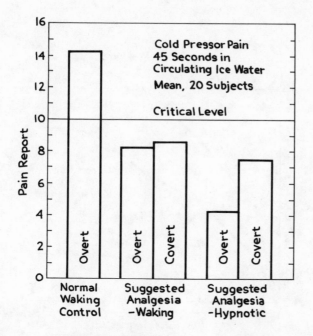

Figure 12. Maximum overt pain reported in the normal waking state, in waking analgesia, in hypnotic analgesia, and maximum covert pain reported in analgesia.

Overt reports were obtained in the usual manner in the waking state and following analgesia suggestions. Covert reports were obtained through the technique of automatic talking, as described in the text. Data from the Stanford laboratory.

covert pain in hypnotic analgesia did not differ significantly from the pain reported, either overtly or covertly, in waking analgesia.

These results imply that pain reduction in hypnosis has at least two components: one of them can be exercised by the nonhypnotized subject through the use of imagination, but the other becomes available to him only when hypnosis has been induced. At the covert level, only the first component appears to be effective; the second component must therefore account for the difference between overt and covert pain in hypnotic analgesia.

Although these average results are significant, they tend to mask the more dramatic results of a few subjects who experienced a vivid distinction between overt and covert pain. Only eight of the twenty subjects had this clear sense of separation between the two systems within themselves that were reporting pain overtly and covertly. The courses of their pain reports in

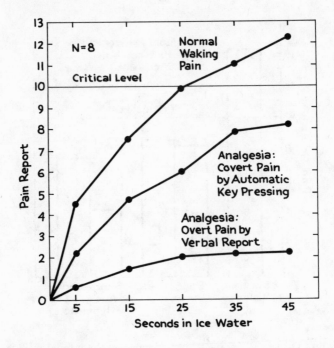

Figure 13. Normal waking pain, and overt and covert pain in hypnotic analgesia.

    Results are for the eight most successful subjects from those twenty whose means are reported in Figure 12. The covert reports were obtained by automatic key-pressing.

normal waking and in hypnotic analgesia, both overt and covert, are shown in Figure 13. Pain in waking analgesia is not shown, but it follows the course of covert hypnotic analgesic pain. These subjects showed the same general effects as for the whole group, but separation between overt and covert pain within hypnotic analgesia was greater.

    An important observation, based on the eight subjects of Figure 13 whose covert pain differed from overt pain, was that there was no distress connected with it; the hidden pain was sensory pain of high intensity, but unaccompanied by suffering. After amnesia for the covert report was lifted, subjects commonly remembered what their covert reports were, but could not remember actually feeling the pain reported in that way.

    Introspective statements made after recovery from amnesia are often confused, especially because the experiences of these subjects were unusual. In ordinary experience outside hypnosis, a memory which has been recovered may seem as if it had been there all along; the ordinary amnesias of daily life are themselves forgotten in this way. For example if you remember what you had for dinner last night after temporarily forgetting, you may say to yourself, " Of course, I remember remarking how tender the beef was." By that time, you have forgotten that you earlier had trouble remembering. In the experimental situation, once the memory for the automatic talking is restored, those who identify a "hidden observer" as responsible for their covert reports, may believe that they were partially aware of this observing part all along. In any case, subjective reports given at the end of the experiment—after the person reflects on what his experience was like before the hidden observer was tapped—vary widely. Here are comments from each of the eight subjects who had clear hidden observer reports in the course of the experiment. These statements are answers to inquiries after all amnesia had been lifted and the subject remembered all the talking that went on.

"... It's as though two things were happening simultaneously; I have two separate memories, as if the two things could have happened to different people. The memory of the hidden observer is more intellectual, but I can't really comprehend or assimilate the two."

"... Both parts were concentrating on what you said—not to feel pain. The water bothered the hidden part a little because it felt it a little, but the hypnotized part was not thinking of my arm at all."

"... The hidden part knew that my hand was in the water, and it hurt as much as it did the other day [in the waking control session]. The hypnotized part was vaguely aware of feeling pain; that's why I had to concentrate really hard." [This subject reported zero overt pain.]

"... When you're hypnotized, there are certain questions that just aren't answered, and you just don't probe them in your mind. I think you're aware that the pain exists, but it's not appropriate to deal with it just then."

"... I don't think I'm totally unaware that there is a hidden observer there, but when you asked me what I had been doing, it was really hard to remember. I don't know if I could have. It was like a block."

"... Today the pain was more general [to the hidden part], and especially the second time I felt it in my shoulder. [The hidden part] knew that my arm was there, but part of me knew it wasn't there. The pain was hidden from the hypnotized part."

"... The hidden part knows the pain is there, but I'm not sure it *feels* it. The hypnotized part doesn't feel it, but I'm not sure if the hypnotized part may have known it was there but didn't say it. The hypnotized part really makes an *effort*."

"... I can separate my mind and my head from the rest of my body. The hidden part—reporting on the keys—was controlling my body. My mind was not counting key-pressing. My mind was reporting what it felt, verbally.

I've always been aware of the difference between the mind and the body when I've been hypnotized."

We shall attempt to interpret these findings later. It may be noted, however, that the presence of the hidden observer was confirmed for a few of the subjects, but not all. Whether covert information does not exist for the others, or whether it is simply not accessible by the methods used, is an unanswered question at this point.

Covert Pain and Suffering in Ischemia. The other laboratory pain we have described is produced by a tourniquet to the upper arm, followed by exercise. To find out more about the pain experienced by some hidden part of the subject, the methods reported for cold pressor pain were also used in connection with ischemic pain. This time, more attention was paid to the suffering component.

Because ischemic pain mounts slowly—in minutes rather than in seconds, as with ice water—the time within the stress is long enough that complex inquiries can be made during the process. We decided to separate as best we could the *sensory-information* aspect of the pain from the *emotional-motivational* component. For this purpose, we instructed the subject to report separately the information, labeled *pain*, from the reactive aspect, labeled as *suffering*.

In the course of the experiments with hypnotic analgesia, verbal covert reports were obtained intermittently during the stress period (ischemia) itself, rather than retrospectively as in the cold pressor experiment. (The intermittent covert reports in the cold pressor experiment were recorded by key-pressing). At approximately 2-minute intervals during the ischemic stress period, four reports were called for: first the subject gave a report on pain and one on suffering, according to the usual overt reports within hypnotic analgesia. Then the experimenter placed his hand on the subject's shoulder in the method of automatic talking and requested a covert report of pain and one on suffering. When the hand was lifted, the subject became immediately amnesic for his covert reports. Such an alternation of conditions in short periods of time has often been demonstrated in other experiments with hypnosis, particularly those of Blum. Although rather remarkable, it is quite feasible with highly selected subjects.

The mean results for eight highly hypnotizable subjects somewhat more experienced in hypnosis than those who participated in the cold pressor experiment, are shown in Figure 14. These subjects were able to control both pain and suffering through hypnotic procedures, as shown by the overt reports of pain and suffering in the figure. The covert reports, obtained through automatic talking, showed a progressive increase in both pain and suffering over time, as indicated. The covert reports revealed more pain and suffering than the overt ones for seven of the eight subjects.

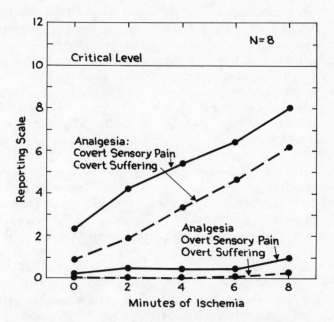

Figure 14. Pain and suffering in ischemia as reported overtly in hypnotic anesthesia, and covertly through automatic talking by the "hidden observer." The horizontal lines at the base of the figure show that these subjects experienced and reported essentially no overt pain or suffering during eight minutes of ischemia in the hypnotic analgesia condition. Through automatic talking, however, both covert pain and suffering were shown to rise progressively during this time. Modified from Knox, Morgan, and Hilgard (1974).

For these eight highly hypnotizable subjects, overt pain and suffering were both essentially absent throughout the time of ischemia, when pain and suffering would normally have been felt. Even at the end, pain had not mounted above the barely noticeable level. Hypnotic analgesia, studied in the usual way, reduces both pain and suffering.

The covert reports, obtained by automatic talking during the period of ischemia, showed steadily rising pain and suffering. Although the levels were below those expected in normal waking pain, the covert reports were significantly higher than the overt reports, for both the pain and the suffering. The suffering was reported being less intense than the pain; however, this was true also in waking ischemic pain, when no hypnosis was involved (Figure 4, Chapter 2).

The failure in this experiment to show more reduction in covert reports of suffering than of sensory pain disagrees with the results of the cold pressor experiment for the more successful subjects. This contradiction remains to be resolved. We have since participated in an experiment, done for another purpose, in which three highly hypnotizable subjects were given analgesia suggestions in the ischemic pain experiment, and were questioned retrospectively by the automatic talking method. Two of them, who overtly reported neither pain nor suffering when hypnotically analgesic, covertly reported a high level of sensory pain but no distress whatever. The differences in methods of inquiry may account for the difference between these results and the experimental results just described.

Anticipations from the Past. Something brought to light as readily as covert pain felt in hypnosis is quite likely to have been noticed in the past, even though no quantitative experiments were performed. Durand de Gros, in 1868, indicated his belief that some sub-ego might suffer when surgery was performed with hypnotic analgesia, even though the conscious ego was ignorant of the suffering. Early in this century, Myers wrote, "A man's nervous system is quite as active and vigorous as ever [when hypnotic suggestion has rendered him incapable of pain]—quite as capable of transmitting and feeling pain—although capable of also inhibiting it altogether." He showed that lack of pain under chemical anesthesia is also no assurance that pain is not felt, for he gave several instances of memories recovered following general anesthesia under chloroform and nitrous oxide. In one such case, the memory of what had happened in the operation was recovered in a dream.

Automatic writing, popular in the late nineteenth century, led to several observations on pain in hypnotically anesthetic arms. One such observation was reported by James, whose account was given in the Proceedings of the American Society for Psychical Research. His subject, one Smith, was a student at the Massachusetts Institute of Technology. Smith had prior experience in automatic writing and was apparently able to prepare himself for the experiment without any formal induction of hypnosis. He sat with his right hand—the writing hand—on the planchette, and his face "averted and buried in the hollow of his left arm," which was lying on the table. After the writing hand had scrawled illegibly for 10 minutes, James pricked the back of it fifteen to twenty times; there was no response to indicate feeling. Following two pricks on the left (normally sensitive) hand, the subject asked, "What did you do that for?" James replied that he wanted to find out whether Smith was going to sleep. Later, as the experiment continued, the anesthetic hand wrote, "Don't you prick me any more." When shown the automatic writing after the session, Smith laughed and said that he had been conscious of only two pricks, those on the left hand. He said of his right hand: "It's working those two pinpricks for all they are worth." In a session two days later, James had Smith write with his left hand. When questioned about the prior session, the hand wrote that he had been pricked "nineteen times on the other hand." James was uncertain whether or not the number was correct, but it was near enough. He summarized the situation as follows: "We have the consciousness of a subject split into two parts, one of which expresses itself through the mouth, and the other through the hand, whilst both are in communication through the ear."

A similar story was told by Estabrooks half a century later. He reported an experiment with a friend who was reading *Oil for the Lamps of China* while his right hand, screened from view by passing it through a cloth curtain, was engaged in automatic writing. The hand was out of awareness because of hypnotic procedures; it was also anesthetic. However, when Estabrooks pricked the hand with a needle, it wrote a stream of profanity "that would have made a top sergeant blush with shame." This went on for five minutes and included an attack on the hypnotist for having pricked him. The subject continued his reading calmly, "without the slightest idea that his good right arm was fighting a private war."

A third case was reported later by Kaplan, a psychiatrist. A deeply hypnotized subject was given the suggestions that his left arm was analgesic and insensitive, and that his right arm would write automatically; the subject would not be aware of what he was writing. When the experimenter pricked the left (anesthetic) arm several times with a hypodermic needle, the other hand wrote, "Ouch, damn it, you're hurting me." After a few minutes had passed, the subject, oblivious to what had transpired, asked Kaplan when he was going to begin the experiment. Kaplan interpreted the result to mean that, although the hypnotic subject was not conscious of his pain, it was being felt at some level, and there experienced as discomfort.

Thus our observations are not alone; the findings, both clinical and experimental, are challenging.

Hypnotic Analgesia Understood as a Split in Consciousness

When suggestions for hypnotic analgesia are successful, the person feels neither pain nor suffering at the conscious level within hypnosis; when the hypnosis is terminated, he remembers only his comfort in what would otherwise have been a painful situation. Although studies show that some types of central stimulation may modify what goes on at the spinal level, it is unlikely that the major influence of central processes within hypnosis occurs at that level. One reason for supposing it lies elsewhere is that, although spinal influence could account for pain reduction, hypnosis can also be used for pain production—for the hallucination of pain without external stimulation. Absence of pain (when physical conditions for pain are present) and hallucinated pain (when physical conditions for pain are absent) are similar to other hallucinatory phenomena within hypnosis in areas not related to pain, such as visual or auditory perception. Hallucinations not related to pain are also responsive to automatic writing or automatic talking, as illustrated in the original demonstration with hypnotic deafness. We have performed similar experiments in other sensory areas; an experience overtly denied in hypnosis may be revealed as having been perceived at a covert level through the automatic procedures.

Hence we seem to be dealing with broader mechanisms than those applicable only to pain and suffering. What goes on is much more likely to be a phenomenon of higher brain centers than a centrifugal influence of the brain upon lower centers. The heart of the problem is explaining how sensory information can be registered and processed even though it is not overtly available, and even though its conscious processing has been distorted by hypnotic suggestion.

Posthypnotic amnesia is the most familiar hypnotic mechanism that has the characteristics of registration and storage along with temporary unavailability to consciousness. The inaccessible information about felt pain in hypnotic analgesia, and about other perceptions concealed by negative hallucinations, must be stored in a manner similar to that in which amnesic memories are stored. If we understood amnesia better, part of our problem would be solved. One additional question would still have to be answered. In the usual posthypnotic amnesia, the original registration of perceptions is overt; only the temporary inability to recall creates the problem. In covert pain an additional first step is involved, in which the perception of the pain is diverted to an amnesic condition *before it has ever entered consciousness.* These two steps of explanation—how the initial experience is deflected from consciousness, and how it is stored in inaccessible form—must be undertaken hypothetically, since amnesia itself, though familiar, is not understood.

In order to deal with two levels of reporting, overt and covert, it is convenient to conceive of alternative control systems that may be split off from each other. At a descriptive level, such alternative control systems are familiar in hypnosis because one effect of hypnosis is to change the ways in which controls operate. What is normally voluntary may become involuntary; what is normally remembered may be forgotten; and what is normally unavailable to recall may be remembered. The dominance of normal waking controls is reduced, though not obliterated. For example, if the hypnotic subject is given a suggestion which violates his self-conception, he is likely to be aroused from hypnosis; we may attribute responsibility for this arousal to the normal waking control system.

If we apply the concept of divided cognitive control systems to our pain experiments, the change in controls may be illustrated as in Figure 15. The

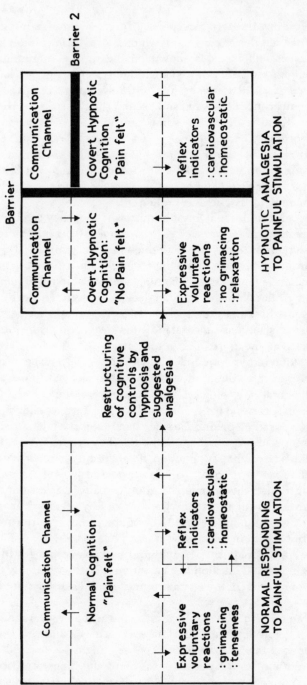
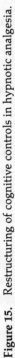

Figure 15. Restructuring of cognitive controls in hypnotic analgesia.

diagram on the left shows the normal response to painful stimulation, with all communication channels open. The way in which restructuring takes place is not indicated, but its end result is shown on the right. Communication barriers have been erected between two cognitive systems: one is available and listed as *Overt Hypnotic Cognition*; the other system records the pain information in some concealed way, and is described as *Covert Hypnotic Cognition*. Between them is *Barrier 1*—something that prevents them from interacting in the ordinary hypnotic analgesia condition. *Barrier 2* keeps the covert cognition from being reported, unless it is broken by a technique such as automatic writing or automatic talking. It should be noted that Barrier 2 can be broken without the Overt Hypnotic Cognition being aware of it; hence Barrier 1 may remain while Barrier 2 is broken.

These barriers are similar to hypnotic amnesia in that they can be made permeable by a prearranged signal, such as the statement to be made after the subject is out of hypnosis: "Now you can remember everything." The main difference from ordinary amnesia is that the covert information about pain is placed behind Barrier 1 without ever becoming conscious. In usual hypnotic amnesia, something once known and attended to is forgotten, to be later recovered; here, something not previously in awareness may later be recovered. Amnesia itself is hard to understand; this deflection from memory prior to perception is all the more difficult to explain.

The interpretation of hypnotic analgesia as a split consciousness (represented by the two separate communication channels) suggests an explanation for the paradox that physiological signs of stress continue, even though the subject consciously feels no pain. These reflex indicators are shown in the right-hand diagram as falling behind the same barriers as the felt pain; hence the subject pays no attention to them even though they occur. The voluntary expressions, to which he might pay attention, do not occur, or occur at greatly reduced values. The fact that covert pain (as shown in the right-hand diagram) is less intense than the normal cognition of pain (the left-hand diagram) may be accounted for in part by the lack of any feedback from the usual "voluntary" expressions of pain. These are present in the normal reaction to pain, but absent in the analgesic situation.

We can now approximate an explanation if we can account for the two steps in amnesia: first, the deflection from awareness at the time of registration; and second, the storing of the memory under an amnesic barrier subject to later recovery.

A serious attempt to account for the first step was made several decades ago by Sears, in a theoretical paper dealing with amnesia and problems of memory. He proposed that anticipatory responses might be aroused when the threat of an emotion-laden experience was imminent. These anticipatory responses could be linked, by conditioning, to alternative responses so that, when the expected stimulus occurred, the normal response would *not* occur. In the case of pain, the sequence would be somewhat as follows. (1) The subject, through prior learning, knows that when given analgesia suggestions he will do something other than feel pain—perhaps engage in fantasy, imagine his arm is numb, or whatever has succeeded in the past. (2) He has experienced pain normally in the past and will respond homeostatically to the pain when it comes; thus the pain will "register," even if it is not consciously perceived. (3) When the pain is threatened, the amnesic sequence is initiated; the alternative to pain takes over and the pain, though registered, is not overtly perceived.

This is all conjectural, but at this state of our knowledge, we have to fall back on conjecture. There is evidence that something important happens before the stress appears, when the subject is preparing to make himself analgesic. Demonstrable rises in both heart rate and blood pressure occur when the ordinarily painful stimulus is threatened, especially if the subject is to be analgesic. That is, the rises in these physiological indicators are greater when analgesia is to follow than when the actual pain is to be overtly experienced. These bodily signs in advance of the stimulus may indicate that some kind of cognitive arousal is taking place as the pain is about to be diverted from consciousness. This is the direction that the solution to the first part of our problem may take—that is, that the pain experience is deflected from consciousness by an anticipatory reaction which conceals it behind a shield of amnesia.

If hypnotic suggestions can shift controls from one system to another, as appears to be the case, then we have an approach to our second question. The question is how the covert material can be made overt. This kind of thing happens whenever hypnotic amnesia is relieved—or, for that matter, when other controls are altered within hypnosis, as when an arm stiffened by suggestion is made normal again.

Assigning the problem of covert pain to a process similar to amnesia places it where it belongs, but it is not a satisfactory explanation because of the difficulties in explaining amnesia. Yet at a phenomenal level, the play of amnesic processes is very evident. An unexpected finding from a recent experiment gives validity to the separation of the overt and covert reporting systems, and to the amnesic relations between them. A subject in an ischemic pain experiment had just had his tourniquet removed; he had felt neither pain nor suffering, but now that he was told his arm would return to normal, he felt the tingling associated with the return of blood into the arm. This tingling was gradually subsiding when the subject was questioned about covert pain by the automatic talking technique; the hidden observer reported that he had felt sensory pain but no suffering. When the experimenter's hand was removed from the subject's shoulder, he made the spontaneous comment: "Strange, there has been a quantum reduction in the tingling just now." It appeared that the hypnotic consciousness had receded and was not aware of the tingling while the hidden observer was talking. Now that the hypnotic consciousness was restored, there was a gap during which the tingling had been steadily reducing; the collapsing of the gap by amnesia made it seem that there had been a sudden step decrease. The experimenter placed his hand on the subject's shoulder again, and the subject spontaneously said he had been wrong about the quantum change—a steady reduction had been taking place while he was talking previously. The experimenter lifted his hand again and, to his surprise, the subject said: "That's funny, there have been two quantum changes in tingling, the one I felt before and another one just now." Quite evidently, the separation between the hidden aspect and the hypnotic aspect was so complete that the same foreshortening had taken place again, and the explanation of the earlier one was not remembered.

A word should be said about the nonhypnotic reduction of pain through suggestion in the waking condition. We indicated earlier that there might be two components to pain reduction by hypnotic analgesia suggestions: first, a component similar to that in waking suggestion, and second, a component added for the highly hypnotizable by the amnesic processes we have been discussing. This separation was made for two reasons: first, for highly hypnotizable subjects waking suggestion was not as successful as the hypnotic suggestion; and second, the covert reports were of pain reduced to about the same level to which it was reduced by waking analgesia. If we assign the hypnotic component of pain reduction to the amnesic effect, what about the nonhypnotic component? One candidate for that is the observed general relaxation and lack of somatic response to the pain. A subject deliberately —and successfully—attempting to imagine that his hand and arm were numb, or trying to distract his attention away from the pain, could be observed to be very quiet and to have the voluntary signs of pain well under control. It may be that when these somatic responses are absent, pain is decreased because of lack of feedback from them, as in the James-Lange theory about the repercussion of emotional responses upon felt emotion. These responses are also absent in hypnotic analgesia, so, according to the same line of thought, the covert experience of pain would be expected to be reduced below its normal sensory level even when pain registers and the memory of it is recoverable.

Some Physiological Possibilities. The brain must be the key to the divisions in consciousness that occur in the control of pain, and to the relative accessibility of overt and covert pain, when the two are distinguishable. The brain is of course complex enough to allow for many ways in which this might occur; unfortunately, it is too complex for anyone to be sure just what the actual processes are that account for the empirical observations in our experiments. However, some directions in which to look are already open.

One possible source of divided consciousness is an actual duality: we have a right and a left hemisphere that act somewhat differently. We do not now know the full implications of the distinctiveness of the two hemispheres, but we might look for a division of function and perhaps a division in memory storage that would account for the division of consciousness.

Another approach to dissociated experiences is the peculiar action of certain drugs upon the retention and reinstatement of learned experiences, leading to what is called *state-dependent* learning. If learning takes place under the influence of an appropriate drug, the memory for that learning may be unavailable in the nondrugged state, but return when the person is again under the influence of the drug. This occasionally happens with alcohol: the drinker forgets what he said or did while intoxicated, only to remember it again when next intoxicated. Because the memory is stored, but unavailable except under special circumstances, this phenomenon has some characteristics of hypnotic amnesia. Presumably, when the site and nature of these effects become known, they may have some bearing on the physiological substratum for hypnosis.

The evolutionary history of the brain provides other clues to splits in awareness. The "old brain" of gray matter around the central parts of the brain has much to do with emotion and motivation, and hence is related to the distress or suffering component of the pain experience. The "new brain" is made up of the cerebral hemispheres, outpouchings from the old brain that are more recent in evolutionary history; their surface (the cerebral cortex) is the most advanced part of the brain. Parts of the cerebral cortex have separate functions: some frontal and prefrontal structures appear to interact with the old brain to integrate the reactions of anguish and distress, and a body-sense area, at the top of the head behind the central fissure, integrates the sensory experience of pain. Such information might help in understanding the experiences of pain and suffering that occur in some of our experiments; the differences between the two systems are recognized in the gate control theory of pain.

New knowledge may be obtained by experimental methods at the human levels that do no violence to the human subject. Because of the importance of verbal reports of pain and distress, animal experiments can give only partial answers to the question of splits in consciousness. The possibilities of experimentation with human subjects can be illustrated by a recent collaborative study done in our laboratory, jointly with an expert on the influence of opiates and their antagonists on the central nervous system. Because we had some subjects who could completely eliminate both overt pain and distress in hypnotic analgesia, while reporting sensory pain but no distress at the covert level, we were able to test a reasonable hypothesis regarding the central location of the control over distress that left the sensory pain intact.

The steps in reaching the hypothesis are several, but they can be followed without familiarity with the anatomical or pharmacological details. There is an area in the central part of the brain that is very sensitive to morphine; morphine injection there tends to reduce distress without affecting the sensory component of pain. A morphine antagonist, naloxone, can bring back the pain by counteracting the morphine. The next step in reasoning is based on empirical evidence, but is somewhat more speculative. It has been found that electrical stimulation at the site where morphine is most effective can also produce analgesia. The speculation is that perhaps this works by releasing a chemical substance with some of the properties of morphine. Many chemical intermediaries of neural activity are known to be produced in the nervous system, so this thought is not too far-fetched. This speculation was tested by using naloxone, the morphine antagonist; it was found that the analgesia produced by electrical stimulation was indeed counteracted, as if a morphine-like substance had been produced. The final step in reasoning is that perhaps hypnotic analgesia, like electrical stimulation, releases such a substance in the centers related to suffering. If so, naloxone might counteract hypnotic analgesia as it counteracts the electrically produced analgesia. The experiment permitted a test of this hypothesis. The results were negative—that is, naloxone had no effect on either pain or distress. Hence the nature of the action of hypnotic analgesia must be looked for elsewhere. Of course a positive result would have been more exciting, but one role of experimentation is to eliminate alternatives, and this experiment served a useful purpose. That purpose could not have been served without using our method for assessing covert pain and suffering, and without the advances in the pharmacology of morphine and its antagonists. In that way, contributions from various sciences operate together in the advancement of knowledge.

Activities related to hypnosis, such as dreaming, sleeptalking, and sleepwalking, involve lack of awareness by one part of the brain of what another part is doing, even though these detached events involve processes normally conscious. The fact that our knowledge of underlying brain mechanisms is incomplete is a challenge to further study. A breakthrough in any one of these areas will increase understanding in the others.

Some Psychological Possibilities.   The questions about splits in consciousness raised in connection with the pain experiments have been asked about consciousness before, in other settings. Splits in personality were prominent in the work of Janet in the last century; he developed a theory of dissociation to account for what he observed when a person seemed to be divided against himself. Studies of multiple personality began at that time by Prince and by others. One of the characteristics shared by multiple personalities and by the splits we have shown in pain is the evident role of an amnesic process. Often, in multiple personality, Personality A will not know about Personality B, even though B may share A's memories.

The most prominent theory to address itself to levels of awareness is, of course, psychoanalysis. In its modern form of ego psychology it provides a means of talking about the kinds of splits shown in the pain experiments. These divided cognitive systems would be considered temporary partial structures within the ego, according to the interpretation of hypnosis offered by Gill and Brenman. It should be noted that the subconscious processes with which we are dealing are not deeply unconscious in the psychoanalytic sense; they belong more nearly to the preconscious than to the unconscious.

Perhaps the role enactment theory of Sarbin could be applied; overt and covert pain reports might represent two levels of role behavior. However, the straightforward labeling of roles does not help to resolve the troublesome problems of amnesia.

Puzzling over these problems has led one of us to propose a neo-dissociation theory, deriving in part from earlier dissociation theory, but not committed to its historical form. Its rationale is that the results of the studies of pain can be generalized beyond the pain setting; and if a more satisfactory general theory can be arrived at, the pain results will also be explained. The distinction between the overt and covert reporting systems suggests the presence of alternate cognitive controls in human consciousness. These controls must have a hierarchical arrangement, because either of them may, on occasion, be in ascendance. A model for the role of hypnosis can be projected from the two reporting systems. It is based on the separation of the two systems, the inhibitory processes that separate them, and the role of hypnosis in enhancing or reducing this amnesic process. As a generalization from this model, hypnotic procedures can be seen as rearranging the hierarchies of control over systems other than those involved in pain. When presented in summary form, this is very abstract; however, it would take us afield to go into more detail. The main point is that the discovery of split cognitive systems in pain has further implications for the study of human consciousness. If a satisfactory understanding emerges, the pain experiments will have contributed to human understanding beyond what they have contributed to the relief of suffering.

Concluding Remarks on Hidden Pain

The fact that some pain is covert does not deny the reality of pain relief by hypnosis. The physiological signs that persist are minor compared to those found in agonizing experiences. The small rises in heart rate and blood pressure within hypnotic analgesia are of theoretical interest in showing that some physiological responsiveness persists within the analgesia, but they are not as pronounced as the changes that occur in only slightly stressful actions, such as running up a flight of stairs.

With respect to hypnotic analgesia, we are left with this conclusion. Both pain and distress are greatly reduced in the overt experience of those who are responsive to hypnotic suggestions. When the hypnosis is terminated, such persons are comfortable; the question of covert pain does not arise any more than it arises after chemical anesthesia, in which there may also be covert pain. Covert pain is of great theoretical interest, however, because it dramatizes the possibility of different levels of cognitive functioning.

Notes

The discovery of the "hidden observer" to account for covert pain was first reported in Hilgard (1973c). The possibility that a technique of "automatic talking" might be equivalent to "automatic writing" was suggested by our associates, Macdonald and Stevenson. The experiments on automatic writing that were being conducted in our laboratory were those of Stevenson (1972) and Knox, Crutchfield, and Hilgard (1975).

Covert Pain in Hypnotic Analgesia

The experiments on cold pressor pain in which automatic key-pressing and automatic talking were employed have been reported briefly in Hilgard (1975c), and in Hilgard, Morgan, and Macdonald (1975).

The corresponding experiments with ischemia were reported by Knox, Morgan, and Hilgard (1974). Rapid reinstatement of amnesia, required in this set of experiments, has been frequently shown to be possible by Blum (1972). The additional experiment, briefly referred to, is that of Goldstein and Hilgard (1975).

Anticipations from the Past

The reference to Durand de Gros (1868) comes from Ellenberger (1970). The quotation regarding the active nervous system is from Myers (1903, p. 179). He was a founder of the Society for Psychical Research, a friend of William James, and a careful observer. Regardless of the spiritualistic title to his two-volume work (*Human Personality and its Survival of Bodily Death*), the first volume is a mine of information upon hypnosis, automatic writing, and related topics. His reference to recovery of memories of things happening under general anesthesia is on p. 473. The experiment by James is reported in detail in James (1889), but is also reported in his textbook (James, 1890, vol. I, p. 208), in a context in which it is readily overlooked. The two later accounts along the same lines are from Estabrooks (1957) and Kaplan (1960).

Hypnotic Analgesia Understood as a Split in Consciousness

Pain hallucinated under hypnosis provides a good illustration of genuinely felt pain without any local source of irritation. Accounts can be found by Barber and Hahn (1964); Dudley and others (1966); Hilgard (1971); and Hilgard and Morgan (1975). The existence of hallucinated pain places limits on any pain theory that requires peripheral stimulation to produce pain.

Reports by automatic talking showing covert perception within other kinds of hypnotic hallucination were obtained in our laboratory by Gettinger (1974). The tasks included selective deafness, a positive music hallucination, anosmia to ammonia, and both positive and negative visual hallucinations. The results varied somewhat from person to person, but for each task some subjects who honestly reported the reality of the overt distortion had covert information based on the physical characteristics (or lack of them) perceived in the midst of the hypnotic distortion.

The theory proposed for diverting something from consciousness before it becomes registered is based on Sears (1936). The arousal of physiological indicators in anticipation of analgesia was reported in Hilgard, Macdonald, Marshall, and Morgan (1974).

The problem of pain reduction in the waking condition is complicated by the exact instructions used. Highly hypnotizable subjects have available to them the pain reduction of selfhypnosis, unless they are specifically instructed to reduce the pain without becoming hypnotized. In the latter case, holding themselves out of hypnosis takes some cognitive effort. The experiments of Spanos, Barber, and Lang (1974) and of Evans and Paul (1970), in which the researchers believed they had found no differences between waking and hypnotic analgesia, are not decisive—both on this score and because they used unselected subjects, many of whom would not be expected to show any differences by any test as a consequence of hypnotic induction. In disagreement with their conclusions, we found significant differences between waking and hypnotic analgesia with highly susceptible subjects. They were able to reduce their pain through waking suggestion, but not as much as through hypnosis (Hilgard, 1975c). The results of Greene and Reyher (1972), in which highly hypnotizable subjects, when not hypnotized, reduced pain less than corresponding subjects who were hypnotized, point in the same direction.

The physiological possibilities opened up by the split brain studies were mentioned in Chapter 1.

State-dependent learning has been widely studied in animals, but only occasionally in man; a good summary is provided by Overton (1972).

The experiment to determine whether or not naloxone would antagonize hypnotic analgesia was done in collaboration with Goldstein, at his suggestion (Goldstein and Hilgard, 1975).

It would take us away from our central concern with pain to discuss what goes on in sleep. Apparently sleeptalking does not occur in the same state as dreaming; night dreams may be recalled when the sleeptalking is forgotten (Arkin and others, 1970).

The possibility of recovering covert memories of experiences within general anesthesia was mentioned by Myers (1903); it is discussed in Chapter 7 of this book. An effort to use hypnosis to break the amnesia produced by thiopental, in which experimenters and subjects from our laboratory participated, had very limited success (Osborn and others, 1967).

The psychological theories mentioned as offering some explanatory possibilities include the dissociation theory of Janet (1887; 1907) and of Prince (1906; 1975). Psychoanalytic ego psychology was applied to hypnotic problems most thoroughly by Gill and Brenman (1959). The role enactment theory of Sarbin has been described over the years, but most completely in Sarbin and Coe (1972). The theory of Sears (1936) was based on aspects of learning, with some reference also to dissociation and psychoanalysis. The modernized form of dissociation theory, under the name of neodissociation theory, was related to the pain studies by Hilgard (1973b; 1973c; 1974). A fuller discussion can be found in a chapter devoted to it (Hilgard, 1976a), and in a forthcoming book (Hilgard, in preparation).

10 The Future of Hypnosis
in Pain Control

It is hazardous to predict the future of hypnosis, particularly in view of past fluctuations in its acceptability and practice. Today, our civilization is in a period of re-assessment of its human values; antiscientific trends appear to be gaining ascendancy. Such intellectual oscillations have occurred in the past, as in the revival of fundamentalist religion in America in the mid-nineteenth century, after a period of very liberal deism. We note the growth of nonestablishment religious groups and of faith-healing sects, as well as the rise of Eastern religions and such offshoots as secular meditation groups. Many of these groups make claims about pain relief.

Interest in consciousness expansion and hidden human potentialities leads some to turn to hypnosis. Such an interest brings attention to hypnosis but threatens its scientific status. In an era in which choice may lie between uncritical commitment and the restraints of a more sober science, we hope to have contributed to the attitudes associated with scientific endeavor.

We do not mean to overplay the role of science. Many legitimate criticisms may be made of science and technology in modern life; the search for other means to satisfy human aspirations is understandable. With respect to the healing arts, however, there is reason for critical caution. The healings that have taken place at shrines and through religious practices attest to the importance of mental factors in illness; in that way folk practices confirm some of the claims made for hypnosis. But the caution is this: *whenever there is no diagnostic procedure and all illnesses are treated by a uniform method or ceremony* the benefits are accompanied by dangers to the health of the person and to the health of others. Examples are readily found in undiagnosed tumors, broken bones, and contagious diseases.

The immediate problem is pain relief, and here we are on firm ground. For a great many people—we cannot say exactly how many—hypnotic procedures can bring relief from sensory pain. Hypnosis does not merely produce relaxation and relief from anxiety and thus make the pain more tolerable; it is capable of reducing the pain itself so it is not felt at all, or is felt at greatly reduced and acceptable levels. The evidence presented in the preceding chapters is clear, and our own experience both with laboratory subjects and with patients in severe pain gives ample assurance of this.

What We have Learned

Our review of pain reduction in the laboratory and the clinic leads to a number of generalizations that could not have been made with as much confidence even as recently as ten years ago. The following assertions, based on evidence already presented, may serve as a kind of summary of the findings.

1. *The more hypnotizable a person is found to be, according to available scales of hypnotic responsiveness, the greater the chance he will be able to reduce pain through hypnotically suggested analgesia.* This relationship has been demonstrated repeatedly under laboratory conditions. It has been shown less frequently in the clinic; however, when assessment of hypnotizability has been attempted in the clinic, the same tendency has been found.

2. *Pain reduction involves both sensory pain and suffering and is not attributable to anxiety reduction.* Hypnosis alone may have a quieting effect, but it does not in itself produce analgesia. Analgesia occurs following specific suggestions for pain reduction, which are usually given directly, although under some circumstances they may be given quite indirectly.

3. *Hypnosis frequently contributes to anxiety reduction, but this effect should be distinguished from pain reduction.* In some situations, as when a patient is anticipating surgery and when he is recovering afterward, pain and anxiety are difficult to separate. Both may affect pain tolerance, making it hard to distinguish between a sedative effect and an analgesic effect. The two major components of pain—sensory pain and suffering—are distinguishable, but tolerance is something beyond these. An heroic person may tolerate both pain and suffering at levels a less heroic person would reject. A chemical tranquilizer may increase tolerance without reducing the primary pain experience. In some cases hypnosis may substitute for such a tranquilizer, but that differs from its role as an analgesic.

4. *Hypnotic pain reduction procedures are equally applicable to many painful conditions.* The same procedures of pain reduction appear to be useful

in many situations: when the pain is short and episodic, as in most dental procedures; when it is longer but with known termination, as in the labor of childbirth and surgery; or even when it is protracted over days or weeks, as in cancer or burns. This means that a clinician in one field of practice can learn from successful methods used in another field. For example, the method of glove anesthesia, with transfer of the insensitivity to another area, appears to be applicable in all of these cases. Similarly, displacement of pain from one area to another and conversion to a more acceptable symptom are widely useful practices. Removal from the scene through fantasy—the reliving of a pleasant event from the past, or the experiencing of an imagined pleasant adventure—appears again and again in reports of successful pain reduction in varied situations.

Another important feature is the preparation of the patient. The rehearsal method has been reported most often in connection with surgical procedures, including caesarean sections; however, it is applicable to other anxiety-producing situations as well, such as normal childbirth and dental procedures.

5. *Induction procedures are changing, with increasing emphasis upon self-hypnosis.* Although they derive in part from a common lore about hypnosis, induction procedures have come increasingly to include more participation by the subject or patient. The subject is active both in selecting areas of fantasy to serve his purposes and in maintaining two-way communication with the hypnotic practitioner. Often some degree of self-hypnosis is involved. The older emphases on relaxation and sleep from earlier practices are maintained because they have their own useful benefits. Some older techniques of induction— swinging pendulums, whirling disks, upward straining eyes—are used less and less. They are unnecessary, and in some cases they distract from the naturalness of the procedures.

6. *The authoritarian hypnotist is giving way to the more permissive guide.* The old stereotype of the hypnotist who orders the patient's symptoms away and controls through authoritarian posthypnotic suggestions no longer fits current practice. Freud saw Bernheim use such nineteenth-century practices, and objected to them. The modern approach is more individualized; the professional clinician using hypnosis in his practice attends to the special needs of the patient, prepares him for what is to come, and enhances the patient's confidence in his own ability to cope.

The foregoing assertions can be made with confidence. They furnish a basis from which to make recommendations regarding the clinical use of hypnosis.

Hypnosis in the Treatment of
Other Painful Conditions

We have demonstrated that hypnotic suggestions can reduce pain with obvious somatic origins, as in cancer, obstetrics, surgery, and dentistry. We hope we have also made it clear that these do not exhaust the applicability of hypnosis to the problems of pain.

A number of cases are at hand in which hypnosis has been used in treating other pains. For example, migraine headaches, estimated to affect about 5 percent of the adult population, frequently have both organic and psychological components. Harding has reported his successes and failures in hypnotic treatment of ninety patients, twenty-six males and sixty-four females, who came to him with intractable migraines. The number of sessions with each patient ranged from 4 to 7; the sessions averaged 30 minutes in length. An inquiry six months to eight years after the hypnotic treatment showed that 38 percent had obtained complete relief; 32 percent found moderate relief; and the remaining 30 percent either had no relief or were lost to follow-up. The degree of success is sufficient to encourage further trials with his method; Harding has in fact continued, and his success rate with 200 patients is at least as great as that reported for the first 90. Anderson, Basker, and Dalton have recently provided additional evidence of the effectiveness of hypnotic treatment of migraine. Ten of twenty-three migraine sufferers treated by hypnotherapy showed complete remission during the last three months of treatment. The hypnotic pain reduction was evidently not a placebo effect, because only three of twenty-four patients treated with an ineffective drug (prochlorperazine) had remission of symptoms.

Another illustration is that of phantom limb pain. Cedercreutz and Uusitalo, investigators in a hospital in Finland, have used hypnosis in more than 100 cases of painful phantoms following amputations. Their results have been so promising that they believe hypnosis should always be attempted before any other treatment. In thirty-seven cases in which the patient had lost either an arm or a leg, twenty claimed that their symptoms disappeared immediately after the hypnosis, and ten more felt that their condition had improved. Unfortunately, as with many treatments for pain by other methods, symptoms may recur; in follow-ups ranging up to eight years, the researchers found only eight of the thirty-seven treated who remained symptom-free, although ten more were still improved. These patients had suffered an average of six years before treatment; the investigators felt they might have been more successful had they seen the patients sooner. They further believe that success is related to hypnotic responsiveness; if the patient is not hypnotized within the first three sessions, the chance of providing symptomatic aid is slight. It was probably unfortunate that the hypnotists in this study did not have access to the patients repeatedly to reinforce the benefits of earlier therapy. Such repetition would be expected in the course of ordinary psychotherapy, and there is no reason to expect hypnosis to operate effectively if limited to a single session or a very brief course of treatment.

These illustrations from migraine and phantom limb pain suffice to show the possibility of subjecting various clinical pain syndromes to treatment by hypnosis. The value of the information gained in clinical studies is enhanced if accompanied by statistics on successes and failures.

Many other painful symptoms have been reduced or eliminated by hypnosis, as evidenced by occasional clinical reports. There are such reports on tic douloureux (trigeminal neuralgia), and on common neck and lower back pains. The range of patients who can be helped by hypnosis is illustrated in a recent study by Melzack and Perry. Twenty-four subjects all had chronic pains incompletely relieved by the drugs that they were taking. Their diagnoses were back pain (10), peripheral nerve injury (4), cancer (3), arthritis (2), phantom limb and stump pain (2), posttraumatic (2), and head pain (1). Because of the small numbers involved, the report gives no indication by category of pain, but overall some 33 percent gained marked relief through hypnosis. The degree of relief on which this success is based was defined as reduction of the initial pain by at least one-third. It is of interest that this proportion is almost identical to that for a whole sample of experimental subjects who were able to reduce laboratory pains one-third or more through hypnosis (see Figure 7 in Chapter 4).

In not discussing many of these pains, we do not mean to imply that hypnosis is inappropriate in their treatment. In some cases it may be appropriate, in others not. Diagnostic procedures need to be thoroughly attended to before a decision is made as to the treatment. Our concern in the earlier chapters has been the reduction of primary somatogenic pain, and we have confined discussion to a few conditions in which such pains are the prominent symptoms.

Psychological and Psychiatric Aspects of Pain

We have definite reservations about extending hypnotic treatment to pains without adequate diagnosis. It might be supposed that a pain of psychological origin would be more readily eliminated by hypnosis than one of organic origin. That is not necessarily the case, because of the differences in meaning to the patients of the two kinds of pain. A pain clearly of somatic origin, such as that from an accident, is one the patient would gladly eliminate; the student who breaks his leg on the ski slope does not welcome the accident, and is pleased to free himself of the pain. On the other hand, pain that has psychological roots is serving some purpose for the individual in pain, and hence may be harder for him to relinquish. In other words, direct pain relief may be more appropriate for pain of focal somatic origin, while multiple psychotherapeutic considerations enter into the control of pain whose origin is primarily psychological.

If a pain is suspected of being primarily psychological in origin, direct symptom removal may or may not be recommended. Diagnostic procedures to determine which treatment is to be used involve the same problems as psychiatry and clinical psychology in general: how to select well from the myriad of treatments available. If pain is the presenting problem, the direct approach is preferred when the condition is essentially monosymptomatic and peripheral to the personality. Many war casualties were of this kind and thus lent themselves well to direct symptom removal; the conditions of warfare and the excessive strains they imposed were so unusual that, even if the pains were in part psychogenic, they corresponded closely to somatic accidents in ordinary life.

We have not dealt with psychiatric aspects of pain in our discussion because of the complexity of pain in patients in need of psychiatric or psychological help. As we have stressed in our clinical reports, we have limited ourselves as much as possible to the organic (somatogenic) sphere. This is the area in which knowledge gained in the laboratory has most bearing upon clinical practice; it has given a base for comparison and integration of the work of the laboratory and the clinic. It is only part of the whole story of pain, however. The existence of a close connection between pain and psychiatric illness is indicated by a number of studies, of which one by Spear is illustrative. He found that of 200 consecutive admissions to a psychiatric clinic, 53 percent had pain as one of their symptoms. Pain occurred, for example, in half the patients who suffered from depression, and in more than half of those grouped as anxiety or hysteria patients. The association of pain with psychological illness is well documented.

In their *Studies in Hysteria*, published in 1895, Breuer and Freud gave detailed case histories of five patients. All four reported by Freud and the one reported by Breuer had pain as one of the presenting symptoms. All five patients were treated by hypnosis, and a psychodynamic foundation for the understanding of hysteria was developed. In this treatment, which antedated psychoanalysis, hypnosis was used as an uncovering technique; Freud found that with it he could unravel ways in which the symptoms, including pain, had resulted from unconscious conflicts.

Although Freud shifted to the method of free association, subsequent workers have developed theories about the psychogenesis of pain on the basis of his earlier and continuing contributions. Pain can in some instances be conceived as a punishment for sexual pleasures and fantasies perceived as forbidden; or, it may occur as an unconscious defense against aggression. An association of pain with hostility, conflict, and guilt has been described by numerous investigators. To relieve headache of the conversion type—in which the headache represents something disturbing in the patient's past —Eisenbud used a rehearsal technique under hypnosis. The disturbing events were first recalled with emotional release in hypnosis; later, they could be comfortably reviewed when awake. Eisenbud also used hypnotic procedures to produce headaches as a consequence of artificially induced complexes. Of six cases in which he produced aggressive or hostile complexes, three resulted in headache. When the complexes involved hetero-sexual erotic conflict, no headaches occurred, although other behavioral derivatives of the implanted complex ensued. Eisenbud was cautious in generalizing from his study, but it gave support to a relation of repressed hostility to some instances of pain.

Engel described twenty patients with atypical facial pain, which he regarded as a hysterical conversion symptom. He thought it most prominent in persons with a masochistic character structure, who become "pain-prone" patients. One patient in our experience was a married woman with periodic atypical facial neuralgia on the left side. A hard slap by her husband on that part of her face, five years earlier, had apparently triggered the onset. After this first occasion, her feelings of hostility and guilt toward her husband following arguments with him precipitated the facial symptom, even though he did not repeat his overt attack. Upon treatment with a combination of conventional psychotherapy and hypnotic therapy, the patient showed sub-stantial improvement.

Pain is associated not only with conversion mechanisms but with a wide variety of conditions such as anxiety, depression, obsessive-compulsive states, addictions, and the psychoses. The problems of gaining a benefit from symptoms—secondary gain—emphasize the role of other persons, whether members of the family, friends and associates, or consulting professionals. These considerations have led to some variants in the psychological theo-rizing about pain and its appropriate treatment. Szasz, for example, has developed a portrait of the person suffering persistent pain as *l'homme dou-loureux*, who needs to occupy the role of the man in pain. Sternbach, too, discusses the chronic pain patient, who frequently makes a career of a variety of "pain games." No matter whether chronic pain is primarily somatogenic or psychogenic, its effect is, as he states it, "to make formerly emotionally stable persons into chronic manipulators." Such patients manipulate their physi-cians to fit into their needs, and their pains persist.

It was in recognition of these complexities that we chose to limit our-selves to pains that had clear organic causes. Nevertheless, even in those selected situations, we sometimes found an overlay of psychological features. They have been mentioned earlier, as in the treatment of pain in cancer patients. The patient may want very much to get rid of the pain, but may have a deeper need to suffer.

The clinician may feel a lingering uneasiness that if pain is a psychogenic symptom, its removal will lead to substitution of a new symptom to serve the same purpose. This is possible, and it occasionally does occur; hence the therapist who uses hypnosis must be well trained in diagnostic procedures and in alternative therapies. Seitz reported some cases in which such substitutions occurred spontaneously; he then showed how hypnosis might exaggerate them. He and Rosen have warned particularly against hypnotic removal of symptoms which serve as defenses against potentially psychotic dissociative reactions. The occurrence of symptom substitution was noted by Harding in his study of migraine patients. Among ninety cases he found seven whose new symptoms might be considered substitutes: three cases of ulcers, and one each of sexual impotence, hay fever, arthritis, and repetitive nightmares.

A number of interesting analogues of familiar defenses are found within the hypnotic control of pain. These days there is a tendency to consider less the negative aspects of defense as irrational and self-deceptive, and to recognize more that defenses may be primarily coping mechanisms.

In traditional dynamic psychiatry, defenses against the anxieties produced by psychological pain or conflict include amnesia (repression), substitution, denial, displacement, and retreat into fantasy. Dynamic methods are designed to probe the underlying reasons for resorting to these defensive maneuvers. The mechanisms of substitution, displacement, and denial are useful tools in hypnotic treatment of pain; in this connection they have been repeatedly illustrated in the experimental and clinical literature. Symptoms may be *substituted*, so what was pain becomes a tingling sensation; symptoms may be *displaced*, so a pain in the abdomen may be felt in a finger; or symptoms may be *denied*, so an arm previously felt to be in pain is now reported as without pain, even though our techniques may show that covert pain is present. Two other forms of denial have been illustrated frequently: amnesia and selective awareness. The amnesic mechanism may erase all memories of a previous experience, as though it never existed. Selective awareness permits the person to divide his consciousness in such a manner that his fantasy may displace the perception of physical reality. A patient may imagine himself watching TV in the next room, leaving his painful body in the bedroom; under these circumstances he may feel no pain.

Although these defensive techniques are initiated at the suggestion of the hypnotist, they nevertheless correspond to ego defenses within psychodynamic theory. Even when the patient comes for pain relief, habitual defenses may operate in hypnosis in other ways than in controlling pain. Many subtle manifestations of defense have been described by Gill and Brenman, who give an interpretation of hypnosis according to contemporary psychoanalytic ego theory. When the problem is essentially psychotherapeutic —as it may be in some pain cases—hypnosis may weaken ego defenses and lead to a display of emotion during induction. We have found such a release of emotion during induction very rare in our experimental work; it is probably more common as an emotional release among those who come for treatment because of personality problems. If hypnosis has produced disturbance by touching a sensitive area, a resistance to hypnosis may develop as a way of strengthening the defense. These complexities are unlikely to arise in the kinds of pain cases we have been discussing, in which pain of organic origin is the primary symptom.

In pain cases in which the diagnosis is baffling—the condition commonly referred to as *intractable pain*—it would be wise if the psychiatrist or psychologist could be brought in during early diagnostic procedures. If psychological factors are pertinent, they should be studied. A psychological or psychiatric diagnosis should not merely emerge as a residual probability when organic factors are ruled out. Furthermore, a past history of organic pain does not eliminate psychological factors in the present complaint: phantom limb pains present a useful illustration, because there has been genuine organic etiology (in the amputation itself), yet the psychological components are evident. As noted earlier, some specialists on phantom pains believe psychological methods should be utilized first, rather than last. If psychological or psychiatric methods are not introduced early, the patient who can be helped by them may embark instead on a prolonged, expensive series of treatments, including repeated surgery, which may leave his main problems unmet and his pain unrelieved.

A great many persons who have pain among their symptoms are being treated by psychotherapy. This is clear from the data on the frequency of pain as found in the psychiatric patient. These patients, however, are usually not reported in the pain literature; hence the effectiveness of psychotherapy in treating pain has not received the attention it deserves.

Hypnosis, Acupuncture, and the Behavior Therapies

In Chapter 3 we considered a variety of nonhypnotic methods for pain relief, including the psychological methods of behavior therapy and biofeedback. The issue is how best to serve the patient through a choice of one or another method, or through several methods in combination. In that respect, combining one psychological method with another is logically similar to combining hypnosis with chemoanalgesia. To the extent that methods overlap, special diagnostic methods may eventually be useful in selecting the most suitable combination for a given patient.

Although acupuncture is proposed as a physical method, and there may be some strictly physiological aspects to its benefits, the effects of suggestion loom so large that we wish to discuss it along with psychological methods of treatment. A correlation between successful treatment with acupuncture and hypnotic susceptibility was demonstrated in a large study by Katz and his associates. Those who participated had all been treated for pain by acupuncture, either successfully or unsuccessfully. Hence success with acupuncture was not influenced by the subjects' attitudes toward hypnosis, because hypnotic responsiveness was tested later. It was found that *those who were not hypnotizable had uniformly failed to profit from their acupuncture treatment.* The prediction did not work as uniformly in the other direction; some subjects who were classified as highly hypnotizable had failed to gain relief from acupuncture. The relationship between hypnotic susceptibility and effective pain relief through acupuncture can be expressed as a correlation of .50. This correlation is equivalent to that found between hypnotic responsiveness and pain relief by hypnotic suggestion (Chapter 4, page 68). Hence the findings of this study can be interpreted as suggesting parallels between hypnosis and acupuncture in pain reduction.

This need not be the whole explanation of acupuncture. Support for the effectiveness of at least some acupuncture points on a physiological basis has come from studies relating these points to the trigger points of Travell, as mentioned in Chapter 2. For example, Travell found many years ago that an area on the back of the hand between the thumb and the forefinger was related to pains in the head and neck region; this turns out to be a favorite acupuncture point also. The dramatic features of acupuncture in surgery do not convincingly demonstrate its advantages over hypnosis; thyroidectomies, caesarean sections, and heart surgery can be demonstrated under hypnosis as well, with the patient equally comfortable and responsive. The uncertain relationships between physiological effects and psychological effects in acupuncture can be cleared up only through further research.

The discussion of acupuncture points up the need for additional studies of the interactions of various methods—in this case, a method avowedly psychological (hypnosis) and one avowedly physical and physiological (acupuncture). We turn now to other methods more strictly psychological or psychophysiological.

Biofeedback is a psychophysiological method in that it depends upon the amplification of physiological responses for the purpose of gaining control over these responses through becoming aware of them. Unfortunately, biofeedback has been so exploited either commercially or by uncritical enthusiasts that at present it is difficult to gauge its therapeutic successes. There is no question that some voluntary control over normally involuntary processes is possible, but the permanence of the control and its consequences for the well-being of the patient have been inadequately demonstrated. Whatever the ultimate findings may be, a difference between biofeedback and hypnosis should be noted. In biofeedback, the person learns to be acutely aware of changes in his bodily functioning, such as changes in heart rate, blood pressure, EEG-alpha. In hypnosis, the effort may be directed in quite a contrary direction, to suppressing awareness of something happening in the body. This is clearly what is done in hypnotic relief of pain from an active source of irritation and stress, as in the main clinical areas we have discussed. It might well turn out that these two approaches are complementary. For the patient whose fantasy life permits him to direct his attention temporarily away from bodily processes, hypnosis might be preferred; for one whose reality ties are so strong that he cannot do this, biofeedback might be preferable.

Since the only reports we have are clinical, it is difficult to distinguish between a true biofeedback effect and what might better be described as placebo effects or suggestion effects, even though the practitioner does not believe himself to be using hypnosis. The possibility of suggestion effects was discussed in connection with the methods of natural childbirth and psychoprophylaxis, in which the overlap with hypnotic procedures is evident. This question was raised also with respect to pain control by peripheral electrical stimulation.

Various relaxation therapies, related in some respects to biofeedback, have had a long vogue; interest in them has risen recently because of widespread practice of meditation as a method of relaxation. There are some uncertainties about what happens in the course of relaxation for therapeutic purposes. Jacobson, who popularized progressive relaxation in the 1930s, was so convinced of the role of tension in consciousness that he asserted that once a person was relaxed he automatically fell asleep. He believed that it required some muscular tonus in order to think. He was probably wrong in this; a curarized animal, though totally relaxed, can still learn avoidance behavior on the basis of an aversive shock. More recent investigators have recognized that *cognitive* and *somatic* relaxation must be distinguished. Sometimes it is cognitively relaxing to engage in violent exercise; correspondingly, when a person lies down, his mind may begin to race so he cannot get to sleep. One experiment in our laboratory gave an indication that much of hypnotic relaxation is cognitive. Subjects were hypnotized standing up, sitting, or lying down; we hypothesized that if somatic relaxation were of the essence, they should respond more readily to hypnotic induction when lying down. It turned out that position did not matter; even though the induction was the standard one—relaxation, drowsiness, and a sleep-like state—subjects responded just as well to the hypnotic responsiveness items in spite of the postural tension required to remain standing.

The cognitive relaxation and the sense of effortlessness in hypnosis are probably more important than the somatic relaxation. In our experiments comparing waking suggestion and hypnotic suggestion for the relief of laboratory pain, we found that subjects partially successful by both methods preferred hypnosis because it involved less effort and strain. The same was noted in the reported study of dental procedures; patients preferred the hypnotic method because of the ease with which hypnosis handled the pain.

The operant conditioning methods of behavior therapy are among the favorites within the pain clinics. Some form of operant conditioning is commonly used with selected patients who have had pain problems for many years, whose repeated surgeries have not helped them, and whose regimen of drug use only partially alleviates their continuing pains. We are not prepared to make any firm assertions about the use of hypnosis with this particular patient population, although we believe that hypnosis should be included in the research going on in multidisciplinary pain clinics. Such clinics provide the best opportunities for experimental study of the interactions among various methods. Hypnotic practitioners are commonly familiar with behavior therapy and incorporate its methods as appropriate in the course of their psychotherapeutic practice; however, we are unaware of their combined use in the treatment of pain. In the practice of operant conditioning in some pain clinics, the attempt to eliminate treatment practices contingent upon felt pain leads to a taboo on mentioning pain at all. Therefore any method that calls attention to the patient's pain, as the glove anesthesia method in hypnosis does, is avoided. We do not believe this avoidance of the mention of pain to be necessary for effective behavior therapy of pain. A record of the patient's pain reduction over time can serve as a reinforcement and a stimulus to progress in much the same manner as a record of the distance he walks each day encourages his improvement.

The foregoing discussion of acupuncture, biofeedback, relaxation, and behavior therapy leaves many questions unanswered. What is needed is careful, dispassionate research free of predilections for any one method over the others that may be available for use alone or in combination.

Needed Research in Laboratory and Clinic

The controversy between basic and applied research has gone on for years without reaching a consensus. At one extreme we have the position that "nothing is so practical as a good theory;" at the other we have "necessity is the mother of invention." Mediators take the position that good research is defined by the adequacy of its methods to the problems faced, not by its subject matter; it can be sound science whether it is called basic research or applied research. However, the constraints upon the scientist in the laboratory and the clinic are recognizably different. The laboratory scientist involved with basic research is able to satisfy his curiosity by changing the direction of his research when a new hypothesis occurs to him. If he is studying pain he may approach the subject from any of several directions: neurophysiological, biochemical, psychological, anthropological, and others. The constraints in the clinic are more severe, in that the clinician must deal with the here-and-now patient who complains of pain. The most important criterion is whether the patient improves, not whether the researcher finds data bearing on a theory. A great deal of lip service is given to the interaction between basic research and its clinical application, but the meeting grounds are not altogether clear. Basic research should furnish knowledge that can be applied in the clinic; the results of the clinic should provide feedback to the laboratory worker. Why does this harmony not find easy and natural expression?

After reviewing both the experimental and the clinical literature on pain, we believe we understand better why a gulf has commonly existed between the laboratory and the clinic. For one accustomed to reading the experimental literature, most clinical studies that have attempted statistical summarization are unsatisfactory in one or more respects. At the same time, if one overlooks some imprecision in the figures of clinical reports, the evidence convinces one that a substantial amount of pain relief has occurred. The exact figures are often not so important for practical purposes, although some ambiguities could readily be resolved if we had a few more careful comparisons. For example, let us suppose that from a statistical standpoint, the Lamaze method and the hypnotic method work equally well for producing a comfortable (if not painless) delivery. It would be very helpful to know if the two methods work for the same women. A simple test of hypnotic susceptibility, given to both those who were to have babies by hypnosis and those by psychoprophylaxis could give an approximate answer to this question and save many futile arguments.

The clinician who reads the experimental literature may be equally baffled by some of the inferences that are drawn. Differences which are trivial from a practical point of view may reach statistical significance. For example, a modeling procedure may increase hypnotic responsiveness by a point or two on a hypnotic responsiveness scale; if the samples are large enough and the study properly conducted, the gain may be statistically significant. If this is interpreted as meaning that individual differences in hypnotizability are unimportant because they can be changed by modeling, the inference is false; the final scores are likely to correlate at a high level with the original ones. But the clinician wants to know whether he can expect to convert a slightly responsive subject into one who can profit by hypnotic treatment. He is not helped by the finding that the person may gain a point or two on a scale of twelve points.

202 · CHAPTER 10   THE FUTURE OF HYPNOSIS IN PAIN CONTROL

Having clearly in mind the problems of mutual understanding and communication between the clinic and the laboratory, we wish to propose some areas of research in which the separation might be bridged.

1. *Hypnotizability scales for clinical use.* Most of the hypnotic responsiveness scales that have been carefully standardized are time-consuming; they are not designed to serve the special purposes of the clinician. If diagnostic procedures are to discriminate who is most likely to reduce pain successfully with hypnosis, a more useful responsiveness scale must be made available. A scale designed for clinical use, known as the Hypnotic Induction Profile, has been developed by Spiegel. The profile is said to be helpful in selecting appropriate psychotherapeutic treatments. We are developing and testing an alternate scale for clinical use, in one form for adults and another for children. Although the new scale is much shorter than the other Stanford scales on which it is based, a preliminary standardization in which 111 students took both the SHSS–Form C and the new clinical scale showed the correlation between the two as a satisfactory .72. The clinical scale is given in the appendix.

Such a scale may be helpful not only in measuring general hypnotic responsiveness, but also in assisting the therapist to choose procedures for use with an individual patient.

2. *Effect of patient motivation on hypnotic responsiveness.* The laboratory studies of motivation as a factor in hypnotic responsiveness are very unsatisfactory. The "task motivation" that has been extensively studied in Barber's laboratory contains such a large component of social compliance that it does not reflect the subject's own desires with respect to hypnosis. It is easy for an experimenter to be misled by statistically significant relationships that are of no practical importance. For example, many slight differences owing to situational factors, such as the hypnotist's manner or the subject's attitude toward hypnosis, led Barber to explain hypnotic responsiveness in terms of such situational influences rather than in terms of more persistent individual differences. Spanos and McPeake, in Barber's laboratory, supported the earlier findings that attitude toward hypnosis was related to hypnotizability; when they put this result in context, however, they showed what a trivial factor it was relative to more persistent differences, such as those involving imaginative absorption outside the hypnotic setting. The persistent subject characteristics correlated .43 with hypnotic suggestibility; when attitude was added in a multiple correlation, the relation was increased only to .46.

Perhaps in the clinic, with the extreme motivation of the patient and his confidence in his physician, a level of motivation beyond that attainable in the laboratory may be reached; and perhaps this has an effect on hypnosis. The impression the clinical literature conveys is that the proportion of cancer patients who can be helped is higher than the corresponding proportion in the laboratory; however, it is extremely difficult to obtain a random sample of patients for comparison. Such studies are very much needed, and their results would be as welcome to the experimenter as to the clinician.

3. *Duration of pain as a problem for hypnotic pain reduction.* The problems of pain reduction in the clinic are so different from those in the laboratory that more imagination will have to be exercised to bring the two together. Typically, the subject in a laboratory experiment comes to the experiment free of pain. He is exposed to a pain of tolerable severity for a few minutes at most, and then the pain is over. That is the control condition in experimental studies. Under hypnotic suggestions, the subject tries to eliminate the pain; if he is sufficiently responsive to hypnosis, he succeeds. Compare this situation with that of a typical clinical patient—for example, a patient with chronic pain from advanced cancer. He already has the pain. Under hypnosis it may be reduced, but what happens when hypnosis is terminated? The patient needs a procedure to make the reinstatement of hypnosis possible, perhaps by self-hypnosis or by playing a tape of the hypnotist's suggestions. Post-hypnotic suggestions may be required. These procedures, so important in the clinic, have not been tested adequately in the laboratory.

To parallel clinical pain, the experimental subject must have a continuous source of pain, such as a tight band about his head to produce a headache. The headache would then be reduced by hypnosis, even while the band remained in place. We doubt that present-day experimenters would care to do this, or that present-day committees on the utilization of human subjects would allow it. However, if chronic pain cannot be studied in the laboratory, the experimenter needs to move his study to the clinic, where such continuing pain occurs naturally. Reports of persistent pain relief from the clinic are common enough, but we need more detail on which methods are most effective for recurrent or persistent pains and by what mechanism the relief occurs. The basic problem is how to make hypnotic analgesia persist in the absence of the hypnotist; surely this is a researchable problem.

4. *The conjoint use of hypnosis and chemical agents in the treatment of pain.* The use of hypnosis and chemical agents together raises some additional problems. It is sensible to reduce the patient's pain by analgesics if the hypnosis is not working. On the other hand, if hypnosis allows dosage of the chemical agents to be reduced, their disadvantages can be minimized or avoided. However, there are problems of interaction between hypnosis and drugs just as there are between several kinds of drugs taken at once. The drug may weaken the hypnosis; it may have no effect; or it may potentiate it. Present evidence on this matter is practically nonexistent. Repeated claims have been made that nitrous oxide inhalation can make a nonhypnotizable person responsive to hypnosis, but evidence to date is unconvincing. There is no evidence that tranquilizers, sedatives, or antianxiety agents enhance hypnotic responsiveness. This does not mean that there is no interaction; it is simply

that drug experiments are carried out only with difficulty in most of the laboratories studying hypnosis, while the clinical settings in which drugs are used seldom employ precise measures of hypnotic responsiveness.

From the foregoing it is clear that those trained in laboratory techniques of control and measurement need to collaborate with those who have clinical experience and expertness, in order to advance the scientific knowledge in many important areas.

Present investigations of both clinician and experimenter are gradually becoming more pertinent and convincing to one another. Collaborative work is essential. It is not enough to ask the clinician to read the experimental literature, or to ask the experimenter to read clinical case reports. Although this sounds like a good recommendation, it might well pull the two groups farther apart rather than bringing them together. They need to work together in mutual understanding to solve common problems, each learning from the experiences and competencies of the others.

If, as investigators ourselves, we express a wish for additional data, we are nonetheless satisfied that the benefits hypnosis can offer to many people in pain are already well documented. Opportunities should be expanded for those with problems of pain to receive these benefits.

Notes

Because of its historical association with magic and mysticism, hypnosis has had to struggle to become disentangled from occult and faith healing methods. The successes of various methods of relieving pain are instructive, but the failures must also be recognized; reliance upon criticized findings is the essence of science. The upsurge of marginal religious movements in contemporary America scarcely needs documentation, but a useful source of details on contemporary movements and practices, is provided by Zaretsky and Leone (1974). When these approaches deal with the alleviation of pain, we ask what diagnostic methods they use and what criteria of success they establish.

What We have Learned

Much of the text discussion consists of reflections on matters that have been discussed earlier. The ability to be moderately hypnotized is very widespread, but the hypnotic virtuoso, who experiences everything the hypnotist suggests, is very rare —perhaps only 1 or 2 percent of an unselected population. Hence we believe it important to make a careful assessment of hypnotic responsiveness to select the most appropriate therapy for a given patient. A low degree of hypnotizability does not mean hypnotic treatment is contraindicated, but it does temper the expectation of what can be done by hypnotic suggestion alone. When it is recognized that the capacity for becoming hypnotized plays such an important role, special techniques of induction become much less important.

Freud's distaste for what he saw Bernheim do is reported in Kline (1958); however, Freud had for a number of years used Bernheim's methods successfully.

Hypnosis and Other Pains

We regret the omission from our more detailed survey of many areas of pain in which we know, from personal experience as well as from case studies, that hypnosis can be successful in reducing pain. These are areas in which the psychological complexities are so great that we would wish for more adequate case studies and summarizations. The cases available at present do not allow for the same kinds of comparison with laboratory procedures that studies of the more somatogenic pains do. We have included citations to the work of Harding (1967) on migraine to show another area in which further work needs to be done. A differential diagnosis of migraine, tension headache, and other types of headaches should be made with great care if hypnosis is to take its place among the other therapeutic approaches. Harding's rate of success with 200 cases was reported in a personal communication from him dated May 17, 1974, for which we express our gratitude to him. The other migraine study mentioned is that of Anderson, Basker, and Dalton (1975).

Phantom limb pain is also an area of great interest; the most extensive hypnotic work has been done by Cedercreutz and Uusitalo (1967). The complex psychological features of this pain, including body-image problems, have been well treated by Kolb (1954). A more recent review is that by Melzack (1971).

The reduction of pain in the study by Melzack and Perry (1975) is attributed to hypnosis, rather than to an interaction between alpha feedback and hypnosis, for the reasons given in Chapter 4.

Psychological and Psychiatric Aspects of Pain

The best review of the psychological and psychiatric aspects of pain is that by Merskey and Spear (1967). Its bibliography of thirty-two pages contains more than 500 references.

That patients with various psychosomatic symptoms during World War II responded well to hypnotic symptom removal is documented by Brenman and Gill (1947). They reported that even in the absence of insight, symptom relief could often be maintained if the disorder had been relatively peripheral to the total personality (p. 90). Such successes were reiterated in their later book (Gill and Brenman, 1959, p. 340). Hypnoanalysis, dealing with many presenting symptoms, has been discussed with case material by Wolberg (1964).

The study of pain in 200 successive admissions to a psychiatric clinic was by Spear (1964). The book by Breuer and Freud (1895) was written during the short period in which they used hypnosis. The Eisenbud study of headache was done at a time when there was great interest in artificial complexes (Eisenbud, 1937). Engel (1951) interpreted atypical facial neuralgia as a hysterical conversion symptom.

The "pain game" approach is developed in Sternbach (1974a; 1974b); the approach of Szasz (1968) is somewhat similar. Szasz and Sternbach criticize both physicians who allow themselves to be manipulated by patients and patients who do the manipulating. Without expressing such criticism, some pain clinics attribute the problems to learning and use learning methods to meet them.

Some clinicians, such as Schafer and Hernandez, (1973), believe that psychogenic pains are more difficult to treat than somatogenic ones. There is also the uneasiness that if a psychogenic pain is removed, a new symptom will emerge to serve the same purpose. The questions about symptom substitution in hypnotic treatment were raised by Seitz (1951; 1953) and Rosen (1960). Studies of the occasional sequelae to hypnosis in the laboratory, were undertaken by Hilgard, Hilgard, and Newman (1961) and extended by J. Hilgard (1974b). Following laboratory hypnosis, some kind of reaction to the induction may persist as long as an hour for about 15 percent of those hypnotized. The symptoms were not found to be severe—often merely drowsiness—but the hypnotist should be aware of them and be sure that hypnosis is fully terminated before the subject leaves him.

The standard treatment of the defenses in the psychoanalytic literature is that of Anna Freud (1937). The reference to Gill and Brenman is to their book (1959).

Hypnosis, Acupuncture, and the Behavior Therapies

The study relating acupuncture to hypnotic susceptibility was reported by Katz, Kao, Spiegel, and Katz (1974). The correlation indicated is one which we computed from their data. The work relating acupuncture points to Travell's trigger points is being carried out by Frost at the Albert Einstein College of Medicine. An informal preliminary report has been prepared (McBroom, 1975). How hard it is to deal with all the interrelationships is shown in a recent report by Stern and others (1975). For the two kinds of laboratory pains we have commonly studied—cold pressor pain and ischemic pain produced by an occlusion cuff—they found that hypnosis produced more pain reduction than acupuncture. However, acupuncture was clearly effective, and it was more effective when the stimulation was done at accepted acupuncture points than at control nonpoints. A further finding was that in all cases, the more highly hypnotizable were more successful than the less hypnotizable in pain reduction, by acupuncture as well as by hypnosis.

Suggestion may well play a part in biofeedback. The setting of a biofeedback experiment is often very similar to that of a hypnosis experiment: the patient sits quietly and is assured that he will gain control over his symptoms. Roberts and others (1975) found, however, that temperature control by biofeedback methods was independent of the degree of hypnotizability. The suggestion components of natural childbirth and psychoprophylaxis were discussed in Chapter 6; the possibility of a suggestion component in electrical stimulation was raised in Chapter 3.

The work of Jacobson, whose relaxation methods provided some of the background for the Read method of natural childbirth, was mentioned in Chapter 6. That somatic relaxation is only one aspect of relaxation has been documented by Davidson and Schwartz (1975). Their theory is that there are two major components of relaxation—somatic and cognitive—which are quite different. They recognize attention as a third component interacting with the other two. To us, however, the third component does not appear to have the same status as the first two. Attentive change seems rather to be a technique by which to gain the advantages of either of the other two components. The experiment on becoming hypnotized standing up, sitting, or lying is that of Ruch and Morgan (1971).

Operant conditioning and other aspects of behavior therapy were discussed more fully in Chapter 3. We have suggested that the pain clinic is the most promising theater for research on various approaches to the diagnosis and treatment of long continued chronic pain. However, we have also pointed out how some features of the pain clinic militate against this desirable outcome. The aim of the pain clinic is to benefit the patients who are admitted; once a satisfactory set of procedures for this particular clientele has been developed, the desire to make the benefits of these practices available rather than trying something new and unknown may cause some aspects of further experimentation to be neglected. This is a familiar history of successful clinical practices. The illustration given in the text—avoidance of the word "pain" in some treatment programs—eliminates not only records with respect to the amount of pain reduction achieved, but prevents exploration of methods that approach the experienced pain more directly. Hence a pain clinic, where multidisciplinary research would be expected, may set its own limits on what can be done. Added evidence that operant programs leading to pain tolerance may succeed despite little reduction in felt pain (unless hypnosis is used) is reviewed in Hilgard (1975a).

Needed Research

Research in clinical settings is unusually difficult. First, there is the sampling problem. Patients come to a clinical service because of its reputation, so there is some self-selection even if consecutive cases are studied. Appropriate control groups are hard to find, and the experimental-control design is often not the preferred design to use. Psychological measurement methods yield unreliable results in the unfamiliar environments in which patients often find themselves. Research that meets conventional standards of data collection and analysis may be limited because the original data are imprecise. In the text we indicated that it would be useful to have a simple study of the hypnotizability of women for whom the Lamaze method had proved either successful or unsuccessful. Since the writing of that statement, such a study has appeared (Samko and Schoenfeld, 1975). The data appear to lead to the conclusion that there is no relationship between hypnotizability and the Lamaze childbirth experience.

Unfortunately, the evidence is unconvincing. The intended sample consisted of 111 women who had delivered their babies with the aid of the Lamaze procedure during the previous year and one-half. For various reasons, this number fell to 55 who participated, and then to 42 whose data were analyzed statistically. We have no way of knowing to what extent this final sample was representative of the women who were having babies by the Lamaze method at that time; nor do we know how they compared with women who were not using the Lamaze method. The sampling problem is nearly universal in clinical studies. The authors reported as fully as they could on the defections from the sample. But because the study was retrospective, it relied on the fallible memories of both patient and physician with respect to variables associated with the Lamaze method. In addition, the measure of hypnotic responsiveness was a score on a fallible scale. The low correlations that resulted cannot be interpreted as evidence that no relationship exists between hypnosis and the success of the Lamaze method, so the desired study remains to be performed.

We return to the problem of measuring hypnotizability in a clinical setting. Whenever measurement has been tried by clinicians, success in hypnotic procedures turns out to be related to measured hypnotizability. Orne and O'Connell (1967) developed a diagnostic rating scale yielding estimates of attained hypnotic depth between 1 for no response, and 5 for profound amnesia effects and posthypnotic response. Unfortunately, norms have not been provided so that it is not possible to ascertain precisely how one group of patients compares with others tested elsewhere. A clinical scale, such as that of Spiegel (Spiegel and Bridger, 1970; Spiegel, 1974) is a move in the right direction; however, some of its statistical features make it an unsatisfactory research device, (Eliseo 1974; Wheeler and others 1974). We have been preparing a scale for clinical use that correlates with previously standardized scales. The new clinical scale is described in Appendix A.

The social compliance feature of Barber's task motivation, leading to lower hypnotic scores was discussed earlier (page 25). Hence the motivation variable remains an uncertain one in the laboratory, although it may be important in the clinic. The experiment of Spanos and McPeake (1975) cited in the text is along the same lines, finding less importance attached to situational variables than to more enduring characteristics of the subjects.

The reference to a continuing headache produced by a tightened band around the head is not a recommendation, but only an illustration of a laboratory pain that would be more like clinical pains actually met. A headache can indeed be produced by such a headband, as shown by Wolff (1963) and by Dudley, Masuda, Martin, and Holmes (1965). Perhaps a better suggestion would be injection of a chemical agent in noninjurious amounts to produce a pain lasting for several hours. As an example, Faires and McCarty (1962) produced an artificial arthritis by injecting sodium urate crystals into their own knees. The pain was more severe than they had intended, and medication was required for its relief, but it did mimic very faithfully the pain of arthritis, and there were apparently no aftereffects. If an appropriate pain were found, the effectiveness of hypnotic suggestion in reducing it throughout the several hours of its duration could be tested.

Weitzenhoffer (1953) reviewed a number of earlier studies on the interaction between drugs and suggestibility. He felt that the best study up to that time was that of Eysenck and Rees (1945), in which they tested the effects of sodium amytal and of nitrous oxide. Subanesthetic doses of either drug increased suggestibility somewhat, but only among those subjects already suggestible. Hence the effect of drugs is similar to the effect of other methods of heightening hypnotic responsiveness.

Orne (1974) reported that he used a combination of drugs and hypnosis in treating the pain of patients with terminal cancer. The phenothiazines were used to permit gradual withdrawal of narcotics rather than to make hypnosis more effective.

The availability of hypnotic services for those in need of them is discussed in Appendix B (page 222).

Stanford Hypnotic
Clinical Scale (SHCS)

We have repeatedly noted that the usefulness of hypnotic procedures with patients depends upon their ability to respond to hypnosis, and that this ability can be tested by means of standard procedures. It seemed important, therefore, to develop a convenient instrument for measuring hypnotic responsiveness in patients; such a scale might also help to guide the selection of particular procedures to be used in therapy. A scale is presented here, in sufficient detail to make it understandable to the responsible professional who wishes to use it.

The original Stanford Hypnotic Susceptibility Scales (SHSS) were developed for research purposes; consequently, they were made extensive enough to provide measures useful in correlational analysis, and to sample a variety of hypnotic performances. Although the SHSS were readily adaptable to clinical use, some features made them less serviceable than they might otherwise have been. Their length was the most common drawback; in other cases the degree of mobility and muscular effort involved made them less suitable for hospitalized patients.

Our experience with patients who may have impediments to sustained motor activity convinced us that we needed a scale combining two characteristics: first, it would be short enough not to tire the patient, and second, it would tap the kinds of processes most likely to be used in therapy. Although there is a common ability reflected in hypnotic responsiveness, special abilities—such as the availability of imagery, the ability to enjoy age regression, and posthypnotic responsiveness—may influence the selection of treatment methods.

We have developed such a scale for use with adults, the Stanford Hypnotic Clinical Scale (SHCS). A similar scale for use with children is in preparation.

The five items selected for the clinical scale were modified from those already tested in the earlier scales, SHSS, forms A, B, and C (Weitzenhoffer and Hilgard, 1959; 1962). The items are: moving hands (an easy motor item, to introduce the patient to response to suggestions); a dream within hypnosis (often useful in interpreting the patient's attitude toward hypnosis); age regression (commonly useful in therapy); a posthypnotic suggestion (possibly related to a capacity for continuation of the hypnotic experience); and posthypnotic amnesia (useful in relation to the experience of pain, among other things). The items were slightly modified from their original form in order to reflect the special purposes of the scale.

Detailed instructions for use of the scale and a specimen scoring pamphlet are given later. The following standardization information relates the results of this shorter scale to the longer scales from which it has been adapted, and suggests the appropriate interpretation of various levels of scoring.

A sample of 111 university undergraduates was selected from the full range of scores (0–10) on a 10-point version of the Harvard Group Scale of Hypnotic Susceptibility, Form A (HGSHS:A; see Shor and Orne, 1962). Individual sessions of the Stanford Hypnotic Clinical Scale and the 12-point Stanford Hypnotic Susceptibility Scale, Form C (SHSS:C) were then administered in balanced order, 56 subjects receiving the clinical scale (SHCS) first, and 55 receiving SHSS:C first. There were no order effects for any item nor for the total score, so the data analyses to be reported are based on the total sample.

Four items (moving hands, dream, age regression, and amnesia) are common to both SHCS and SHSS:C. The HGSHS:A contains a posthypnotic suggestion item (touching an ankle at a pencil tap), for comparison with the SHCS posthypnotic suggestion of coughing or clearing the throat at a pencil tap.

Score distributions for the new clinical scale are given in Table 1. The means for male and female subjects were not significantly different. The average score of 2.75 means that half the subjects were able to perform correctly more than two of the five items but fewer than three. As a rough guide, a subject who passes four or five is in the upper third of responsiveness, one who passes two or three is in the middle third, and one who passes none or one is in the lowest third.

The subjects tested in this standardization were normal university students; norms for patients are not yet available, but they will be important also. Preliminary work with a few patients shows that the intent of the scale has been achieved: it can be performed by patients who are ill, with restricted strength, restricted movement, or very little stamina.

That the items drawn from the earlier, longer scales have not been distorted in difficulty by using them in the shorter clinical scale is indicated

Table 1. Norms for Stanford undergraduates on the Stanford Hypnotic Clinical Scale.

Susceptibility Level	Raw Scores	Number of Cases			Percent of Cases
		Male	Female	Total	
High	5 ⎱	9	5	14 ⎱ 42	12 ⎱ 37
	4 ⎰	17	11	28 ⎰	25 ⎰
Medium	3 ⎱	15	11	26 ⎱ 41	23 ⎱ 37
	2 ⎰	10	5	15 ⎰	14 ⎰
Low	1 ⎱	9	6	15 ⎱ 28	14 ⎱ 26
	0 ⎰	9	4	13 ⎰	12 ⎰
Cases		69	42	111	100%
Mean		2.71	2.81	2.75	
S. D.		1.60	1.52	1.56	

by the results shown in Table 2. The same subjects attempted the same items in two contexts, that of a longer scale and that of the shorter, clinical one. The percents passing on the two scales were very nearly alike; such differences as appear are nonsignificant from a statistical standpoint.

That some common hypnotic ability is reflected in each item is shown in the correlations given in the last column, all of which are positive. A factor analysis would show a common first factor, because each item reflects some ability that is measured by the total set of items.

A reliability estimate for SHCS can be obtained from the product-moment correlation between the total score on this scale and the total score on SHSS:C. This correlation was .72. The corresponding correlation between the four items common to both SHCS and SHSS:C was .81. Thus the SHCS appears to be a reliable estimate of hypnotic responsiveness as measured by the longer standardized procedures.

The moving hands and dream items are scored in SHCS exactly as in SHSS:C. The scoring of the age regression item has been modified from that of SHSS:C, in which it is scored on the basis of a clear handwriting change in one of two regressed ages. Writing was eliminated from the item in the new clinical scale, because it may be difficult for patients to write who are weakened by their illness or in bed, and also because the subjective aspects of regression confirm sufficiently the reality of what is reported. Thus, in the new scale, age regression is scored partly on the basis of what the patient himself reports as his experience. In one sense, this makes the item "easier" to pass, though the scoring criterion adopted resulted in comparable scores on the two tests.

Table 2. Percent passing each item of the Stanford Hypnotic Susceptibility Scale, Form C (SHSS:C) and the Stanford Hypnotic Clinical Scale (SHCS).

N = 111

	Percent Passing		Correlation with Total Score minus this item, SHCS
Item	SHSS:C	SHCS	Biserial r's
Moving hands	84	81	.57
Dream	69	60	.77
Age regression	67	66	.54
Posthypnotic suggestion	32*	27	.36
Amnesia	44	40	.61

* The posthypnotic item percent is from HGSHS:A rather than SHSS:C, which lacks such an item.

In the longer SHSS:C the subject could recall three of the twelve items and still pass amnesia; in the shorter SHCS he could not recall more than two of the five items and pass amnesia. These criteria yielded essentially the same proportion of subjects passing in the two tests. The posthypnotic suggestion item was the one most different in content between the two tests. However, roughly a third of the subjects passed the item in both instances.

The Stanford Hypnotic Clinical Scale requires approximately 20 minutes for administration, including the standard hypnotic induction; this is about half the time required by the longer SHSS:C.

With this background, the administration protocol of the scale follows. After it is a specimen scoring form, which in practice is prepared as a booklet.

Protocol for Administering the Stanford Hypnotic Clinical Scale (SHCS)*

(*Patient may be seated in any kind of chair with arms, or may be in bed, sitting or lying.*)

Introductory Remarks
In a moment I shall hypnotize you and suggest to you a number of experiences which you may or may not have, and a number of effects which you may or may not produce. Not everyone can have the same experiences or produce the same effects when hypnotized. People vary greatly. We need to know which experiences you can

*The scale was prepared and standardized by Arlene H. Morgan and Josephine R. Hilgard.

have so we can build on them and know how to make hypnosis best serve you. Please remember always to respond to what you are *feeling*, so we can use hypnosis in ways that are natural for you.

Induction
Please close your eyes and listen carefully to what I say. As we go on, you will find yourself becoming more and more relaxed. . . . Begin to let your whole body relax. . . . Let all the muscles go limp. . . . Now you will be able to feel special muscle groups relaxing even more. If you pay attention to your right foot, you can feel the muscles in it relax . . . feel the muscles in the right lower leg relaxing . . . in the right upper leg relaxing. . . . Now on the left side, concentrate on the way that the left foot is relaxing . . . and the left leg, how the lower part and the upper part are both relaxing more. . . . Next, you'll be able to feel the muscles of the right hand relaxing, the right lower arm and the right upper arm relaxing. . . . Now direct your attention to your left hand. Let it relax, let the lower arm and the upper arm relax. . . . As you have become relaxed, your body begins to feel rather heavy. Just think of the chair (bed) as being strong, sink into it, and let it hold you . . . Your shoulders . . . neck . . . and head, more and more relaxed. . . . The muscles of your scalp and forehead, just let them relax even more. . . . All of this time you have been settling more deeply and more comfortably into the chair (bed).

Your mind has relaxed, too, along with your body. It is possible to set all worries aside. Your mind is calm and peaceful. You are getting more and more comfortable. . . . You will continue to feel pleasantly relaxed as you continue to listen to my voice. . . . Just keep your thoughts on what I am saying . . . more and more deeply relaxed and perhaps drowsy but at no time will you have any trouble hearing me. You will continue in this state of great relaxation until I suggest that it is time for you to become more alert. . . . Soon I will begin to count from one to twenty. As I count, you will feel yourself going down further and further into this deeply relaxed hypnotic state. You will be able to do all sorts of things that I suggest, things that will be interesting and acceptable to you. You will be able to do them without breaking the pattern of complete relaxation that is gradually coming over you. . . . one — you are becoming more deeply relaxed . . . two — down, down into a deeper, tranquil state of mind . . . three — four — more and more relaxed . . . five — six — seven — you are sinking deeper and deeper. Nothing will disturb you. You are finding it easy just to listen to things that I say . . . eight — nine — ten — halfway there . . . always deeply relaxed . . . eleven — twelve — thirteen — fourteen — fifteen — although deeply relaxed, you can hear me clearly. You will always hear me distinctly no matter how hypnotized you are . . . sixteen — seventeen — eighteen — deeply relaxed. Nothing will disturb you . . . nineteen — twenty — *completely relaxed*.

You can change your position any time you wish. Just be sure you remain comfortable and relaxed.

You are very relaxed and pleasantly hypnotized. While you remain confortably listening to my words, I am going to help you learn more about how thinking about something affects what you do. Just experience whatever you can. Pay close attention to what I tell you, and think about the things I suggest. Then let happen whatever you find is happening, even if it surprises you a little. Just *let it happen by itself*.

1. *Moving hands together* [*or, if one arm is immobile, go to 1a, Hand lowering*]
   All right, then . . . please hold both hands straight out in front of you, palms facing inward, hands about a foot apart. Here, I'll help you. [*Take hold of hands and position them about a foot apart.*] Now I want you to imagine a force attracting your hands toward each other, pulling them together. Do it any way that seems best to you—think of rubber bands stretched from wrist to wrist, pulling your hands together, or imagine magnets held in each hand pulling them together—the closer they get the stronger the pull. . . . As you think of this force pulling your hands together, they will move together, slowly at first, but they will move closer together, closer and closer together as though a force is acting on them . . . moving . . . moving . . . closer, closer. . . .

   [*Allow ten seconds without further suggestion, and note extent of motion.*]

   That's fine. Everything is back to normal now. Just place your hands in their resting position and relax.

   (Score + if hands move slowly toward each other, and are not more than six inches apart at end of ten seconds.)

1a. *Hand lowering* (alternative to *Moving hands together*)
    (If one hand is immobile for any reason, we recommend substituting a hand lowering suggestion, similar to that given as Item I in SHSS:C. The arm is held straight out at shoulder height, with the palm of the hand up. The suggestion is given to imagine something heavy in the hand pressing it down. After a few suggestions of downward movement, if the arm is not completely down, a 10-second wait is introduced. The item is passed if the hand has lowered at least six inches by the end of the 10 seconds.)

2. *Dream*
   Now I am going to ask you to keep on relaxing, and this time you are going to have a dream . . . a real dream . . . much like the kind you have when you sleep at night. When I stop talking to you very shortly, you will begin to dream. Any kind of dream may come. . . . Now it is as though you are falling asleep, deeper and deeper asleep. You can sleep and dream about anything you want to. As soon as I stop talking, you will begin to dream. When I speak to you again in a minute or so, you will stop dreaming if you are still dreaming, and you will listen to me just as you have been doing. If you stop dreaming before I speak to you again, you will remain pleasantly and deeply hypnotized. Now just sleep and have a dream.

   [*Allow 1 minute. Then say:*]

   The dream is over, but you can remember it very well and clearly, very clearly. . . . I want you now to tell me about your dream, while remaining deeply hypnotized. Please tell me about your dream . . . right from the beginning. Tell me all about it. [*Record verbatim.*]

   [*If subject has no dream:*] That's all right. Not everyone dreams.
   [*If subject hesitates or reports vaguely, probe for details.*]

Inquiry: How real would you say your dream was?

Termination: That's all for the dream. Remain as deeply hypnotized as you have been.

(Score + if subject has an experience comparable to a dream . . . not just vague fleeting experiences or just feelings or thoughts. The dream should show imagery, some reality, and not give evidence of being under voluntary control.)

3. *Age regression*

Something very interesting is about to happen. In a little while you are going back to a happy day in elementary school. If you had a choice to return to the third, fourth, or fifth grade, would you prefer one of these to the other?

[*If yes:*] Which grade?

[*If no preference, use fourth grade.*]

All right then, I would like you now to think about when you were in the [*selected*] grade of school, and in a little while, you are going to start to *feel* like you are growing younger and smaller, going back to the time you were in the [*selected*] grade. . . . *one,* you are going back into the past. It is no longer [*state present year*], nor [*state an earlier year*], nor [*state a still earlier year*], but much earlier . . . *two,* you are becoming much younger and smaller . . . in a moment you will be back in the [*selected*] grade, on a very nice day. *Three,* getting younger and younger, smaller and smaller all the time. Soon you will be back in the [*selected*] grade, and you will feel an experience exactly as you did once before on a nice day when you were in school. *Four,* very soon you will be there. . . . Once again a little boy (girl) in the [*selected*] grade. Soon you will be right back there. *Five!* You are now a small boy (girl) in school. . . . Where are you? . . . . What are you doing? . . . . Who is your teacher? . . . . How old are you? . . . . What are you wearing? . . . . Who is with you? . . . .

[*Ask additional questions as appropriate. Record answers.*]

That's fine. . . . Now you can grow up again. You are no longer in the [*selected*] grade but getting older, growing up. You are now your correct age, this is [*current day and date*], and you are in [*locale of testing*]. You are no longer a little boy (girl), but an adult, sitting in a chair (bed) deeply hypnotized. How old are you? . . . . And what is today? . . . . Where are you? . . . . Fine. Today is [*correct date*] and you are [*correct age*] and this is [*name place where subject is being tested*]. Everything is back as it was. Just continue to be comfortably relaxed. . . .

(Postpone scoring until inquiry at end.)

4. *Posthypnotic suggestion (clearing throat or cough);*
5. *Amnesia*

Stay completely relaxed, but listen carefully to what I tell you next. In a little while I shall begin counting backwards from ten to one. You will gradually come out of hypnosis, but you will be the way you are now for most of the count. When

I reach "five" you will open your eyes, but you will not be fully awake. When I get to "one" you will be entirely roused, as awake as you usually are. You will have been so relaxed, however, that you will have trouble recalling the things I have said to you and the things you did. It will take so much effort to think of these that you will prefer not to try. It will be much easier just to forget everything until I tell you that you can remember. You will forget all that has happened until I say to you: "Now you can remember everything!" You will not remember anything until then. After you wake up you will feel refreshed. I shall now count backwards from ten, and at "five," not sooner, you will open your eyes, but not be fully aroused until I reach "one." At "one" you will be fully awake. A little later I shall tap my pencil on the table like this. [*Demonstrate with two taps.*] When I do, you will feel a sudden urge to clear your throat or to cough. And then you will clear your throat or cough. You will find yourself doing this but *you will forget that I told you to do so*, just as you will forget the other things, until I tell you, "Now you can remember everything." All right, ready — ten — nine — eight — seven — six — *five* — four — three — two — one.

[*If subject has eyes open:*] How do you feel? Do you feel alert?
[*If groggy:*] The feeling will go away soon. You feel alert now!

[*If subject keeps eyes closed:*] Please open your eyes. How do you feel?
[*If groggy:*] You are beginning to feel more alert and refreshed. . . . You feel alert now!

[*Hypnotist now taps pencil against table twice. Wait ten seconds.*]

(Score + if patient clears throat or coughs after pencil tap.)

Now I want to ask you a few questions about your experience. Please tell me in your own words everything that has happened since I asked you to close your eyes.

[*Record subject's responses verbatim. If blocked, ask, "Anything else?" and record answers until subject reaches a further impasse.*]

Listen carefully to my words. *Now you can remember everything.* Anything else now?

[*Again record subject's responses verbatim. Remind subject of any items not recovered; note these also.*]

(Score + if subject recalls no more than two items before memory is restored.)

[*If subject is awake and comfortable:*] That's all now. You are completely out of hypnosis, feeling alert and refreshed. Any tendency that you may have to clear your throat or to cough is now completely gone.

FOR CORRECTING DIFFICULTIES WHEN NECESSARY:
[*If there is residual difficulty, e.g., difficulty in restoring alertness or persistence of a cough, proceed as follows with appropriate suggestions:*] Please close your eyes and drift back into hypnosis as I count to five. One — two — three — four — five. . . . Now I am about to arouse you by counting backwards from five to one. You will feel alert, refreshed, with no tendency to cough. [*Wait ten seconds.*] Five — four — three — two — one. Fully aroused!

SCORING BOOKLET
STANFORD HYPNOTIC CLINICAL SCALE (SHCS)

Subject Name _____ Date _____ Total Score _____

Hypnotist _____

Summary of Scores

Details on the pages that follow		Score
1. Moving hands together (or 1a. Hand lowering, as an alternate)		
2. Dream		
3. Age regression		
4. Posthypnotic suggestion (clearing throat or cough)		
5. Amnesia	No. items recalled _____ No. items recovered after memory restored _____	
Total Score		

Special circumstances (medicated? in pain? movement handicap?)

1

ITEM	SCORE
1. MOVING HANDS TOGETHER (or 1a. HAND LOWERING) Describe movement: (At end of session, probe for type of experience if movement is very fast:) Score (+) if movement is slow and hands are not more than six inches apart by end of 10 seconds.	(1) _____
2. DREAM Record dream, or report thoughts, fantasies, etc.: Score (+) if subject has an experience comparable to a dream, not just vague fleeting experiences or just feelings or thoughts. The dream should show imagery, some reality, and not give evidence of being under voluntary control.	(2) _____

2

ITEM	SCORE

3. AGE REGRESSION (SCHOOL)
 	
Selected grade: _____
 	
Where are you? _____
 	
What are you doing? _____
 	
_____
 	
Who is your teacher? _____
 	
How old are you? _____
 	
What are you wearing? _____
 	
Who is with you? _____
 	
a. Hypnotist's rating: _____ : _____ : _____
                   No   Fair   Good
                   regression	

b. Subjective rating by subject (TO BE DETERMINED AT END OF SESSION): (Read to subject and ask him to select the statement that best describes his experience:) ____1) I did not go back at all. ____2) I was thinking about when I was that age, but had no visual experiences. ____3) Although I did not go back, I could see myself as a young child reliving a past experience. ____4) I knew I was really my present age, but I felt in part as though I was reliving an experience. ____5) I actually felt as though I was back at the suggested age, and reliving a past experience.	
Score (+) if hypnotist's rating is good, *or* if the subjective rating is 4 or 5.	(3) ____

3

ITEM	SCORE
4. POSTHYPNOTIC SUGGESTION (Clearing throat or coughing) Note nature and degree of response. a. Hypnotist's rating: ——————— ——————— ——————————— Absent Present Exceptionally Clear	
b. Subjective rating by subject (TO BE DETERMINED AT END OF SESSION IF SUBJECT RESPONDED): You coughed (or cleared your throat) during the session. 1) Do you remember why? ———————————— 2) Did you know why at the time? —————————— ———————————————————————— ·3) If you remembered that I said you would do this, why did you carry out the suggestion? ———————————————————————— ———————————————————————— 4) Would you say it was voluntary or involuntary? ———————————————————————— Score (+) if hypnotist's rating is Present or Exceptionally Clear, unless subject declares response voluntary.	(4) ————

ITEM	SCORE
5. POSTHYPNOTIC AMNESIA a. Please tell me now in your own words everything that has happened from the time you closed your eyes. (List items in order of mention; record descriptions of induction sensations, etc., also. If subject blocks, ask, "Anything else?" until subject reaches a further impasse.) _____ _____ _____ _____ _____ _____ _____ _____ Anything else? _____ _____ _____ _____ b. Listen carefully to my words. NOW YOU CAN REMEMBER EVERYTHING. Anything else now? (List in order of mention.) _____ _____ _____ _____ _____ _____ Remind subject of omitted items. List these also, and add any remarks on nature of amnesic experience. _____ _____ _____ Score (+) if subject recalls no more than two items before memory is restored.	(5) _____
(Complete inquiry on items 3 and 4 at end of session.) TOTAL SCORE	_____

5

The Availability of Hypnotic Services

It is awkward to tell an expectant mother that it would be fine for her to have her baby with the aid of hypnosis, and then have her unable to find an obstetrician sympathetic to its use. The same applies to dentistry and to other problems for which hypnosis might be of value. Unless the services are widely available and in the hands of respected professionals, supplemented by hospital staffs ready to give supporting services, the optimal use of hypnosis is unlikely to occur.

A reputable hypnotic practitioner is one well established in his specialty, be it medicine, dentistry, psychiatry, or psychology. He is trained in those aspects of his profession which lie outside hypnosis, and he conforms to the ethical practices of his profession. Unfortunately, there are not at present too few hypnotists, but only too few who are reputable according to these standards.

The problems of specialization within the healing professions have many facets, such as definition of the field, specification of appropriate training, accrediting and licensing, recognition of specialty boards, and inclusion within medical insurance arrangements. The eventual decisions are in many cases based on social history rather than purely rational considerations. For example, how many people can state precisely the difference between an optometrist and an ophthalmologist? What are the areas of distinctiveness among the psychiatrist, psychoanalyst, and clinical psychologist? These difficulties are relevant to the problems of hypnotic practice, because hypnosis is ill-defined, training facilities are not clearly demarcated, and the social history has not been coherent enough to establish who is and who is not a reputable hypnotist.

The establishment of societies with standards of membership is a first step toward greater protection of the public. Requirements for membership include, in addition to hypnotic competence, appropriate standing within his own profession of medicine, dentistry, or psychology. To better attest hypnotic competence, specialty boards have been established as the American Boards of Clinical Hypnosis, with subspecialties in medicine, dentistry, and psychology. These do not yet have sufficiently large memberships to be very serviceable as sources of credentialed hypnotists except in larger cities, but the move is in the right direction. It is difficult for state legislatures to enact wise standards for recognition of hypnotists until sufficient criteria are established by those who are practicing reputably.

In the United States, two societies and a division of the American Psychological Association are involved in efforts to upgrade the clinical and experimental aspects of hypnosis. If local sources are insufficient to provide adequate guidance, the individual seeking hypnotic services may inquire of these organizations. The addresses of their headquarters are:

American Society of Clinical Hypnosis
2400 E. Devon Avenue, Suite 218
Des Plaines, Illinois 60018

Society for Clinical and Experimental Hypnosis
250 West End Avenue, Suite 1P
New York, New York 10023

American Psychological Association
Division 30, Psychological Hypnosis
1200 Seventeenth Street N. W.
Washington, D.C. 20036

There are other societies with high-sounding names operative in the field of hypnosis, but some of their members have uncertain credentials, so it is a matter of discretion to remain in communication with the two societies and the division mentioned.

Outside the United States, the hypnotic societies which correspond most closely to those listed above are affiliated with the International Society of Hypnosis. A new directory of its affiliated societies and its current members is about to be issued and will be available from:

International Society of Hypnosis
c/o Unit for Experimental Psychiatry
111 North 49th Street
Philadelphia, Pennsylvania 19139

Local sources of information, such as hospitals, medical societies, and departments of psychology in colleges or universities, can provide membership information regarding those who offer their services as hypnotists. The authors of this book cannot act as a referral service.

References and Index to Authors of Works Cited

The bold-face numerals following each reference indicate the pages in the text or notes on which the reference provides a background for the discussion. Citations in the notes are made by date of publication.

AARONSON, G. A., *see* Schibley and Aaronson (1966).

ABELOFF, M. D., *see* Craig and Abeloff (1974).

ABRAMSON, M., and HERON, W. T. (1950) An objective evaluation of hypnosis in obstetrics: Preliminary Report. *American Journal of Obstetrics and Gynecology*, 59: 1069–1074. **110, 118**

ADLER, C., *see* Budzynski, Stoyva, and Adler (1970).

AKESON, W. H., *see* Sternbach and others (1974).

AKIL, H., *see* Liebeskind, Mayer, and Akil (1974).

ANDERSON, J. A. D.; BASKER, M. A.; and DALTON, R. (1975) Migraine and hypnotherapy. *International Journal of Clinical and Experimental Hypnosis*, 23: 48–58. **192, 205**

ANDERSON, M. N. (1957) Hypnosis in anesthesia. *Journal of the Medical Association of the State of Alabama*, 27: 121–125. **129, 140, 142, 143**

ARKIN, A. M.; TOTH, M.; BAKER, J.; and HASTEY, J. M. (1970) The degree of concordance between the content of sleep-talking and mentation recalled in wakefulness. *Journal of Nervous and Mental Disease*, 151: 375–393. **187**

ASKEN, M. J. (1975) Psychoemotional aspects of mastectomy: A review of recent literature. *American Journal of Psychiatry*, 132: 56–59. **101**

ATKINSON, G. *see* Tellegen and Atkinson (1974).

AUGUST, R. V. (1961) *Hypnosis in obstetrics*. New York: McGraw-Hill. **112, 114, 118, 119**

BACON, J. G., *see* Roberts and others (1975).

BAKAN, D. (1968) *Disease, pain, and sacrifice*. Chicago: University of Chicago Press. **29, 44**

BAKAN, P. (1969) Hypnotizability, laterality of eye movements, and functional brain asymmetry. *Perceptual and Motor Skills*, 28: 927–932. **24**

BAKER, J., *see* Arkin and others (1970).

BANDURA, A. L. (1969) *Principles of behavior modification*. New York: Holt, Rinehart, and Winston. **55, 61**

BARBER, T. X. (1963) The effects of "hypnosis" on pain: A critical review of experimental and clinical findings. *Psychosomatic Medicine*, 24: 303–333. **81**

BARBER, T. X. (1969) *Hypnosis: A scientific approach*. New York: Van Nostrand Reinhold. **14, 24, 25**

BARBER, T. X. (1972) Suggested "hypnotic" behavior: The trance paradigm versus an alternative paradigm. *In* Fromm and Shor (1972), 115–182. **14, 24**

BARBER, T. X., and CALVERLEY, D. S. (1963a) Toward a theory of hypnotic behavior: Effects on suggestibility of task motivating instructions and attitudes toward hypnosis. *Journal of Abnormal and Social Psychology*, 67: 557–565. **15, 25**

BARBER, T. X., and Calverley, D. S. (1963b) "Hypnotic-like" suggestibility in children and adults. *Journal of Abnormal and Social Psychology*, 66: 589–597. **24**

BARBER, T. X., and Cooper, B. J. (1972) Effects on pain of experimentally induced and spontaneous distraction. *Psychological Reports*, 31: 647–651. **67, 81**

BARBER, T. X., and GLASS, L. B. (1962) Significant factors in hypnotic behavior. *Journal of Abnormal and Social Psychology*, 64: 222–228. **15, 25**

BARBER, T. X., and HAHN, K. W., JR. (1962) Physiological and subjective responses to pain-producing stimulation under hypnotically suggested and waking-imagined "analgesia." *Journal of Abnormal and Social Psychology* 65: 411–415. **75, 81**

BARBER, T. X., and HAHN, K. W., JR. (1964) Experimental studies in "hypnotic" behavior: Physiological and subjective effects of imagined pain. *Journal of Nervous and Mental Disease*, 139: 416–425. **177, 187**

BARBER, T. X., SPANOS, N. P., and CHAVES, J. F. (1974) *Hypnosis, imagination, and human potentialities*. New York: Pergamon Press. **81**

BARBER, T. X., *see also* SPANOS and BARBER (1968; 1974); SPANOS, BARBER, and LANG (1974).

BARKER, J. L., and LEVITAN, H. (1974) Studies on mechanisms underlying non-narcotic analgesia. *In* Bonica (1974a), 503–511. **60**

BARRETT, R. H., and VON DEDENROTH, T. E. A. (1967) Problems of deglutition. *American Journal of Clinical Hypnosis*, 9: 161–165. **159, 163**

BARTLETT, E. E. (1971) Hypnoanesthesia for bilateral oophorectomy: A case report. *American Journal of Clinical Hypnosis*, 14: 122–124. **134**

BARTLETT, M. K., *see* Egbert and others (1964).

BASKER, M. A., *see* Anderson, Basker, and Dalton (1975).

BATTIT, G. E., *see* Egbert and others (1963; 1964).

BEECHER, H. K. (1956) Relationship of significance of wound to pain experienced. *Journal of the American Medical Association*, 161: 1609–1613. **45**

BEECHER, H. K. (1959) *Measurement of subjective responses: Quantitative effects of drugs.* New York: Oxford University Press. **44, 49, 60**

BEECHER, H. K. (1968) The measurement of pain in man: A re-inspection of the work of the Harvard group. In Soulairac and others (1968), 201–213. **46**

BEECHER, H. K. (1969) Anxiety and pain. *Journal of the American Medical Association,* 209: 1080. **79**

BEECHER, H. K., *see also* Egbert and others (1963); Smith and others (1966).

BELOZERSKI, G. G., *see* Katchan and Belozerski (1940).

BERNICK, S. M. (1972) Relaxation, suggestion, and hypnosis in dentistry. *Pediatric Dentistry,* 11: 72–75. **147, 161**

BERNSTEIN, M. R. (1965a) Observations on the use of hypnosis with burned children on a pediatric ward. *International Journal of Clinical and Experimental Hypnosis,* 13: 1–10. **142**

BERNSTEIN, M. R. (1965b) Significant value of hypnoanesthesia: Three clinical examples. *American Journal of Clinical Hypnosis,* 7: 259–260. **131, 134, 142**

BETCHER, A. M. (1958) Hypno-induction techniques in pediatric anesthesia. *Anesthesiology,* 19: 279–281. **123, 141**

BETCHER, A. M. (1960) Hypnosis as an adjunct in anesthesiology. *New York State Journal of Medicine,* 60: 816–822. **124, 142**

BING, E. (1969) *Six practical lessons for an easier childbirth: The Lamaze method.* New York: Bantam Books. **117**

BLITZ, B. *see* Dinnerstein, Lowenthal, and Blitz (1966).

BLUM, G. S. (1972) Hypnotic programming techniques in psychological experiments. *In* Fromm and Shor (1972), 359–385.

BONELLO, F. J., *see* Papermaster and others (1960).

BONICA, J. J. (1959) *Clinical applications of diagnostic and therapeutic nerve blocks.* Springfield, Ill.: Thomas. **50, 60**

BONICA, J. J., ed. (1974a) International symposium on pain. *Advances in Neurology,* Vol. 4. New York: Raven Press. **44**

BONICA, J. J. (1974b) Current role of nerve blocks in diagnosis and therapy of pain. *In* Bonica (1974a), 445–453. **50, 51, 60**

BONICA, J. J. (1974c) Organization and function of a pain clinic. *In* Bonica (1974a), 433–443. **58, 62**

BONILLA, K. B.; QUIGLEY, W. F.; and BOWERS, W. F. (1961) Experience with hypnosis on a surgical service. *Military Medicine,* 126: 364–370. **134, 142**

BORING, E. G. (1950) *A history of experimental psychology.* 2d ed. New York: Appleton-Century-Crofts. **80**

BOWEN, D. E. (1973) Transurethral resection under self-hypnosis. *American Journal of Clinical Hypnosis,* 16: 132–134. **131, 132, 134, 142**

BOWERS, K. S. (1967) The effects of demands for honesty on reports of visual and auditory hallucinations. *International Journal of Clinical and Experimental Hypnosis*, 15: 31–36. **15, 25**

Bowers, W. F., *see* Bonilla, Quigley, and Bowers (1961).

Braid, J. (1843) *Neurypnology.* Revised as *Braid on hypnotism,* 1889. New York: Julian Press, reprinted 1960. **4, 23**

Bramwell, J. M. (1903) *Hypnotism: Its history, practice and theory.* New York: Julian Press, reprinted 1956. **23**

Brenman, M., and Gill, M. (1947) *Hypnotherapy: A survey of the literature.* New York: International Universities Press. **205**

Brenman, M., *see also* Gill and Brenman (1959).

Breuer, J., and Freud, S. (1895) *Studies in hysteria.* New York: Basic Books, 1957. **5, 23, 194, 205**

Bridger, A. A., *see* Spiegel and Bridger (1970).

Bromfield, E., *see* Schwartz and others (1973).

Brooks, C. H. (1922) *The practice of autosuggestion by the method of Emile Coué.* New York: Dodd, Mead. **25**

Brown, M., *see* Stern and others (1975).

Budzynski, T.; Stoyva, J.; and Adler, C. (1970) Feedback-induced muscle relaxation. *In* Barber, T.; DiCara, L.; Kamiya, J.; Miller, N.; Shapiro, D.; and Stoyva, J., eds. *Biofeedback and self-control.* Chicago: Aldine-Atherton. **57, 61**

Bunker, J. P., *see* Osborn and others (1967).

Butler, B. (1954a) The use of hypnosis in the care of the cancer patient. *Cancer,* 7: 1–14. **97, 102**

Butler, B. (1954b) The use of hypnosis in the care of the cancer patient. (Part I). *British Journal of Medical Hypnotism,* 6:2: 2–12. **97, 102**

Butler, B. (1955a) The use of hypnosis in the care of the cancer patient. (Part II). *British Journal of Medical Hypnotism,* 6: 3: 2–12. **97, 102**

Butler, B. (1955b) The use of hypnosis in the care of the cancer patient. (Part III). *British Journal of Medical Hypnotism,* 6: 4: 9–17. **97, 102**

Buxton, L. (1962) *A study of psychophysical methods for relief of childbirth pain.* Philadelphia: Saunders. **118**

Buytendijk, F. J. J. (1962) *Pain: Its modes and functions.* Chicago: University of Chicago Press. **29, 44**

Cahn, J., *see* Soulairac, Cahn, and Charpentier (1968).

Calverley, D. S., *see* Barber and Calverley (1963a; 1963b).

Campbell, C., *see* Rock, Shipley, and Campbell (1969).

Campbell, J. N., *see* Taub and Campbell (1974).

Cangello, V. W. (1961) The use of the hypnotic suggestion for relief in malignant disease. *International Journal of Clinical and Experimental Hypnosis,* 9: 17–22. **97–99, 102**

CANGELLO, V. W. (1962) Hypnosis for the patient with cancer. *American Journal of Clinical Hypnosis*, 4: 215–226. **97–99, 102**

CAROLAN, M. T., *see* Long and Carolan (1974).

CASEY, K. L. (1970) Some current views on the neurophysiology of pain. *In* Crue, B. L., ed. *Pain and suffering.* Springfield, Ill.: Thomas, 168–175. **37, 46**

CASEY, K. L. (1973) Pain: A current view of neural mechanisms. *American Scientist*, 61: 194–200. **37, 46**

CASEY, K. L., *see also* Melzack and Casey (1968; 1970).

CEDERCREUTZ, C., and UUSITALO, E. (1967) Hypnotic treatment of phantom sensations in 37 amputees. *In* Lassner, J., ed. *Hypnosis and psychosomatic medicine.* New York: Springer-Verlag, 65–66. **192, 205**

CHAPMAN, C. R., and FEATHER, B. W. (1973) Effects of diazepam on human pain tolerance and pain sensitivity. *Psychosomatic Medicine*, 35: 330–340. **77, 78, 82**

CHAPPLE, P. A. L., *see* Furneaux and Chapple (1964).

CHARPENTIER, J., *see* Soulairac, Cahn, and Charpentier (1968).

CHAVES, J. F., *see* Barber, Spanos, and Chaves (1974).

CHEEK, D. B. (1959) Unconscious perception of meaningful sounds during surgical anesthesia as revealed in hypnosis. *American Journal of Clinical Hypnosis*, 1: 101–113. **143**

CHEEK, D. B. (1964) Surgical memory and reaction to careless conversation. *American Journal of Clinical Hypnosis*, 6: 237–240. **122, 137, 141, 143**

CHEEK, D. B. (1966) The meaning of continued hearing sense under general chemo-anesthesia: A progress report and report of a case. *American Journal of Clinical Hypnosis*, 8: 275–280. **143**

CHEEK, D. B., and LE CRON, L. M. (1968) *Clinical hypnotherapy.* New York: Grune and Stratton. **110, 111, 118, 119, 122, 141**

CHERTOK, L. (1959) *Psychosomatic methods in painless childbirth: History, theory, and practice.* New York: Pergamon Press. **117, 119**

CHERTOK, L. (1973) *Motherhood and personality: Psychosomatic aspects of childbirth.* New York: Harper and Row. **106, 117, 118**

CHONG, T. M. (1963) Childbirth under hypnosis. *Medical Journal of Malaya*, 18: 83–86. **117**

CHONG, T. M. (1964) The use of hypnosis as an adjunct in surgery. *Medical Journal of Malaya*, 19: 154–160. **134**

CHONG, T. M. (1968) The use of hypnosis in the management of patients with cancer. *Singapore Medical Journal*, 9: 211–214. **99, 102**

CHOUGOM, E. A. *see* Velvovski and others (1960).

CHOW, K. L., *see* Nissen, Chow, and Semmes (1951).

CLARK, R. E., and FORGIONE, A. G. (1974) Gingival and digital vasomotor response to thermal imagery in hypnosis. *Journal of Dental Research*, 53: 792–796. **158, 163**

COE, W. C., *see* Sarbin and Coe (1972).

COHEN, A. R., *see* Zimbardo and others (1966).

COOPER, B. J., *see* Barber and Cooper (1972).

COOPER, L., and ERICKSON, M. H. (1959) *Time distortion in hypnosis.* Baltimore: Williams and Wilkins. **96, 101**

COOPER, L. M., *see* London and Cooper (1969); Osborn and others (1967).

COPANS, S. A., *see* Standley and others (1974).

COPPOLINO, C. A. (1965) *Practice of hypnosis in anesthesiology.* New York: Grune and Stratton. **141, 143**

COPPOLINO, C. A., *see also* Wallace and Coppolino (1960).

COUÉ, E. (1923) *How to practice suggestion and autosuggestion.* New York: American Library Service. **16, 25**

CRAIG, J. T., and ABELOFF, M. D. (1974) Psychiatric symptomatology among hospitalized cancer patients. *American Journal of Psychiatry,* 131: 1323–1327. **101**

CRASILNECK, H. B., and HALL, J. A. (1973) Clinical hypnosis in problems of pain. *American Journal of Clinical Hypnosis,* 15: 153–161. **100, 102, 113, 119, 143**

CRASILNECK, H. B., and JENKINS, M. T. (1958) Further studies in the use of hypnosis as a method of anesthesia. *Journal of Clinical and Experimental Hypnosis,* 6: 152–158. **130, 134, 142**

CRASILNECK, H. B.; McCRANIE, E. J.; and JENKINS, M. T. (1956) Special indications for hypnosis as a method of anesthesia. *Journal of the American Medical Association,* 162: 1606–1608. **133, 134, 143, 150, 151, 162**

CRITCHLEY, M. (1956) Congenital indifference to pain. *Annals of Internal Medicine,* 45: 737–747. **28, 44**

CRUTCHFIELD, L. *see* Knox, Crutchfield, and Hilgard (1975).

DALLENBACH, K. M. (1939) Pain: History and present status. *American Journal of Psychology,* 52: 331–347. **45**

DALTON, R., *see* Anderson, Basker, and Dalton (1975).

DANIELS, E. (1962) The hypnotic approach in anesthesia for children. *American Journal of Clinical Hypnosis,* 4: 244–248. **142**

DAVIDSON, J. A. (1962) Assessment of the value of hypnosis in pregnancy and labor. *British Medical Journal,* 2, No. 5310: 951–953. **115, 119**

DAVIDSON, R. J., and SCHWARTZ, G. E. (1976) The psychobiology of relaxation and related states. *In* Mostofsky, D., ed. *Behavior control and modification of physiological activity.* Engelwood Cliffs, N.J.: Prentice-Hall (in press). **199, 206**

DAVIDSON, R. J., *see also* Schwartz and others (1973).

DE LATEUR, B. J. (1974) The role of physical medicine in problems of pain. *In* Bonica (1974a), 495–497. **53, 61**

DE LATEUR, B. J. *see also* Fordyce and others (1973).

DE LEE, S. T., *see* Kroger and De Lee (1957).

DESSOIR, M. (1887) *Bibliographie der modernen Hypnotismus.* Berlin: Carl Duncker Verlag. 23

DESSOIR, M. (1890) *Erster Nachtrag zur Bibliographie des modernen Hypnotismus.* Berlin: Carl Duncker Verlag. 23

DIAMOND, M. J. (1974) The modification of hypnotizability: A review. *Psychological Bulletin*, 81: 180–198. 24

DICK-READ, G., *see* Read, G. D.

DINNERSTEIN, A.; LOWENTHAL, M.; and BLITZ, B. (1966) The interaction of drugs with placebos in the control of pain and anxiety. *Perspectives in Biology and Medicine*, 10: 103–117. 60

DOBERNECK, R. C., *see* Papermaster and others (1960).

DORCUS, R. M. (1963) Fallacies in predictions of susceptibility to hypnosis based on personality characteristics. *American Journal of Clinical Hypnosis*, 5: 163–170. 26

DRAKE, R. L., *see* MacCarty and Drake (1956).

DRIPPS, R. D.; ECKENHOFF, J. E.; and VANDAM, L. D. (1967) *Introduction to anesthesia.* 3d ed. Philadelphia: Saunders. 143

DUCHOWNY, M. S., *see* Standley and others (1974).

DUDLEY, D. L.; HOLMES, T. H.; MARTIN, C. J.; and RIPLEY, H. S. (1966) Hypnotically induced facsimile of pain. *Archives of General Psychiatry*, 15: 198–204. 177, 187

DUDLEY, D. L.; MASUDA, M.; MARTIN, C. J.; and HOLMES, T. H. (1965) Psychophysiological studies of experimentally induced action oriented behavior. *Journal of Psychosomatic Research*, 9: 209–221. 208

DURAND DE GROS, J. P. (1868) *Polyzoisme ou pluralité animale chez l'homme.* Paris: Imprimerie Hennuyer. 176, 186

DURRANI, Z., *see* Winnie, Ramamurphy, and Durrani (1974).

DWORKIN, L., *see* Zimbardo and others (1966).

ECCLES, D., *see* LaBaw and others (1975).

ECKENHOFF, J. E. *see* Dripps, Eckenhoff, and Vandam (1967).

ECKER, H. A. (1959) Medical hypnosis in maxillofacial and plastic surgery. *American Journal of Surgery*, 98: 826–829. 140, 143

EGBERT, L. D.; BATTIT, G. E.; TURNDORT, H.; and BEECHER, H. K. (1963) The value of the preoperative visit by an anesthetist. *Journal of the American Medical Association*, 185: 553. 135, 143

EGBERT, L. D.; BATTIT, G. E.; WELCH, C. E.; and BARTLETT, M. K. (1964) Reduction of postoperative pain by encouragement and instruction of patients. *New England Journal of Medicine*, 270: 825–827. 82, 126, 142

EGBERT, L. D., *see also* Smith and others (1966).

EISENBUD, J. (1937) The psychology of headache. *Psychiatric Quarterly*, 11: 592:619. 195, 205

ELISEO, T. S. (1974) The hypnotic induction profile and hypnotic susceptibility. *International Journal of Clinical and Experimental Hypnosis*, 22: 320–326. **208**

ELLENBERGER, H. F. (1970) *The discovery of the unconscious.* New York: Basic Books. **23, 80, 186**

ENGEL, G. L. (1951) Primary atypical facial neuralgia: An hysterical conversion symptom. *Psychosomatic Medicine*, 13: 375–396. **195, 205**

ERICKSON, M. H. (1959) Hypnosis in painful terminal illnesses. *American Journal of Clinical Hypnosis*, 2: 117–122. **95, 101**

ERICKSON, M. H. (1967) An introduction to the study and application of hypnosis for pain control. *In* Lassner, J., ed. *Hypnosis and psychosomatic medicine.* New York: Springer-Verlag. **93, 95, 101**

ERICKSON, M. H.; HERSHMAN, S.; and SECTER, I. I. (1961) *The practical application of medical and dental hypnosis.* New York: Julian Press. **157, 163**

ERICKSON, M. H., *see also* Cooper and Erickson (1959).

ERVIN, F. R., *see* Mark, Ervin, and Yakovlev (1963).

ESDAILE, J. (1846) *Hypnosis in medicine and surgery.* New York: Julian Press, reprinted 1957. **4, 23**

ESTABROOKS, G. H. (1957) *Hypnotism.* New York: Dutton. **177, 186**

EVANS, F. J. (1974) The placebo response in pain reduction. *In* Bonica (1974a), 289–296. **50, 60**

EVANS, F. J., *see also* McGlashan, Evans, and Orne (1969).

EVANS, M. B., and PAUL, G. L. (1970) Effects of hypnotically suggested analgesia on physiological and subjective responses to cold stress. *Journal of Consulting and Clinical Psychology*, 35: 362–371. **68, 71, 81, 82, 187**

EYSENCK, H. J., and FURNEAUX, W. D. (1945) Primary and secondary suggestibility: An experimental and statistical study. *Journal of Experimental Psychology*, 35: 485–503. **74, 81**

EYSENCK, H. J., and REES, W. L. (1945) States of heightened suggestibility: Narcosis. *Journal of Mental Science*, 91: 301–310. **208**

FAIRES, J. S., and McCARTY, D. J., Jr. (1962) Acute arthritis in man and dog after intrasynovial injection of sodium urate crystals. *Lancet*, 2: 682–685. **208**

FARKAS, H., *see* Mandy and others (1952).

FEATHER, B. W., *see* Chapman and Feather (1973).

FERGUSON, V. S., *see* Freedman and Ferguson (1950).

FERNANDEZ, A., *see* Ruiz and Fernandez (1960).

FIELDS, H. L. *see* Meyer and Fields (1972).

FINER, B. L. (1967) Hypnosis as a psychosomatic weapon in the anesthesiologist's armory. *In* Lassner, J. (Ed.) *Hypnosis and psychosomatic medicine.* New York: Springer-Verlag, 96–99. **142**

FINER, B. L., and Nylén, B. O. (1961) Cardiac arrest in the treatment of burns, and report on hypnosis as a substitute for anesthesia. *Plastic Reconstructive Surgery*, 27: 49–55. **142**

FINKELMAN, A., *see* Lucas, Finkelman, and Tocantins (1962).

FLANARY, H. B., *see* Hill and others (1952).

FORDYCE, W. E. (1973) An operant conditioning method for managing chronic pain. *Postgraduate Medicine*, 53: 123–128. **56, 57, 61**

FORDYCE, W. E. (1974a) Pain viewed as learned behavior. *In* Bonica (1974a), 415–422. **56, 57, 61**

FORDYCE, W. E. (1974b) Treating chronic pain by contingency management. *In* Bonica (1974a), 583–589. **56, 57, 61**

FORDYCE, W. E.; FOWLER, R. S., JR.; LEHMANN, J. F.; DeLATEUR, B. J.; SAND, P. L.; and TRIESCHMANN, R. B. (1973) Operant conditioning in the treatment of chronic pain. *Archives of Physical Medicine and Rehabilitation*, 54: 399–408. **59, 62**

FORGIONE, A. G., *see* Clark and Forgione (1974).

FOWLER, R. S. *see* Fordyce and others (1973).

FRANK, G. S., *see* Osborn and others (1967).

FREEDMAN, L. Z., and FERGUSON, V. S. (1950) The question of "painless childbirth" in primitive cultures. *American Journal of Orthopsychiatry*, 20: 363–372. **103, 117**

FREEMAN, W., and WATTS, J. W. (1950) *Psychosurgery in the treatment of mental disorders and intractable pain*. Springfield, Ill.: Thomas. **30, 44**

FREUD, A. (1937) *The ego and the mechanisms of defense*. London: Hogarth Press. **206**

FREUD, S. (1888) Preface to translation of Bernheim's *Suggestion. Standard Edition of Collected Works*. London: Hogarth Press, 1966, vol. I, pp. 75–85. **23**

FREUD, S., *see also* Breuer and Freud (1895).

FRIEDMAN, H.; NASHOLD, B. S., JR.; and SOMJEN, G. (1974) Physiological effects of dorsal column stimulation. *In* Bonica (1974a), 769–773. **61**

FRIEDMAN, M. M. (1960) Hypnotherapy in advanced cancer. *Rocky Mountain Medical Journal*, 57: 6: 33–37. **90, 91, 94, 101**

FROMM, E., and SHOR, R. E., eds. (1972) *Hypnosis: Research developments and perspectives*. Chicago: Aldine-Atherton. **23**

FURNEAUX, W. D., and CHAPPLE, P. A. L. (1964) Some objective and subjective characteristics of labor influenced by personality, and their modification by hypnosis and relaxation. *Proceedings of the Royal Society of Medicine*, 57: 261–262. **111, 118**

FURNEAUX, W. D., *see also* Eysenck and Furneaux (1945).

GAGGE, A. P., and STEVENS, J. C. (1968) Thermal sensitivity and comfort. *In* Kenshalo, D. R., ed. *The skin senses*. Springfield, Ill.: Thomas, 345–364. **45**

GANNON, L., and STERNBACH, R. A. (1971) Alpha enhancement as a treatment for pain: A case study. *Journal of Behavior Therapy and Experimental Psychiatry*, 2: 209–213. **61**

GARDNER, G. G. (1975) Childhood, death, and human dignity. *International Journal of Clinical and Experimental Hypnosis* (In press). **94, 102**

GAZZANIGA, M. S. (1970) *The bisected brain.* New York: Appleton-Century-Crofts. **12, 24**

GETTINGER, D. (1974) Levels of awareness in hypnosis: A preliminary study. Unpublished senior honors thesis, Stanford University. **187**

GILL, M., and BRENMAN, M. (1959) *Hypnosis and related states.* New York: International Universities Press. **185, 188, 196, 205, 206**

GILL, M., *see also* Brenman and Gill (1947).

GLASS, L. B., *see* Barber and Glass (1962).

GOLAN, H. P. (1971) Control of fear reaction in dental patients by hypnosis: Three case reports. *American Journal of Clinical Hypnosis,* 13: 279–284. **145, 160, 161, 163**

GOLDIE, L. (1956) Hypnosis in the casualty department. *British Medical Journal,* 2: 1340–1342. **134, 143**

GOLDSCHEIDER, A. (1894) *Über den Schmerz in physiologischer und klinischer Hinsicht.* Berlin: Hirschwald. **34, 45**

GOLDSTEIN, A., and HILGARD, E. R. (1975) Lack of influence of the morphine antagonist naloxone on hypnotic analgesia. *Proceedings of the National Academy of Sciences,* 72: 2041–2043. **176, 183, 184, 186, 187**

GOLDSTEIN, M. N., *see* Satran and Goldstein (1973).

GONDA, T. A. (1962) The relation between complaints of persistent pain and family size. *Journal of Neurology, Neurosurgery, and Psychiatry,* 25: 277–281. **33, 45**

GOTTFREDSON, D. K. (1973) Hypnosis as an anesthetic in dentistry. Doctoral dissertation, Department of Psychology, Brigham Young University. *Dissertation Abstracts International,* 33: 7–B: 3303. **152–157, 162, 163**

GRAHAM, G. (1974) Hypnoanalysis in dental practice. *American Journal of Clinical Hypnosis,* 16: 178–187. **159, 163**

GREEN, E. E., *see* Sargent, Walters, and Green (1973).

GREENE, R. J., and REYHER, J. (1972) Pain tolerance in hypnotic analgesic and imagination states. *Journal of Abnormal Psychology,* 79: 29–38. **70, 77, 82, 187**

GREENHOOT, J. H., and STERNBACH, R. A. (1974) Conjoint treatment of chronic pain. *In* Bonica (1974a), 595–603. **62**

GREENHOOT, J. H., *see also* Sternbach and others (1974).

GRIFFEN, W. O., *see* Papermaster and others (1960).

GROSS, H., and POSNER, N. A. (1963) An evaluation of hypnosis for obstetric delivery. *American Journal of Obstetrics and Gynecology,* 87: 912–920. **119**

GRUPSMITH, E., *see* Wheeler and others (1974).

GUR, R. C., *see* Gur and Gur (1974).

GUR, R. E., and GUR, R. C. (1974) Handedness, sex, and eyedness as moderating variables in the relationship between hypnotic susceptibility and functional brain asymmetry. *Journal of Abnormal Psychology,* 83: 635–643. **13, 24**

HAGFORS, N., *see* Long and Hagfors (1975).

HAHN, K. W., JR., *see* Barber and Hahn (1962; 1964).

HALL, J. A., *see* Crasilneck and Hall (1973).

HARDING, H. C. (1967) Hypnosis in the treatment of migraine. *In* Lassner, J., ed. *Hypnosis and psychosomatic medicine.* New York: Springer-Verlag, 131–134. **192, 196, 205**

HARDY, J. D., *see* Wolf and Hardy (1941).

HARNETT, W. E., *see* Roberts and others (1953).

HARTLAND, J. (1971) *Medical and dental hypnosis.* 2d ed. Baltimore: Williams and Wilkins. **111, 118**

HARTMANN, W., and RAWLINS, C. M. (1960) Hypnosis in the management of a case of *placenta abruptio. International Journal of Clinical and Experimental Hypnosis,* 8: 103–119. **119**

HASTEY, J. M., *see* Arkin and others (1970).

HELLMAN, L. M., *see* Hingson and Hellman (1956).

HERNANDEZ, A., *see* Schafer and Hernandez (1973).

HERON, W. T., *see* Abramson and Heron (1950).

HERSHMAN, S., *see* Erickson, Hershman, and Secter (1961).

HIGGINS, J. D.; TURSKY, B.; and SCHWARTZ, G. E. (1971) Shock elicited pain and its reduction by concurrent tactile stimulation. *Science,* 172: 866–867. **46**

HIGHTOWER, P. R. (1966) The control of pain. *American Journal of Clinical Hypnosis,* 9: 67–70. **100, 102**

HILGARD, E. R. (1965a) *Hypnotic susceptibility.* New York: Harcourt Brace Jovanovich. (Shorter version in paperback, under title *The experience of hypnosis,* 1968). **24, 25**

HILGARD, E. R. (1965b) Hypnosis. *Annual Review of Psychology,* 16:157–180. **23**

HILGARD, E. R. (1967) A quantitative study of pain and its reduction through hypnotic suggestion. *Proceedings of the National Academy of Sciences,* 57: 1581–1586. **46, 68, 81, 82**

HILGARD, E. R. (1969) Pain as a puzzle for psychology and physiology. *American Psychologist,* 24: 103–113. **40, 43, 46, 71, 81, 82**

HILGARD, E. R. (1971) Pain: Its reduction and production under hypnosis. *Proceedings of the American Philosophical Society,* 115: 470–476. **46, 177, 187**

HILGARD, E. R. (1973a) The domain of hypnosis, with some comments on alternative paradigms. *American Psychologist,* 28: 972–982. **81**

HILGARD, E. R. (1973b) Dissociation revisited. *In* Henle, M.; Jaynes, J.; and Sullivan, J., eds. *Historical conceptions of psychology.* New York: Springer, 205–219. **185, 188**

HILGARD, E. R. (1973c) A neodissociation interpretation of pain reduction in hypnosis. *Psychological Review,* 80: 396–411. **166, 185, 186, 188**

HILGARD, E. R. (1974) Toward a neodissociation theory: Multiple cognitive controls in human functioning. *Perspectives in Biology and Medicine,* 17: 301–316. **185, 188**

HILGARD, E. R. (1975a) The alleviation of pain by hypnosis. *Pain,* 1 (in press) **207**

HILGARD, E. R. (1975b) Hypnosis. *Annual Review of Psychology,* 26: 19–44. **23, 24**

HILGARD, E. R. (1975c) Hypnosis in the relief of pain. *In* Weisenberg, M., ed. *The control of pain.* New York: Psychological Dimensions (in press). **46, 72, 81, 170, 186**

HILGARD, E. R. (1976a) Pain perception in man. *In* Held, R. M.; Leibowitz, H. W.; and Teuber, H-L., eds. *Handbook of sensory physiology,* vol. 8. New York: Springer-Verlag (in press). **46**

HILGARD, E. R. (1976b) Neodissociation theory of multiple cognitive controls. *In* Schwartz, G. E. and Shapiro, D., eds. *Consciousness and self regulation.* New York: Plenum Press (in press). **185, 188**

HILGARD, E. R. (in preparation) *A neodissociation theory of human cognitive controls.* New York: Wiley. **185, 188**

HILGARD, E. R.; MACDONALD, H.; MARSHALL, G. D.; and Morgan, A. H. (1974) The anticipation of pain and pain control under hypnosis: Heart rate and blood pressure responses in the cold pressor test. *Journal of Abnormal Psychology,* 83: 561–568. **79, 181, 187**

HILGARD, E. R., and MORGAN, A. H. (1975) Heart rate and blood pressure in the study of laboratory pain in man under normal conditions and as influenced by hypnosis. *Acta Neurobiologiae Experimentalis* (in press). **46, 69, 76, 177, 187**

HILGARD, E. R.; MORGAN, A. H.; LANGE, A. F.; LENOX, J. R.; MACDONALD, H.; MARSHALL, G. D.; and SACHS, L. B. (1974). Heart rate changes in pain and hypnosis. *Psychophysiology,* 11: 692–702. **76, 82**

HILGARD, E. R.; MORGAN, A. H.; and MACDONALD, H. (1975) Pain and dissociation in the cold pressor test: A study of hypnotic analgesia with "hidden reports" through automatic key-pressing and automatic talking. *Journal of Abnormal Psychology* (in press). **46, 66, 81, 170–174, 186**

HILGARD, E. R.; RUCH, J. C.; LANGE, A. F.; LENOX, J. R.; MORGAN, A. H.; and SACHS, L. B. (1974) The psychophysics of cold pressor pain and its modification through hypnotic suggestion. *American Journal of Psychology,* 87: 17–31. **46, 81**

HILGARD, E. R., *see also* Goldstein and Hilgard (1975); Hilgard, J., Hilgard, and Newman (1961); Knox, Crutchfield, and Hilgard (1975); Knox, Morgan, and Hilgard (1974); Morgan and Hilgard (1973); Morgan, Johnson, and Hilgard (1974); Osborn and others (1967); Ruch, Morgan, and Hilgard (1973); Weitzenhoffer and Hilgard (1959; 1962).

HILGARD, J. R. (1965) Personality and hypnotizability: Inferences from case studies. *In* E. R. Hilgard (1965a), 343–374. **11, 24**

HILGARD, J. R. (1970) *Personality and hypnosis: A study of imaginative involvement.* Chicago: University of Chicago Press. **11, 24**

HILGARD, J. R. (1971) How the subject perceives the hypnotist: A study of the hypnotist-subject relationship. (Unpublished). Frieda Fromm-Reichmann Lecture, Stanford Medical School. **18, 20, 25**

HILGARD, J. R. (1974a) Imaginative involvement: Some characteristics of the highly hypnotizable and the non-hypnotizable. *International Journal of Clinical and Experimental Hypnosis*, 22: 138–156. **11, 24**

HILGARD, J. R. (1974b) Sequelae to hypnosis. *International Journal of Clinical and Experimental Hypnosis*, 22: 281–298. **206**

HILGARD, J. R.; HILGARD, E. R.; and NEWMAN, M. (1961) Sequelae to hypnotic induction with special reference to earlier chemical anesthesia. *Journal of Nervous and Mental Disease*, 133: 461–478. **206**

HILL, H. E.; KORNETSKY, C. H.; FLANARY, H. B.; and WIKLER, A. (1952) Effects of anxiety and morphine on discrimination of intensities of painful stimuli. *Journal of Clinical Investigation*, 31: 473–480. **82**

HINGSON, R. A., and HELLMAN, L. M. (1956) *Anesthesia for obstetrics*. Philadelphia: Lippincott. **117**

HOFFMAN, E. (1959) Hypnosis in general surgery. *American Surgeon*, 25: 163–169. **142**

HOFFMAN, G. L., JR.; and KOPENHAVER, D. B. (1961) Medical hypnosis and its use in obstetrics. *American Journal of Medical Sciences*, 241: 788–810. **117**

HOLMES, T. H., *see* Dudley and others (1965; 1966).

HOLTON, C., *see* LaBaw and others (1975).

HULL, C. L. (1929) Quantitative methods of investigating waking suggestion. *Journal of Abnormal and Social Psychology*, 24: 153–169. **23**

HULL, C. L. (1930) Quantitative methods of investigating hypnotic suggestion. Part I. *Journal of Abnormal and Social Psychology*, 25: 200–223. **23**

HULL, C. L. (1931) Quantitative methods of investigating hypnotic suggestion. Part II. *Journal of Abnormal and Social Psychology*, 25: 390–417. **23**

HULL, C. L. (1933) *Hypnosis and suggestibility: An experimental approach*. New York: Appleton-Century-Crofts. (Paperbound edition, 1968). **5, 23, 25, 81**

HULL, C. L. (1962) Psychology of the scientist: IV. Passages from the 'idea books' of Clark L. Hull. *Perceptual and Motor Skills*, 15: 807–882. **23**

JACOBSON, E. (1929) *Progressive relaxation*. Chicago: University of Chicago Press. **117, 199, 206**

JACOBSON, E. (1954) Relaxation in labor: A critique of current techniques in natural childbirth. *American Journal of Obstetrics and Gynecology*, 67: 1035–1048. **117**

JACOBSON, E. (1965) *How to relax and have your baby*. New York: McGraw-Hill. **117**

JACOBY, J. D. (1960) Statistical report on general practice; hypnodontics; tape recorder conditioning. *International Journal of Clinical and Experimental Hypnosis*, 3: 115–119. **152, 162**

JAMES, L. S. (1960) The effect of pain relief for labor and delivery on the fetus and newborn. *Anesthesiology*, 21: 405–430. **118**

JAMES, L. S., *see also* Moya and James (1960).

JAMES, W. (1889) Automatic writing. *Proceedings of the American Society for Psychical Research*, 1: 548–564. **176, 186**

JAMES, W. (1890) *Principles of psychology.* 2 volumes. New York: Holt. **5, 176, 186**

JANET, P. (1889) *L'Automatisme psychologique.* Paris: Alcan. **184, 188**

JANET, P. (1907) *The major symptoms of hysteria.* New York: Macmillan. **184, 188**

JANET, P. (1925) *Psychological healing.* 2 volumes. London: George Allen and Unwin. **5, 23**

JENKINS, M. T., *see* Crasilneck and Jenkins (1958); Crasilneck, McCranie, and Jenkins (1956).

JOHNSON, D. L., *see* Morgan, Johnson, and Hilgard (1974).

JOSPE, M. L. (1974) *The placebo effect.* Unpublished doctoral dissertation, University of Minnesota. **60**

KALENDGIEV, T. Z., *see* Petrov, Traikov, and Kalendgiev (1964).

KAMIYA, J. (1969) Operant control of the EEG alpha rhythm and some of its reported effects on consciousness. In Tart, C. T. ed. *Altered states of consciousness.* New York: Wiley, 507–517. **61**

KANE, K., and TAUB, A. (1975) A history of local electrical analgesia. *Pain,* 1: 125–138. **61**

KANE, K. M., *see* Roberts and others (1953).

KAO, C. Y., *see* Katz and others (1974).

KAPLAN, E. A. (1960) Hypnosis and pain. *A.M.A. Archives of General Psychiatry,* 2: 567–568. **177, 186**

KARLOVSKY, E., *see* Thoms and Karlovsky (1954).

KATCHAN, F. A., and BELOZERSKI, G. G. (1940) Obstetrical analgesia by hypnosis and suggestion. (In Russian) *Sborn. Tsent. nauch. issled. acouch-guinek., Inst. Leningrad,* 6: 19–89. *From* Chertok (1959), ref. 262. **114, 119**

KATZ, G. L., *see* Katz, R. L., and others (1974).

KATZ, R. L.; KAO, C. Y.; SPIEGEL, H.; and KATZ, G. J. (1974) Pain, acupuncture, hypnosis. *In* Bonica (1974a), 819–825. **198, 206**

KEWMAN, D. G., *see* Roberts, Kewman, and Macdonald (1973).

KLINE, M. V. (1958) *Freud and hypnosis.* New York: Julian Press. **205**

KNOX, V. J.; CRUTCHFIELD, L.; and HILGARD, E. R. (1975). The nature of task interference in hypnotic dissociation. *International Journal of Clinical and Experimental Hypnosis,* 23: 305–323. **186**

KNOX, V. J.; MORGAN, A. H.; and HILGARD, E. R. (1974) Pain and suffering in ischemia: The paradox of hypnotically suggested anesthesia as contradicted by reports from the "hidden observer". *Archives of General Psychiatry,* 30: 840–847. **42, 46, 70, 81, 174–176, 186**

KOLB, L. C. (1954) *The painful phantom.* Springfield, Ill.: Thomas. **205**

KOLOUCH, F. T. (1962) Role of suggestion in surgical convalescence. *Archives of Surgery,* 85: 304–315. **127, 142**

KOLOUCH, F. T. (1964) Hypnosis and surgical convalescence: A study of subjective factors in postoperative recovery. *American Journal of Clinical Hypnosis*, 7: 120–129. **127, 142**

KOLOUCH, F. T. (1968) The frightened surgical patient. *American Journal of Clinical Hypnosis*, 11: 89–98. **127, 128, 142**

KOPENHAVER, D. B., *see* Hoffman and Kopenhaver (1961).

KORNETSKY, C. H., *see* Hill and others (1952).

KOSAMBI, D. D. (1967) Living prehistory in India. *Scientific American*, 216: 105–114. **47, 60**

KROGER, W. S. (1953) "Natural childbirth": Is Read's method of "natural childbirth" waking hypnotism? *British Journal of Medical Hypnotism*, 4, No. 4: 29–43. **105, 117**

KROGER, W. S. (1957) Introduction and supplemental report. *In* Esdaile, J., ed. *Hypnosis in medicine and surgery*. New York: Julian Press. **138, 143**

KROGER, W. S. (1959) Film: *Thyroidectomy under hypnoanesthesia*. Wexler Film Co., 802 Seward, Hollywood, California. **134**

KROGER, W. S., ed. (1962) *Psychosomatic obstetrics, gynecology and endocrinology*. Springfield, Ill.: Thomas. **118**

KROGER, W. S. (1963) *Clinical and experimental hypnosis*. Philadelphia: Lippincott. **99, 102, 111, 118, 122, 133, 134, 141**

KROGER, W. S., and DE LEE, S. T. (1957) Use of hypnoanesthesia for caesarean section and hysterectomy. *Journal of the American Medical Association*, 163: 442–444. **133, 134**

KROLL, R. G. (1962) Hypnosis for the poor risk dental patient. *American Journal of Clinical Hypnosis*, 5: 142–144. **147, 161**

LABAW, W. L. (1969) Terminal hypnosis in lieu of terminal hospitalization: An effective alternative in fortunate cases. *Gerontologia Clinica*, 11: 312–320. **92, 101**

LABAW, W. L.; HOLTON, C.; ECCLES, D.; and TEWELL, K. (1975) The use of self-hypnosis by children with cancer. *American Journal of Clinical Hypnosis*, 17, 233–238. **102**

LAMAZE, F., and VELLAY, P. (1957) *Psychologic analgesia in obstetrics*. New York: Pergamon Press. **103, 117**

LANG, G., *see* Spanos, Barber, and Lang (1974).

LANGE, A. F., *see* Hilgard, Morgan, and others (1974); Hilgard, Ruch and others (1974).

LASSNER, J., ed. (1964) *Hypnosis in anesthesiology*. New York: Springer-Verlag. **141**

LAUX, R. (1953) An investigation of the analgesic effects of hypnosis on postoperative pain resulting from urological surgery. Unpublished doctoral dissertation, University of Southern California. **142**

LEA, P., WARE, P., and MONROE, R. (1960) The hypnotic control of intractable pain. *American Journal of Clinical Hypnosis*, 3: 3–8. **97, 102**

LECRON, L. M., *see* Cheek and LeCron (1968).

LEHMANN, J. F. *see* Fordyce and others (1973).

LENOX, J. R. (1970) Effect of hypnotic analgesia on verbal report and cardiovascular responses to ischemic pain. *Journal of Abnormal Psychology*, 75: 199–206. **72, 76, 81, 82**

LENOX, J. R., *see also* Hilgard, Morgan, and others (1974); Hilgard, Ruch, and others (1974).

LEONE, M. P., *see* Zaretsky and Leone (1975).

LEVANDER, S., *see* Schalling and Levander (1964).

LEVINSON, B. W. (1967) States of awareness during general anesthesia. *In* Lassner, J., ed. *Hypnosis and psychosomatic medicine.* New York: Springer-Verlag, 200–207. **136, 137, 143**

LEVINSON, J. *see* Winkelstein and Levinson (1959).

LEVINSON, P. (1975) Obstacles in the treatment of dying patients. *American Journal of Psychiatry*, 132: 28–32. **101**

LEVITAN, H., *see* Barker and Levitan (1974).

LEWIN, I. (1965) The effect of reward on the experience of pain. *Dissertations in cognitive processes.* Detroit: Center for Cognitive Processes, Wayne State University. **33, 45**

LIEBESKIND, J. C.; MAYER, D. J.; and AKIL, H. (1974) Central mechanisms of pain inhibition: Studies of analgesia from focal brain stimulation. *In* Bonica (1974), 261–268. **37, 46**

LIM, R. K. S. (1970) Pain. *Annual Review of Physiology*, 32: 269–288. **37, 46**

LOGAN, W. C. (1963) Delay of premature labor by hypnosis. *American Journal of Clinical Hypnosis*, 5: 209–211. **119**

LONDON, P. (1962) *The Children's Hypnotic Susceptibility Scale.* Palo Alto, Calif.: Consulting Psychologists Press. **24**

LONDON, P., and COOPER, L. M. (1969) Norms of hypnotic susceptibility in children. *Developmental Psychology*, 1: 113–124. **24**

LONG, D. M., and CAROLAN, M. T. (1974) Cutaneous afferent stimulation in the treatment of chronic pain. *In* Bonica (1974a), 755–759. **61**

LONG, D. M., and HAGFORS, N. (1975) Electrical stimulation of the nervous system: The current status of electrical stimulation of the nervous system for relief of pain. *Pain*, 1: 109–123. **61**

LOWENTHAL, M., *see* Dinnerstein, Lowenthal, and Blitz (1966).

LUCAS, O. N.; FINKELMAN, A.; and TOCANTINS, L. M. (1962) Management of tooth extractions in hemophiliacs by the combined use of hypnotic suggestion, protective splint, and packing of sockets. *Journal of Oral Surgery, Anesthesia, and Hospital Dental Service*, 20: 488–500. **150, 158, 163**

LUCAS, O. N., and TOCANTINS, L. M. (1964) Problems in hemostasis in hemophiliacs undergoing dental extraction. *Annals of the New York Academy of Sciences*, 115: 470–480. **158, 163**

LUTHE, W., *see* Schultz and Luthe (1969).

McBROOM, P. (1975) Acupuncture pain relief patterns linked to referred pain syndromes. *Hospital Tribune*, 9, No. 4: 1, 18–19. **206**

MacCarty, C. S., and Drake, R. L. (1956) Neurosurgical procedures for the control of pain. *Proceedings of the Staff Meetings, Mayo Clinic*, 31: 208–214. **52**

McCarty, D. J., Jr., *see* Faires and McCarty (1962).

McCay, A. R. (1963) Dental extraction under self-hypnosis. *Medical Journal of Australia*, 1, No. 22: 820–822. **150**

McCranie, E. J., *see* Crasilneck, McCranie, and Jenkins (1956).

Macdonald, H., *see* Hilgard, Macdonald, and others (1974); Hilgard, Morgan, and others (1974); Hilgard, Morgan, and Macdonald (1975); Roberts, Kewman, and Macdonald (1973).

McDougall, W. (1926) *Outline of abnormal psychology*. New York: Scribner's. **23**

McGlashan, T. H.; Evans, F. J.; and Orne, M. T. (1969) The nature of hypnotic analgesia and the placebo response to experimental pain. *Psychosomatic Medicine*, 31: 227–246. **74, 75, 81**

McMurray, G. A. (1950) Experimental study of a case of insensitivity to pain. *Archives of Neurology and Psychiatry*, 64: 650–667. **28, 44**

McPeake, J. D., *see* Spanos and McPeake (1975).

MacWilliam, J. A., and Webster, W. J. (1923) Some applications of physiology to medicine; sensory phenomena associated with defective blood supply to working muscle. *British Medical Journal*, 1: 51–53. **46**

Maer, F., *see* Schwartz and others (1973).

Mandy, A. J.; Mandy, T. E.; Farkas, H.; and Scher, E. (1952) Is natural childbirth natural? *Psychosomatic Medicine*, 14: 432–438. **117**

Mandy, T. E., *see* Mandy, A. J., and others (1952).

Marcuse, F. L., ed. (1964) *Hypnosis throughout the world*. Springfield, Ill.: Thomas. **23**

Mark, V. H.; Ervin, F. R.; and Yakovlev, P. I. (1963) Stereotactic thalamotomy. *Archives of Neurology* (Chicago), 8: 528–538. **30, 44**

Markowitz, R. A., *see* Smith and others (1966).

Marmer, M. J. (1959a) Hypnoanalgesia and hypnoanesthesia for cardiac surgery. *Journal of the American Medical Association*, 171: 512–517. **134, 142**

Marmer, M. J. (1959b) Hypnosis as an adjunct to anesthesia in children. *American Journal of Diseases of Children*, 97: 314–317. **122, 123, 142**

Marmer, M. J. (1959c) *Hypnosis in anesthesiology*. Springfield, Ill.: Thomas. **124, 141, 142**

Marmer, M. J. (1961) Present applications of hypnosis in anesthesiology. *Western Journal of Surgery*, 69: 260–263. **139, 142, 143**

Marmer, M. J. (1963) Hypnosis in anesthesiology and surgery. *In* Schneck, J. M., ed. *Hypnosis in modern medicine*. Springfield, Ill.: Thomas. **138, 142, 143**

Marmer, M. J. (1969) Unusual applications of hypnosis in anesthesiology. *International Journal of Clinical and Experimental Hypnosis*, 17: 199–208. **124, 142**

Marshall, G. D., *see* Hilgard, Macdonald, and others (1974); Hilgard, Morgan, and others (1974); Maslach, Marshall, and Zimbardo (1972).

MARTIN, C. J., *see* Dudley and others (1965; 1966).

MASLACH, C.; MARSHALL, G. D.; and ZIMBARDO, P. G. (1972) Hypnotic control of peripheral skin temperature: A case report. *Psychophysiology*, 9: 600–605. **158, 163**

MASON, A. A. (1955) Surgery under hypnosis. *Anesthesia*, 10: 295–299. **134**

MASUDA, M., *see* Dudley and others (1965).

MAYER, D. J., *see* Liebeskind, Mayer, and Akil (1974).

MELZACK, R. (1971) Phantom limb pain: Implications for treatment of pathological pain. *Anesthesiology*, 35: 409–419. **45, 205**

MELZACK, R. (1973) *The puzzle of pain.* New York: Basic Books. **32, 44, 45, 46, 54, 60, 61**

MELZACK, R. (1974) *Acupuncture and pain mechanisms.* Invited address at meeting of Society for Clinical and Experimental Hypnosis, Montreal, October 13. **48, 60**

MELZACK, R., and CASEY, K. L. (1968) Sensory, motivational, and central control mechanisms of pain: A new conceptual model. *In* Kenshalo, D., ed. *The skin senses.* Springfield, Ill.: Thomas, 423–439. **36, 46**

MELZACK, R., and CASEY, K. L. (1970) The affective dimension of pain. *In* Arnold, M., ed. *Feelings and emotions.* New York: Academic Press, 55–68. **36, 46**

MELZACK, R., and PERRY, C. (1975) Self-regulation of pain: Use of alpha feedback and hypnotic training for control of chronic pain. *Experimental Neurology*, 46: 452–469. **45, 61, 193, 205**

MELZACK, R., and SCOTT, T. H. (1957) The effects of early experience on the response to pain. *Journal of Comparative and Physiological Psychology*, 50: 155–161. **33, 45**

MELZACK, R., and TORGERSON, W. S. (1971) On the language of pain. *Anesthesiology*, 34: 50–59. **31, 45**

MELZACK, R., and WALL, P. D. (1965) Pain mechanisms: A new theory. *Science*, 150: 971–979. **34, 45, 46**

MELZACK, R., and WALL, P. D. (1968) Gate control theory of pain. *In* Soulairac, Cahn, and Charpentier (1968), 11–31. **46**

MELZACK, R., and WALL, P. D. (1970) Psychophysiology of pain. *International Anesthesiology Clinics*, 8: 3–34. **34, 46**

MELZACK, R.; WEISZ, A. Z.; and SPRAGUE, L. T. (1963) Stratagems for controlling pain: Contributions of auditory stimulation and suggestion. *Experimental Neurology*, 8: 239–247. **54, 61**

MERSKEY, H. (1965) Psychiatric patients with persistent pain. *Journal of Psychosomatic Research*, 9: 299–309. **45**

MERSKEY, H., and SPEAR, F. C. (1967) *Pain: Psychological and psychiatric perspectives.* London: Baillière, Tindall and Cassel; Baltimore: Williams and Wilkins. **45, 205**

MEYER, G. A., and FIELDS, H. L. (1972) Causalgia treated by selective large fibre stimulation of peripheral nerve. *Brain*, 95: 163–168. **61**

MILLET, J. B., *see* Wolfe and Millet (1960).

MINISTRY OF HEALTH, SOVIET UNION (1951) *Temporary directions on the practice of the psychoprophylaxis of the pains of childbirth.* (In Russian) No. 142, February 13. From Chertok (1959), p. 92. **106, 118**

MOLL, A. (1890) *The study of hypnosis: Historical, clinical and experimental research in the techniques of hypnotic induction.* New York: Julian Press, reprinted 1958. **23**

MONROE, R., *see* Lea, Ware, and Monroe (1960).

MOORE, R. K. (1964) Susceptibility to hypnosis and susceptibility to social influence. *Journal of Abnormal and Social Psychology,* 68: 282–294. **73, 81**

MORDKOFF, A. M., *see* Wheeler and others (1974).

MORGAN, A. H. (1973) The heritability of hypnotic susceptibility in twins. *Journal of Abnormal Psychology,* 82: 55–61. **10, 24**

MORGAN, A. H., and HILGARD, E. R. (1973) Age differences in susceptibility to hypnosis. *International Journal of Clinical and Experimental Hypnosis,* 21: 78–85. **24**

MORGAN, A. H.; JOHNSON, D. L.; and HILGARD, E. R. (1974) The stability of hypnotic susceptibility: A longitudinal study. *International Journal of Clinical and Experimental Hypnosis,* 22: 249–257. **24**

MORGAN, A. H.; *see also* Hilgard, Macdonald, and others (1974); Hilgard and Morgan (1975); Hilgard, Morgan, and others (1974); Hilgard, Morgan, and Macdonald (1975); Hilgard, Ruch, and others (1974); Knox, Morgan, and Hilgard (1974); Ruch and Morgan (1971); Ruch, Morgan, and Hilgard (1973).

MORPHIS, O. L. (1961) Hypnosis and its use in controlling patients with malignancy. *American Journal of Roentgenology,* 85: 897–900. **99, 102**

MOSS, A. A. (1963a) Hypnosis for pain management in dentistry. *Journal of Dental Medicine,* 18: 110–112. **149, 162**

MOSS, A. A. (1963b) Hypnodontics: Hypnosis in dentistry. *In* Kroger (1963), 279–290. **152, 161, 162**

MOSTELLER, F., *see* Smith and others (1966).

MOYA, F., and JAMES, L. S. (1960) Medical hypnosis for obstetrics. *Journal of the American Medical Association,* 174: 2026–2032. **113, 118**

MURPHY, R. W., *see* Sternbach and others (1974).

MYERS, F. W. H. (1903) *Human personality and its survival of bodily death.* 2 volumes. New York: Longmans Green. (Reprinted, New Hyde Park, New York: University Books, 1961). **176, 186, 187**

NASHOLD, B. S., JR., *see* Friedman, Nashold, and Somjen (1974).

NATHAN, P. W. (1956) Reference of sensation at the spinal level. *Journal of Neurology, Neurosurgery, and Psychiatry,* 19: 88–100. **45**

NEWMAN, M. (1971) The role of amnesia in dentistry: A case report. *American Journal of Clinical Hypnosis,* 14: 127–130. **158, 163**

NEWMAN, Martha, *see* Hilgard, Hilgard, and Newman (1961).

NIBOYET, J. E. H. (1973) *L'anesthésie par l'acupuncture,* Sainte-Ruffine, France: Maisonneuve. **54, 61**

NISSEN, H. W.; CHOW, K. L.; and SEMMES, J. (1951) Effects of restricted opportunity for tactual, kinesthetic, and manipulative experience on the behavior of a chimpanzee. *American Journal of Psychology*, 64: 485–507. **33, 45**

NOGIER, P. F. M. (1972) *Treatise of auriculotherapy.* Sainte-Ruffine, France: Maisonneuve. **54, 55, 61**

NYLÉN, B. O., *see* Finer and Nylén (1961).

O'CONNELL, *see* Orne and O'Connell (1967).

ORNE, E. C., *see* Shor and Orne (1962).

ORNE, M. T. (1972) On the simulating subject as a quasi-control group in hypnosis research: What, why, and how. *In* Fromm and Shor (1972), 399–443. **16, 25**

ORNE, M. T. (1974) Pain suppression by hypnosis and related phenomena. *In* Bonica (1974a), 563–582. **208**

ORNE, M. T., and O'CONNELL, D. N. (1967) Diagnostic ratings of hypnotizability. *International Journal of Clinical and Experimental Hypnosis*, 15, 125–133. **142, 208**

ORNE, M. T., *see also* McGlashan, Evans, and Orne (1969); Shor and Orne (1965).

OSBORN, A. G.; BUNKER, J. P.; COOPER, L. M.; FRANK, G. S.; and HILGARD, E. R. (1967) Effects of thiopental sedation on learning and memory. *Science*, 157: 574–576. **188**

OVERTON, D. A. (1972) State-dependent learning produced by alcohol and its relevance to alcoholism. *In* Kissin, B., and Begleiter, H., eds. *The biology of alcoholism.* Vol. 2. New York: Plenum Press, 193–217. **183, 187**

OWENS, H. E. (1970) Hypnosis and psychotherapy in dentistry: Five case histories. *International Journal of Clinical and Experimental Hypnosis*, 18: 181–193. **148, 150, 162**

PAPERMASTER, A. A.; DOBERNECK, R. C.; BONELLO, F. J.; GRIFFEN, W. O.; and WANGENSTEEN, O. H. (1960) Hypnosis in surgery: II. Pain. *American Journal of Clinical Hypnosis*, 2: 220–224. **142**

PATTERSON, R., *see* Roberts and others (1975).

PATTON, I. B. (1969) Report on thyroidectomy performed under hypnosis. *Journal of the Medical Association of the State of Alabama*, 38: 617–619. **134**

PAUL, G. L., *see* Evans and Paul (1970).

PAVLOV, I. P. (1927) *Conditioned reflexes.* New York: Oxford University Press. **50, 60**

PEARSON, R. E. (1961) Responses to suggestions given under general anesthesia. *American Journal of Clinical Hypnosis*, 4: 106–114. **126, 127, 142**

PERRY, C., *see* Melzack and Perry (1975).

PETROV, P.; TRAIKOV, D.; and KALENDGIEV, T. Z. (1964) A contribution to psychoanesthetization through hypnosis in some stomatological manipulations. *British Journal of Medical Hypnotism*, 15: 8–16. **150**

PIXA, B. (1975) A therapy where the hurt may help. *San Francisco Sunday Examiner and Chronicle*, February 2. **53, 61**

PLATONOV, K. I. (1959) *The word as a physiological and therapeutic factor.* 2d ed. Moscow: Foreign Languages Publishing House. **26**

PLATONOV, K. I., *see also* Velvovski and others (1960).

PLOTITCHER, V. A., *see* Velvovski and others (1960).

PODMORE, F. (1902) *Modern spiritualism*. London: Methuen. Vol. I, pp. 154–176. **23**

POLLACK, S. (1966) Pain control by suggestion. *Journal of Oral Medicine*, 21: 89–95. **152, 162**

POSNER, N. A., *see* Gross and Posner (1963).

PRILL, H. J. (1956) Das Autogene Training zur Geburtsschmerzleichterung. (Autogenic training for lessening the pain of childbirth). *Psychotherapie*, 1: 165–177. **118**

PRINCE, M. (1906) *The dissociation of a personality*. New York: Longmans Green. **185, 188**

PRINCE, M. (1975) *Psychotherapy and multiple personality: Selected essays*. Edited with an introductory essay by N. G. Hale, Jr. Cambridge: Harvard University Press. **185**

QUIGLEY, W. F., *see* Bonilla, Quigley, and Bowers (1961).

RADIN, H. (1972) Extractions using hypnosis for a patient with bacterial endocarditis. *British Journal of Clinical Hypnosis*, 3: 32–33. **150, 151, 162**

RAMAMURTHY, S., *see* Winnie, Ramamurthy, and Durrani (1974).

RAWLINS, C. M., *see* Hartmann and Rawlins (1960).

READ, G. D. (1933) *Natural childbirth*. London: Heinemann. **103, 117**

READ, G. D. (1944) *Childbirth without fear*. New York: Harper. (Second edition, 1953). **105, 117**

READ, G. D. (1962) Thoughts upon the use of hypnosis in pregnancy and labor. *In* Kroger (1962), 203–208. **117**

REES, W. L., *see* Eysenck and Rees (1945).

REIS, H. T., *see* Wheeler and others (1974).

REYHER, J., *see* Greene and Reyher (1972).

REYNOLDS, D. V. (1969) Surgery in the rat during electrical analgesia. *Science*, 164: 444–445. **34, 46**

RICE, F. G. (1961) The hypnotic induction of labor: Six cases. *American Journal of Clinical Hypnosis*, 4: 119–131. **119**

RINZLER, S. H., *see* Travell and Rinzler (1952).

RIPLEY, H. S., *see* Dudley and others (1966).

ROBERTS, A. H. (1975) Private communication. **59, 62**

ROBERTS, A. H.; KEWMAN, D. G.; and MACDONALD, H. (1973) Voluntary control of skin temperature: Unilateral changes using hypnosis and feedback. *Journal of Abnormal Psychology*, 82: 163–168. **158, 163**

ROBERTS, A. H., SCHULER, J., BACON, J. G., ZIMMERMAN, R. L., and PATTERSON, R. (1975) Individual differences and autonomic control: Absorption, hypnotic susceptibility, and the unilateral control of skin temperature. *Journal of Abnormal Psychology*, 84: 272–279. **158, 163**

ROBERTS, H.; WOOTEN, I. D. P.; KANE, K. M.; and HARNETT, W. E. (1953) The value of antenatal preparation. *Journal of Obstetrics and Gynecology*, (British Empire) 60, 404–408. **117**

ROCK, N.; SHIPLEY, T.; and CAMPBELL, C. (1969) Hypnosis with untrained, nonvolunteer patients in labor. *International Journal of Clinical and Experimental Hypnosis*, 17: 25–36. **115, 116, 119**

RODBARD, S. (1970) Pain associated with muscle contraction. *Headache*, 10: 105–115. **46**

ROSEN, H. (1960) Hypnosis: Applications and misapplications. *Journal of the American Medical Association*, 172: 683–687. **196, 206**

RUCH, J. C. (1972) *A study of self-hypnosis under alternative procedures*. Unpublished doctoral dissertation, Stanford University. **15, 25**

RUCH, J. C., and MORGAN, A. H. (1971) Subject posture and hypnotic susceptibility: A comparison of standing, sitting, and lying-down subjects. *International Journal of Clinical and Experimental Hypnosis*, 19: 100–108. **199, 207**

RUCH, J. C.; MORGAN, A. H.; and HILGARD, E. R. (1973) Behavioral predictions from hypnotic responsiveness scores with and without prior induction procedures. *Journal of Abnormal Psychology*, 82: 543–546. **15, 25**

RUCH, J. C., *see also* Hilgard, Ruch, and others (1974).

RUIZ, O. R. G., and FERNANDEZ, A. (1960) Hypnosis as an anesthetic in ophthalmology. *American Journal of Ophthalmology*, 50: 163. **132, 134, 142**

SACERDOTE, P. (1965) Additional contributions to the hypnotherapy of the advanced cancer patient. *American Journal of Clinical Hypnosis*, 7: 308–319. **92, 102**

SACERDOTE, P. (1970) Theory and practice of pain control in malignancy and other protracted or recurring painful illnesses. *International Journal of Clinical and Experimental Hypnosis*, 18: 160–180. **93, 99, 102**

SACERDOTE, P. (1972) Some individualized psychotherapeutic techniques. *International Journal of Clinical and Experimental Hypnosis*, 20: 1–14. **102**

SACERDOTE, P. (1974) Convergence of expectations: An essential component of successful hypnotherapy. *International Journal of Clinical and Experimental Hypnosis*, 22: 95–115. **102**

SACHS, L. B. (1970) Comparison of hypnotic analgesia and hypnotic relaxation during stimulation by a continuous pain source. *Journal of Abnormal Psychology*, 76: 206–210. **76, 81, 82**

SACHS, L. B. (1975) Training moderately susceptible hypnotic subjects to reduce pain by hypnotic analgesia suggestions. (Manuscript in preparation.) **73, 81**

SACHS, L. B., *see also* Hilgard, Morgan, and others (1974); Hilgard, Ruch, and others (1974).

SAMKO, M. R., and SCHOENFELD, L. S. (1975) Hypnotic susceptibility and Lamaze childbirth experience. *American Journal of Obstetrics and Gynecology*, 121, 631–636. **207**

SAMPIMON, R. L. H., and WOODRUFF, M. F. A. (1946) Some observations concerning the use of hypnosis as a substitute for anesthesia. *Medical Journal of Australia*, 1: 393–395. **144, 161**

SAND, P. L., *see* Fordyce and others (1973).

SARBIN, T. R., and COE, W. C. (1972) *Hypnosis: A social psychological analysis of influence communication*. New York: Holt, Rinehart, and Winston. **14, 18, 24, 185, 188**

SARGENT, J. D.; WALTERS, E. D.; and GREEN, E. E. (1973) Psychosomatic self-regulation of migraine headaches. *Seminars in Psychiatry*, 5: 415–428. **57, 61**

SATRAN, R., and GOLDSTEIN, M. N. (1973) Pain perception: Modification of threshold of intolerance and cortical potentials by cutaneous stimulation. *Science*, 180: 1201–1202. **46**

SCHAFER, D. W. (1975) Hypnosis on a burn unit. *International Journal of Clinical and Experimental Hypnosis*, 23: 1–14. **142**

SCHAFER, D. W., and HERNANDEZ, A. (1973) *Hypnosis, pain, and the context of therapy.* Paper presented at the 25th Annual Meeting of the Society for Clinical and Experimental Hypnosis, December. **206**

SCHALLING, D., and LEVANDER, S. (1964) Ratings of anxiety-proneness and responses to electrical pain stimulation. *Scandinavian Journal of Psychology*, 5: 1–9. **82**

SCHER, E., *see* Mandy and others (1952).

SCHIBLY, W. J., and AARONSON, G. A. (1966) Hypnosis: Practical in obstetrics? *Medical Times*, 94: 340–343. **112, 118**

SCHNECK, J. M., ed. (1963) *Hypnosis in modern medicine*. Springfield, Ill.: Thomas. **141**

SCHOENFELD, L. S., *see* Samko and Schoenfeld (1975).

SCHULER, J., *see* Roberts and others (1975).

SCHULTZ, J. H., and LUTHE, W. (1969) *Autogenic therapy: I. Autogenic methods*. New York: Grune and Stratton. **16, 118**

SCHWARCZ, B. E. (1965) Hypnoanalgesia and hypnoanesthesia in urology. *Surgical Clinics of North America*, 45: 1547–1555. **134**

SCHWARTZ, G. E.; DAVIDSON, R. J.; MAER, F.; and BROMFIELD, E. (1973) *Patterns of hemispheric dominance in musical, emotional, verbal, and spatial tasks*. Paper presented at Society for Psychophysiological Research, October. **12, 24**

SCHWARTZ, G. E., *see also* Davidson and Schwartz (1975); Higgins, Tursky, and Schwartz (1971).

SCHWARTZ, M. M. (1963) Cessation of labor using hypnotic techniques. *American Journal of Clinical Hypnosis*, 5, 211–213. **119**

SCOTT, D. L. (1973) Hypnoanalgesia for major surgery: A psychodynamic process. *American Journal of Clinical Hypnosis*, 16: 84–91. **134**

SCOTT, T. H., *see* Melzack and Scott (1957).

SEARS, R. R. (1932) Experimental study of hypnotic anesthesia. *Journal of Experimental Psychology*, 15: 1–22. **75, 81**

SEARS, R. R. (1936) Functional abnormalities of memory with special reference to amnesia. *Psychological Bulletin*, 33: 229–274. **180, 187, 188**

SECTER, I. I. (1964) Dental surgery in a psychiatric patient. *American Journal of Clinical Hypnosis*, 6: 363–364. **150**

SECTER, I. I., *see also* Erickson, Hershman, and Secter (1961).

SEITZ, P. F. D. (1951) Symbolism and organ choice in conversion reactions: An experimental approach. *Psychosomatic Medicine*, 13: 254–259. **196, 206**

SEITZ, P. F. D. (1953) Experiments in the substitution of symptoms in hypnosis: II. *Psychosomatic Medicine*, 15: 405–424. **196, 206**

SEMMES, J., *see* Nissen, Chow, and Semmes (1951).

SHEALY, C. N. (1974) Six years' experience with electrical stimulation for control of pain. *In* Bonica (1974a), 775–782. **61**

SHERMAN, S. E. (1971) Very deep hypnosis: An experimental and electroencephalographic investigation. Unpublished doctoral dissertation, Stanford University. **26**

SHEVACH, B. J., *see* White and Shevach (1942).

SHIPLEY, T., *see* Rock, Shipley, and Campbell (1969).

SHOR, R. E. (1959a) *Explorations in hypnosis: A theoretical and experimental study.* Doctoral dissertation, Brandeis University. **68, 69, 77, 81, 82**

SHOR, R. E. (1959b) Hypnosis and the concept of generalized reality-orientation. *American Journal of Psychotherapy*, 13: 582–602. **18, 25**

SHOR, R. E. (1962a) Three dimensions of hypnotic depth. *International Journal of Clinical and Experimental Hypnosis*, 10: 23–38. **25**

SHOR, R. E. (1962b) Physiological effects of painful stimulation during hypnotic analgesia under conditions designed to minimize anxiety. *International Journal of Clinical and Experimental Hypnosis*, 10: 183–202. **75, 77, 81, 82**

SHOR, R. E. (1970) The three-factor theory of hypnosis as applied to the book-reading fantasy and the concept of suggestion. *International Journal of Clinical and Experimental Hypnosis*, 18: 89–98. **25**

SHOR, R. E., and ORNE, E. C. (1962) *The Harvard Group Scale of Hypnotic Susceptibility, Form A.* Palo Alto, Calif.: Consulting Psychologists Press. **210**

SHOR, R. E., and ORNE, M. T. (1965) *The nature of hypnosis: Selected basic readings.* New York: Holt, Rinehart, and Winston. **23**

SHOR, R. E., *see also* Fromm and Shor (1972).

SJOBERG, B. M., *see* Weitzenhoffer and Sjoberg (1961).

SLETTEN, I., *see* Stern and others (1975).

SMITH, G. M.; EGBERT, L. D.; MARKOWITZ, R. A.; MOSTELLER, F.; and BEECHER, H. K. (1966) An experimental pain method sensitive to morphine in man: The submaximum effort tourniquet technique. *Journal of Pharmacology and Experimental Therapeutics*, 154: 324–332. **41, 46**

SMITH, H. W. (1970) Some medicolegal aspects of pain, suffering, and mental anguish in American law and culture. *In* Crue, B. L., ed. *Pain and suffering.* Springfield, Ill: Thomas, 186–204. **29, 44**

SOLDENHOF, R. de (1956) The assessment of relaxation in obstetrics. *Practitioner,* 176: 410–415. **117**

SOMJEN, G., *see* Friedman, Nashold, and Somjen (1974).

SOULAIRAC, A. (1968) An experimental approach to pain. *In* Soulairac, Cahn, and Charpentier (1968), 3–7. **28, 44**

SOULAIRAC, A.; CAHN, J.; and CHARPENTIER, J., eds. (1968) *Pain.* New York: Academic Press.

SOULE, A. B., III, *see* Standley and others (1974).

SPANOS, N. P., and BARBER, T. X. (1968) "Hypnotic" experiences as inferred from subjective reports: Auditory and visual hallucinations. *Journal of Experimental Research in Personality,* 3: 136–150. **15, 25**

SPANOS, N. P., and BARBER, T. X. (1974) Toward a convergence in hypnosis research. *American Psychologist,* 29: 500–511. **25**

SPANOS, N. P.; BARBER, T. X.; and LANG, G. (1974) Cognition and self-control: Cognitive control of painful sensory input. *In* London, H., and Nisbett, R. E., eds. *Thought and feeling: Cognitive alteration of feeling states.* Chicago: Aldine, 141–158. **80, 187**

SPANOS, N. P., and McPEAKE, J. D. (1975) Involvement in everyday imaginative activities, attitudes toward hypnosis, and hypnotic suggestibility. *Journal of Personality and Social Psychology,* 31: 594–598. **202, 208**

SPANOS, N. P., *see also* Barber, Spanos, and Chaves (1974).

SPEAR, F. G. (1964) *A study of pain as a symptom in psychiatric illness.* Unpublished M.D. thesis, Bristol University. **194, 205**

SPEAR, F. G., *see also* Merskey and Spear (1967).

SPIEGEL, H. (1974) *Manual for Hypnotic Induction Profile.* New York: Soni Medica. **202, 208**

SPIEGEL, H., and BRIDGER, A. A. (1970) *Manual for Hypnotic Induction Profile.* New York: Soni Medica. **202, 208**

SPIEGEL, H., *see also* Katz and others (1974).

SPRAGUE, L. T., *see* Melzack, Weisz, and Sprague (1963).

STANDLEY, K.; SOULE, A. B., III; COPANS, S. A.; and DUCHOWNY, M. S. (1974) Local-regional anesthesia during childbirth: Effect on newborn behaviors. *Science,* 186: 634–635. **118**

STERN, J. A.; BROWN, M.; SLETTEN, I.; and ULETT, G. (1975) Hypnosis, acupuncture, and "chemotherapy": Their influence on experimental pain perception and physiological responses. (Unpublished). Paper presented at the National Institutes of Health Acupuncture Conference, Bethesda, Maryland. **206**

STERNBACH, R. A. (1963) Congenital insensitivity to pain: A critique. *Psychological Bulletin,* 60: 252–264. **28, 44**

STERNBACH, R. A. (1965) Autonomic responsivity and the concept of sets. In Green-field, N. S., and Lewis, W. C., eds. *Psychoanalysis and current biological thought.* Madison: University of Wisconsin Press. **82**

STERNBACH, R. A. (1968) *Pain: A psychophysiological analysis.* New York: Academic Press. **33, 44, 45**

STERNBACH, R. A. (1970) Strategies and tactics in the treatment of patients with pain. In Crue, B. L., ed. *Pain and suffering.* Springfield, Ill.: Thomas, 176–185. **61**

STERNBACH, R. A. (1974a) Varieties of pain games. In Bonica (1974a), 423–430. **195, 205**

STERNBACH, R. A. (1974b) *Pain patients: Traits and treatment.* New York: Academic Press. **82, 195, 205**

STERNBACH, R. A.; MURPHY, R. W.; TIMMERMANS, G.; GREENHOOT, J. H.; and AKESON, W. H. (1974) Measuring the severity of clinical pain In Bonica (1974a), 281–288. **46**

STERNBACH, R. A., *see also* Gannon and Sternbach (1971); Greenhoot and Sternbach (1974).

STEVENS, J. C., *see* Gagge and Stevens (1968).

STEVENSON, J. H. (1972) *The effect of hypnotic and posthypnotic dissociation on the performance of interfering tasks.* Unpublished doctoral dissertation, Stanford University. **186**

STEWARD, J. H. (1946) *Handbook of South American Indians.* Vol. 1. Washington, D. C.: Smithsonian Institution, Bureau of American Ethnology Bulletin 143. **48, 60**

STOLZENBERG, J. (1961) Age regression in the treatment of two instances of dental phobia. *American Journal of Clinical Hypnosis,* 4: 122–123. **146, 161**

STOYVA, J., *see* Budzynski, Stoyva, and Adler (1970).

SUTCLIFFE, J. P. (1961) "Credulous" and "skeptical" views of hypnotic phenomena: Experiments in esthesia, hallucination, and delusion. *Journal of Abnormal and Social Psychology,* 62: 189–200. **75, 81**

SWEET, W. H., and WEPSIC, J. G. (1968) Treatment of chronic pain by stimulation of fibers of primary afferent neuron. *Transactions of the American Neurological Association,* 93: 103–107. **61**

SWEET, W. H., and WEPSIC, J. G. (1974) Stimulation of pain suppressor mechanisms: A critique of some current methods. In Bonica (1974a), 737–747. **61**

SWEET, W. H., *see also* Wall and Sweet (1967).

SZASZ, T. S. (1968) The psychology of persistent pain: A portrait of l'homme doul-oureux. In Soulairac and others (1968), 93–113. **195, 205**

TART, C. T. (1970) Self-report scales of hypnotic depth. *International journal of Clinical and Experimental Hypnosis,* 18: 105–125. **21, 22, 25**

TART, C. T. (1972) Measuring the depth of an altered state of consciousness, with special reference to self-report scales of hypnotic depth. In Fromm and Shor (1972), 445–477. **21, 22, 25**

TAUB, A., and CAMPBELL, J. N. (1974) Percutaneous local electrical analgesia: Peripheral mechanisms. In Bonica (1974a), 727–732. **61**

TAUB, A., *see also* Kane and Taub (1975).

TAUGHER, V. J. (1958) Hypnoanesthesia. *Wisconsin Medical Journal,* 57: 95–96. **132, 134, 142**

TELLEGEN, A., and ATKINSON, G. (1974) Openness to absorbing and self-altering experiences ("absorption"), a trait related to hypnotic susceptibility. *Journal of Abnormal Psychology,* 83: 268–277. **11, 24**

TEWELL, K., *see* LaBaw and others (1975).

THOMPSON, K. F. (1963) A rationale for suggestion in dentistry. *American Journal of Clinical Hypnosis,* 5: 181–186. **148, 162**

THOMS, H. (1950) *Training for childbirth: A program of natural childbirth with rooming-in.* New York: McGraw-Hill. **105, 117**

THOMS, H., and KARLOVSKY, E. (1954) Two thousand deliveries under a training for childbirth program. *American Journal of Obstetrics and Gynecology,* 68: 279–284. **117**

TIMMERMANS, G., *see* Sternbach and others (1974).

TINBERGEN, N. (1951) *The study of instinct.* London: Oxford University Press. **24**

TINTEROW, M. M. (1960) The use of hypnotic anesthesia for major surgical procedures. *American Surgeon,* 26: 732–737. **134**

TINTEROW, M. M. (1970) *Foundations of hypnosis.* Springfield, Illinois: Thomas. **84**

TOCANTINS, L. M., *see* Lucas, Finkelman, and Tocantins (1962); Lucas and Tocantins (1964).

TORGERSON, W. S., *see* Melzack and Torgerson (1971).

TOTH, M., *see* Arkin and others (1970).

TRAIGER, H. (1952) Children and hypnodontics. *British Journal of Medical Hypnotism,* 4: 42–43. **150**

TRAIKOV, D., *see* Petrov, Traikov, and Kalendgiev (1964).

TRAVELL, J., and RINZLER, S. H. (1952) The myofascial genesis of pain. *Postgraduate Medicine,* 11: 425–434. **45, 198**

TRIESCHMANN, R. B. *see* Fordyce and others (1973).

TURNDORT, H., *see* Egbert and others (1963).

TURSKY, B. (1976) Laboratory approaches to the study of pain. *In* Mostofsky, D., ed. *Behavior modification and control of physiological activity.* Englewood Cliffs, N. J.: Prentice-Hall (in press). **46**

TURSKY, B., *see also* Higgins, Tursky, and Schwartz (1971).

ULETT, G., *see* Stern and others (1975).

UUSITALO, E., *see* Cedercreutz and Uusitalo (1967).

VANDAM, L. D., *see* Dripps, Eckenhoff, and Vandam (1967).

VAN DYKE, P. B. (1970) Some uses of hypnosis in the management of the surgical patient. *American Journal of Clinical Hypnosis,* 12: 227–235. **134**

VELLAY, P., *see* Lamaze and Vellay (1957).

VELVOVSKI, I. Z.; PLATONOV, K. I.; PLOTITCHER, V. A.; and CHOUGOM, E. A. (1960) *Painless childbirth through psychoprophylaxis.* Moscow: Foreign Languages Publishing House. **103, 106, 117**

VON DEDENROTH, T. E. A., *see* Barrett and von Dedenroth (1967).

VON FREY, M. (1896) *Untersuchungen über die Sinnensfunctionen der menschlichen Haut.* Leipzig: Hirzel. **34, 45**

WALL, P. D. (1969) The physiology of controls of sensory pathways with special reference to pain. *In* Chertok, L., ed. *Psychophysiological mechanisms of hypnosis.* New York: Springer Verlag, 107–111. **82**

WALL, P. D. (1972) An eye on the needle. *New Scientist,* July 20, 129–181. **61**

WALL, P. D. (1974) The future of attacks on pain. *In* Bonica (1974a), 301–308. **46**

WALL, P. D., and SWEET, W. H. (1967) Temporary abolition of pain in man. *Science,* 155: 108–109. **46, 53, 61**

WALL, P. D., *see also* Melzack and Wall (1965; 1968; 1970).

WALLACE, G., and COPPOLINO, C. A. (1960) Hypnosis in anesthesiology. *New York Journal of Medicine,* 60: 3258–3273. **138, 143**

WALTERS, E. D., *see* Sargent, Walters, and Green (1973).

WANGENSTEEN, O. H., *see* Papermaster and others (1960).

WARE, P., *see* Lea, Ware, and Monroe (1960).

WATTS, J. W., *see* Freeman and Watts (1950).

WEBSTER, W. J., *see* MacWilliam and Webster (1923).

WEDDELL, G. (1955) Somesthesis and the chemical senses. *Annual Review of Psychology,* 6: 119–136. **45**

WEISENBERG, M., *see* Zimbardo and others (1966).

WEISZ, A. Z., *see* Melzack, Weisz, and Sprague (1963).

WEITZENHOFFER, A. M. (1953) *Hypnotism: An objective study in suggestibility.* New York: Wiley. (Paperbound edition, 1963). **5, 23, 208**

WEITZENHOFFER, A. M. (1957) *General techniques of hypnotism.* New York: Grune and Stratton. **24**

WEITZENHOFFER, A. M., and HILGARD, E. R. (1959) *Stanford Hypnotic Susceptibility Scale, Forms A and B.* Palo Alto, Calif.: Consulting Psychologists Press. **210**

WEITZENHOFFER, A. M., and HILGARD, E. R. (1962) *Stanford Hypnotic Susceptibility Scale, Form C.* Palo Alto, Calif.: Consulting Psychologists Press. **210**

WEITZENHOFFER, A. M., and SJOBERG, B. M. (1961) Suggestibility with and without "induction of hypnosis." *Journal of Nervous and Mental Disease,* 132: 204–220. **15, 25**

WELCH, C. E., *see* Egbert and others (1964).

WEPSIC, J. G., *see* Sweet and Wepsic (1968; 1974).

WERBEL, E. W. (1967) Hypnosis in serious surgical problems. *American Journal of Clinical Hypnosis*, 10: 44–47. **129, 130, 142**

WEYANDT, J. A. (1972) Three case reports in dental hypnotherapy. *American Journal of Clinical Hypnosis*, 15: 49–55. **149, 150, 157, 162**

WHEELER, L.; REIS, H. T.; WOLFF, E.; GRUPSMITH, E.; and MORDKOFF, A. M. (1974) Eye-roll and hypnotic susceptibility. *International Journal of Clinical and Experimental Hypnosis*, 22: 327–334. **208**

WHITE, J. C. (1968) Operations for the relief of pain in the torso and extremities: Evaluation of their effectiveness over long periods. *In* Soulairac, Cahn, and Charpentier (1968), 503–519. **52, 60**

WIKLER, A., *see* Hill and others (1952).

WILLKENS, R. F. (1974) The mechanisms of anti-inflammatory agents in the control of pain. *In* Bonica (1974a), 547–555. **60**

WINKELSTEIN, L. B., and LEVINSON, J. (1959) Fulminating pre-eclampsia with caesarean section performed under hypnosis. *American Journal of Obstetrics and Gynecology*, 78: 420–423. **128, 129, 142**

WINNIE, A. P.; RAMAMURTHY, S.; and DURRANI, Z. (1974) Diagnostic and therapeutic nerve blocks: Recent advances in technique. *In* Bonica (1974a) 455–460. **60**

WOLBERG, L. R. (1964) *Hypnoanalysis.* 2d ed. New York: Grune and Stratton. **205**

WOLF, S., and HARDY, J. D. (1941) Studies on pain. Observations on pain due to local cooling and on factors involved in the "cold pressor" effect. *Journal of Clinical Investigation*, 20: 521–533. **46**

WOLF, S., *see also* Wolff and Wolf (1958).

WOLFE, L. S., and MILLET, J. B. (1960) Control of postoperative pain by suggestion under general anesthesia. *American Journal of Clinical Hypnosis*, 3: 109–111. **126, 142**

WOLFF, E., *see* Wheeler and others (1974).

WOLFF, H. G. (1963) *Headache and other head pain.* 2d ed. New York: Oxford University Press. **208**

WOLFF, H. G., and WOLF, S. (1958) *Pain.* 2d ed. Springfield, Ill.: Thomas. **28, 44**

WOODRUFF, M. F. A., *see* Sampimon and Woodruff (1946).

WOOTEN, I. D. P., *see* Roberts and others (1953).

YAKOVLEV, P. I., *see* Mark, Ervin, and Yakovlev (1963).

ZARETSKY, I. I., and LEONE, M. P., eds. (1974) *Religous movements in contemporary America.* Princeton, N. J.: Princeton University Press. **204**

ZBOROWSKI, M. (1952) Cultural components in responses to pain. *Journal of Social Issues*, 8: 16–30. **45**

ZBOROWSKI, M. (1969) *People in pain.* San Francisco: Jossey-Bass. **45, 60**

ZIMBARDO, P. G.; COHEN, A. R.; WEISENBERG, M.; DWORKIN, L.; and FIRESTONE, I. (1966) Control of pain motivation by cognitive dissonance. *Science*, 151: 217–219. **34, 45**

ZIMBARDO, P. G., *see also* Maslach, Marshall, and Zimbardo (1972).

ZIMMERMAN, R. L., *see* Roberts and others (1975).

Subject Index